Movement Disorders in Sleep

Editor

DIEGO GARCIA-BORREGUERO

SLEEP MEDICINE CLINICS

www.sleep.theclinics.com

Consulting Editor
TEOFILO LEE-CHIONG Jr

June 2021 • Volume 16 • Number 2

ELSEVIER

1600 John F. Kennedy Boulevard • Suite 1800 • Philadelphia, Pennsylvania, 19103-2899

http://www.theclinics.com

SLEEP MEDICINE CLINICS Volume 16, Number 2
June 2021, ISSN 1556-407X, ISBN-13: 978-0-323-81367-9

Editor: Joanna Collett
Developmental Editor: Axell Ivan Jade M. Purificacion

Sleep Medicine Clinics (ISSN 1556-407X) is published quarterly by Elsevier Inc., 360 Park Avenue South, New York, NY 10010-1710. Months of issue are March, June, September and December. Business and Editorial Offices: 1600 John F. Kennedy Blvd., Ste. 1800, Philadelphia, PA 19103-2899. Customer Service Office: 3251 Riverport Lane, Maryland Heights, MO 63043. Periodicals postage paid at New York, NY and additional mailing offices. Subscription prices are $225.00 per year (US individuals), $100.00 (US and Canadian students), $625.00 (US institutions), $272.00 (Canadian individuals), $252.00 (international individuals) $135.00 (International students), $656.00 (Canadian and International institutions). Foreign air speed delivery is included in all *Clinics* subscription prices. All prices are subject to change without notice. **POSTMASTER:** Send change of address to *Sleep Medicine Clinics*, Elsevier Health Sciences Division, Subscription Customer Service, 3251 Riverport Lane, Maryland Heights, MO 63043. Customer Service: **Tel: 1-800-654-2452 (U.S. and Canada); 314-447-8871 (outside U.S. and Canada). Fax: 314-447-8029. E-mail: journalscustomerservice-usa@elsevier.com (for print support); journalsonline-support-usa@elsevier.com (for online support).**

Reprints. For copies of 100 or more of articles in this publication, please contact the Commercial Reprints Department, Elsevier Inc., 360 Park Avenue South, New York, NY 10010-1710. Tel.: 212-633-3874; Fax: 212-633-3820; E-mail: reprints@elsevier.com.

Sleep Medicine Clinics is covered in *MEDLINE/PubMed (Index Medicus)*.

SLEEP MEDICINE CLINICS

FORTHCOMING ISSUES

September 2021
Sleep Medicine: Current Challenges and its Future
Barbara Gnidovec Strazišar, *Editor*

December 2021
Measuring Sleep
Erna Sif Arnardóttir, *Editor*

RECENT ISSUES

March 2021
Piecing Together the Puzzle of Adherence in Sleep Medicine
Jessie P. Bakker, *Editor*

December 2020
Noninvasive Ventilation
Lisa F. Wolfe and Amen Sergew, *Editors*

September 2020
Telehealth in Sleep Medicine
Dennis Hwang and Jean-Louis Pépin, *Editors*

SERIES OF RELATED INTEREST

Clinics in Chest Medicine
Available at: https://www.chestmed.theclinics.com/

Contributors

CONSULTING EDITOR

TEOFILO LEE-CHIONG, Jr., MD
Professor of Medicine, National Jewish Health,
Professor of Medicine, University of Colorado,
Denver, Colorado, USA; Chief Medical Liaison,
Philips Respironics, Pennsylvania, USA

EDITOR

DIEGO GARCIA-BORREGUERO, MD, PhD
Director, Sleep Research Institute, Madrid,
Spain

AUTHORS

RICHARD P. ALLEN, PhD
Department of Neurology, Johns Hopkins
University, Johns Hopkins Bayview Medical
Center, Baltimore, Maryland, USA

SAMANTHA S. ANGUIZOLA E, MD
European Sleep Institute, Panamá City,
Panama

ALON Y. AVIDAN, MD, MPH
Director, UCLA Sleep Disorders Center,
Professor, UCLA Department of Neurology,
David Geffen School of Medicine at UCLA, Los
Angeles, California, USA

LUCA BALDELLI, MD
Department of Biomedical and NeuroMotor
Sciences (DiBiNeM), University of Bologna,
Bologna, Italy

THOMAS BORNHARDT, DDS, MSc
Assistant Professor, Department of Integral
Adult Care Dentistry, Temporomandibular
Disorder and Orofacial Pain Program, Sleep
and Pain Research Group, Faculty of
Dentistry, Universidad de La Frontera,
Temuco, Chile

LAURA M. BOTTA P, MD
European Institute of Sleep, Santiago, Chile

IRENE CANO-PUMAREGA, MD, PhD
Sleep Research Institute, Sleep Unit,
Respiratory Department, Hospital Ramón y
Cajal, IRYCIS, CIBERES, Madrid, Spain

FRANCESCA CASONI, MD, PhD
Department of Clinical Neurosciences, Sleep
Disorders Center, IRCCS San Raffaele Scientific
Institute, San Raffaele Hospital, Milan, Italy

ANDREA CASTRO-VILLACAÑAS, MD
Director, Sleep Unit, Sleep Research Institute,
Madrid, Spain

LOURDES M. DELROSSO, MD, FAASM
Associate Professor, Department of Pediatrics,
Division of Pulmonary Sleep Medicine,
University of Washington, Seattle Children's
Hospital, Seattle, Washington, USA

CHRISTOPHER J. EARLEY, MBBCh, PhD
Department of Neurology, Johns Hopkins
University, Johns Hopkins Bayview Medical
Center, Baltimore, Maryland, USA

JEROME ENGEL, JR., MD, PhD
Director, UCLA Seizure Disorder Center,
Jonathan Sinay Distinguished Professor of
Neurology, Neurobiology, and Psychiatry and
Biobehavioral Sciences, Brain Research

Institute, David Geffen School of Medicine at UCLA, Los Angeles, California, USA

SERGI FERRÉ, MD, PhD
Integrative Neurobiology Section, Intramural Research Program, National Institute on Drug Abuse, National Institutes of Health, Baltimore, Maryland, USA

RAFFAELE FERRI, MD
Scientific Director, Oasi Research Institute – IRCCS, Troina, Italy

STEPHANY FULDA, PhD
Sleep Medicine unit, Neurocenter of Southern Switzerland, Lugano, Switzerland

ANDREA GALBIATI, PhD
School of Psychology, Department of Clinical Neurosciences, Sleep Disorders Center, IRCCS San Raffaele Scientific Institute, San Raffaele Hospital, Università Vita-Salute San Raffaele, Milan, Italy

DIEGO GARCIA-BORREGUERO, MD, PhD
Director, Sleep Research Institute, Madrid, Spain

CELIA GARCIA-MALO, MD
Sleep Research Institute, Madrid, Spain

XAVIER GUITART, PhD
Integrative Neurobiology Section, Intramural Research Program, National Institute on Drug Abuse, National Institutes of Health, Baltimore, Maryland, USA

BIRGIT HÖGL, MD
Professor of Neurology, Head of the Sleep Disorders Unit, Head of Sleep Research Group, Department of Neurology, Medical University of Innsbruck, Innsbruck, Austria

ALEX IRANZO, MD
Neurology Service, Sleep Disorders Center, Hospital Clinic de Barcelona, CIBERNED, IDIBAPS, University of Barcelona, Spain

VERONICA ITURRIAGA, DDS, MSc, PhD
Assistant Professor, Department of Integral Adult Care Dentistry, Temporomandibular Disorder and Orofacial Pain Program, Sleep and Pain Research Group, Faculty of Dentistry, Universidad de La Frontera, Temuco, Chile

SABELA NOVO, MD
Instituto de Investigaciones del Sueño, Madrid, Spain; Hospital Universitario Puerta de Hierro, Majadahonda, Spain

FEDERICA PROVINI, MD, PhD
Department of Biomedical and NeuroMotor Sciences (DiBiNeM), University of Bologna, IRCCS Istituto delle Scienze Neurologiche di Bologna, Bologna, Italy

CÉSAR QUIROZ, PhD
Integrative Neurobiology Section, Intramural Research Program, National Institute on Drug Abuse, National Institutes of Health, Baltimore, Maryland, USA

LINA AGUDELO RAMOS, MD
Neurology Service, Instituto Neurológico de Colombia (INDEC), Medellín, Colombia

WILLIAM REA, MA
Integrative Neurobiology Section, Intramural Research Program, National Institute on Drug Abuse, National Institutes of Health, Baltimore, Maryland, USA

SOFIA ROMERO-PERALTA, MD
Sleep Research Institute, Madrid, Spain; Sleep Unit, Respiratory Department, Hospital de Guadalajara, Guadalajara, Spain

ROSALIA SILVESTRI, MD
Associate Professor of Neurology, Department of Clinical and Experimental Medicine, Sleep Medicine Center, University of Messina, Messina, Messina, Italy

AMBRA STEFANI, MD
Department of Neurology, Medical University of Innsbruck, Innsbruck, Austria

JOHN W. WINKELMAN, MD, PhD
Sleep Disorders Clinical Research Program, Departments of Psychiatry and Neurology, Massachusetts General Hospital, Harvard Medical School, Boston, Massachusetts, USA

BENJAMIN WIPPER, BA
Sleep Disorders Clinical Research Program, Massachusetts General Hospital, Harvard Medical School, Boston, Massachusetts, USA

TING WU, MD
Neurophysiology and Epilepsy Fellow, Ronald Reagan Medical Center, David Geffen School of Medicine at UCLA, Los Angeles, California, USA

MARCO ZUCCONI, MD
Department of Clinical Neurosciences, Sleep Disorders Center, IRCCS San Raffaele Scientific Institute, San Raffaele Hospital, Milan, Italy

Contents

disorders. Nowadays, it is recommended that first-line treatment should be alpha-2 ligands, which are more effective in the absence of previous DT. As a second-line treatment, opioids, such as oxycodone extended-release with naloxone, are approved in Europe. Brain iron should be monitored before and during treatment and corrected if necessary. Two new promising non-DTs are being developed: perampanel and dipyridamole. More research is needed.

Restless legs syndrome (RLS) is a sensory-motor neurological disorder that is associated with high levels of distress and sleep disturbance. Cross-sectional and longitudinal evidence suggests that individuals suffering from RLS may be at an increased risk of certain psychiatric illnesses and cardiovascular diseases. There also is evidence for increased mortality rates in RLS patients, although contrasting results do exist. Periodic limb movements of sleep (PLMS), repetitive leg movement observed in most RLS patients, and sleep disturbance may mediate the relationship between RLS and long-term morbidity. This article summarizes the literature investigating the potential consequences of both RLS and PLMS.

Periodic leg movements during sleep (PLMS) are a frequent finding in nocturnal sleep registrations that include tibialis anterior electromyographic signals. Different PLMS scoring rules exist and can have a major impact on PLMS frequency, which tends to be underappreciated. There is no consistent evidence that frequent PLMSs are a causal risk factor for clinically significant outcomes. Several critical open questions are identified that need to be addressed, including but not limited to the consideration of the full range of all sleep-related leg movement activity.

 Video content accompanies this article at http://www.sleep.theclinics.com.

Early-onset restless legs syndrome has a relatively high prevalence in pediatrics, is highly familial, and is often preceded by a diagnosis of periodic limb movement disorder or childhood insomnia. Diagnostic criteria are derived but not equal to those of the adult syndrome and are adapted according to children's age and linguistic competence. Diagnosis requires parents or caregivers to participate; video-polysomnographic nocturnal recording, although not mandatory, may help confirm dubious cases. The syndrome severely impacts children's sleep and cognitive-behavioral abilities. Iron supplementation is currently the most used and viable therapeutic option.

Sleep-related rhythmic movements disorder (SRRMD), typically considered a benign pediatric sleep disorder, comprise a group of movement disorders that occur predominantly early in childhood with an average age of onset of 9 months of age. Although it usually resolves spontaneously as the child ages, it can persist into adulthood. In this article, the authors review the identification, diagnosis, and management of SRRMD in children and adults.

Sleep Disorders in Parkinson Disease   323

Ambra Stefani and Birgit Högl

Sleep disorders in Parkinson disease have attracted the attention of clinicians and researchers for decades. Recently, major advances in their clinical characterization, polysomnographic description, pathophysiologic understanding, and treatment took place. Parkinson disease encompasses the whole spectrum of sleep medicine: every category of sleep disorder can be observed in these patients. Video polysomnography frequently is indicated, sometimes followed by multiple sleep latency/maintenance of wakefulness tests. Additional studies may include actigraphy, cardiorespiratory polygraphy, and dim light melatonin assessment. Treatment needs to be specific to the underlying sleep disorder and can include medications and nondrug treatments, for example, behavioral therapy and light therapy.

The Isolated Form of Rapid Eye Movement Sleep Behavior Disorder: The Upcoming Challenges   335

Alex Iranzo, Lina Agudelo Ramos, and Sabela Novo

The diagnosis of rapid eye movement (REM) sleep behavior disorder (SBD) requires videopolysomnography detection of excessive electromyographic activity during REM sleep, which is time consuming and difficult. An easier, faster, reliable, and reproducible methodology is needed for its diagnosis. The isolated form of RBD represents an early manifestation of the synucleinopathies Parkinson disease and dementia with Lewy bodies. There is a need to find neuroprotective drugs capable of preventing parkinsonism and dementia onset in isolated RBD. Clonazepam and melatonin ameliorate the RBD symptoms, but therapeutic alternatives are needed when these medications fail or show produce side effects.

Fragmentary Hypnic Myoclonus and Other Isolated Motor Phenomena of Sleep   349

Luca Baldelli and Federica Provini

Excessive fragmentary hypnic myoclonus, hypnic jerks, hypnagogic foot tremor, alternating leg muscle activation, and sleep-related cramps are less known sleep-related motor disorders (SRMDs). These manifestations are frequently missed or misinterpreted polygraphic findings that can be frequently confused with the more frequent SRMDs. These symptoms can present as isolated motor symptoms but can be also the cause of otherwise cryptogenic insomnias and somnolence. Expanding the knowledge on these isolated symptoms and defining their polygraphic and clinical features are essential for their identification. However, clear cut-offs to discern between the isolated phenomenon and the disorder are still to be found.

Propriospinal Myoclonus   363

Marco Zucconi, Francesca Casoni, and Andrea Galbiati

Propriospinal myoclonus (PSM) consists of paroxysmal and sudden jerks involving axial flexion trunk and hip muscles, conditioning sudden myoclonias of the trunk and arms/limbs, both spontaneous and triggered by sensory stimulations, emerging in relaxed wakefulness typically during the transition between wake and sleep. Generally, PSM originates from a thoracic myelomere and spreads caudally and rostrally, provoking flexion and/or extension movements, leading to jumps or trunk jerks. They appear triggered by the lying-down position and disappear when the subject stands up. The main consequences are the difficulties in sleep start and the reappearance during the period of wakefulness after sleep onset.

Preface

Sleep Related Movement Disorders: Introduction to an Evolving New Field

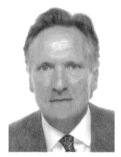

Diego Garcia-Borreguero, MD, PhD
Editor

Traditionally, sleep was considered a period of brain inactivity characterized by an overall reduction of the main neural functions. However, this concept changed following the discovery of rapid eye movement (REM) sleep in the middle of the last century. During REM sleep, the brain is active while the rest of the body is paralyzed: sleep is not a uniform state, but a dual state of REM and non-REM sleep. As sleep deepens, muscle tone gradually decreases, becoming markedly diminished during REM sleep. Failure to do so can lead to pathologic conditions, such as in certain REM parasomnias.

The close functional relationship between wakefulness with motor activity and sleep with motor inactivity, can, under certain pathologic conditions, lead to abnormal movement during sleep or an absence of movement during wakefulness. For example, intermittently, excitatory postsynaptic potentials break through the generalized muscle inhibition and cause myoclonus, mainly in the limbs. During pathologic states, or even during the normal wake-sleep transition, this can give rise to abnormal movements during sleep.

The interaction between sleep and movement disorders is reciprocal. The movement disorder per se, as well as the underlying pathologic state causing the movement disorder or its treatment, can affect sleep. Sleep also suppresses and can transform movement disorders that occur mainly during wakefulness. Thus, either directly or indirectly, the movement disorders may act upon sleep, and their treatments can cause further sleep/wake difficulties.

Some of the movement disorders occurring predominantly or exclusively during sleep are common and are treated by both sleep and movement disorder specialists. Thus, the understanding of the interplay between sleep and the motor system is important for both specialists.

Within sleep medicine, the presence of movement disorders occurring during sleep is common and frequently disrupt and may worsen other concomitant sleep disorders (ie, obstructive sleep apnea).

The purpose of this issue is to provide an overview for the sleep specialist of the different movement disorders occurring during sleep and to address the difficulties encountered in understanding and distinguishing different types of abnormal movement during sleep. We also discuss recent advances in the pathophysiologic

Sleep Med Clin 16 (2021) xi–xii
https://doi.org/10.1016/j.jsmc.2021.03.004
1556-407X/21/© 2021 Published by Elsevier Inc.

understanding of sleep and movement disorders, as recent years have seen a substantial increase in knowledge. Movement disorders in sleep are evolving as a special field of interest for both sleep experts and movement disorder specialists.

By bringing together international experts in the field who share their experience and knowledge, this special issue covers most aspects of abnormal movements during sleep. We hope that the reader will widen their understanding of these sometimes complex interactions that interfere with normal sleep.

Diego Garcia-Borreguero, MD, PhD
Sleep Research Institute
C/ Padre Damián 44
28036 Madrid, Spain

E-mail address:
dgb@iis.es

The Clinical Evaluation of Sleep-Related Movement Disorders

Samantha S. Anguizola E, MD[a], Laura M. Botta P, MD[b],
Andrea Castro-Villacañas, MD[c], Diego Garcia-Borreguero, MD, PhD[c],*

KEYWORDS

- Sleep • Sleep-related movement disorders • Parasomnias • Disorders of arousal
- REM sleep behavior disorder • Restless legs syndrome • Nocturnal epilepsy

KEY POINTS

- Sleep-related movement disorders are typically characterized by involuntary, abnormal movements, and behaviors during sleep.
- Abnormal motor phenomena can lead to sleep interference, impaired daytime function, or self-inflicted bodily injury.
- The evaluation is based on a retrospective description of the events from the point of view of the patient and ideally from an observer, including recognition of any other clinical features, such as family history, past medical history, and predisposing factors.
- Physicians need to recognize which nocturnal events may imply underlying neurologic abnormalities or benign age-appropriate episodes.
- Sleep-related movement disorders are classified into 4 main groups: motor parasomnias, nocturnal seizures, involuntary movement disorders, and sleep-related movement disorders owing to other causes, with the last group being those disorders that are unable to fit the characteristics of the previous three groups.

INTRODUCTION

Rapid eye movement (REM) and non–rapid eye movement (NREM) sleep are associated with neuronal firings, which lead to changes in the control of motor functions. Usually, as the process of sleep starts, muscle tone is gradually suppressed during NREM sleep, primarily the neck, trunk, and proximal legs muscles, that is, the muscles implicated in postural control. Subsequently, during REM sleep, muscles are characterized by hypotonia or atonia. This close relation between motor regulation and sleep-wake control explains why movement disorders and disturbances of motor control primarily manifest during sleep or shortly before a person falls asleep.[1]

DEFINITION

Sleep-related movement disorders (SRMD) are typically characterized by involuntary, abnormal movements, with positive motor phenomena activation or negative motor phenomena inhibition, which increase or decrease muscle tone during sleep. Abnormal motor activity during sleep may also lead to abnormal behaviors during sleep. It is important to recognize these abnormal motor phenomena because not only may they be responsible for sleep fragmentation, injury, and impaired daytime functioning but also they may indicate an underlying neurologic disease.[1,2]

a European Sleep Institute, Edif. Habitats Plaza, Calle 51, Panama City, Panama; b European Institute of Sleep, Luis Pasteur 5607, Vitacura, Santiago, Chile; c Sleep Unit, Sleep Research Institute, Calle Padre Damián 44 Madrid 28036, Spain
* Corresponding author.
E-mail address: dgb@iis.es

Sleep Med Clin 16 (2021) 223–231
https://doi.org/10.1016/j.jsmc.2021.02.001
1556-407X/21/© 2021 Elsevier Inc. All rights reserved.

EVALUATION OF A PATIENT WITH A MOVEMENT DISORDER

The clinical evaluation should be performed through a comprehensive sleep history, including questions about sleep habits and abnormal movements or behaviors during sleep; the patient history should also focus on recognizing predisposing factors within the patient's previous medical background and family history (especially neurologic and psychiatric history), including consumption of alcohol and drugs (**Fig. 1**).[2]

CLINICAL HISTORY

The sleep history should cover the entire 24-hour span, not only complaints during sleep at night. A detailed history, including a clear description of the events and their frequency, from the patient and the bed partner or other family members/caregivers if possible, is the cornerstone of establishing clues about the underlying cause. The event description should be obtained from a bed partner when possible, although many of these events can be remembered by both the patient and the bed partner/caregiver. The patient's bed partner/caregiver should be asked about the patient's sleeping habits, any changes in these habits, and the use of drugs or coexisting psychosocial problems. It is important to inquire if the behaviors are simple or complex (eating-related, sleepwalking, or even driving). Patients and bed partners/caregivers should also be asked if the sleep-related events have caused any harm to themselves or others (eg, wounds or injuries).[2]

Other information that may help distinguish the type of event includes the time of onset, which provides a clue about the sleep phase during which the events occur. Some of these events take place in the first part of the night, presenting as a presleep condition, like hypnagogic jerks or restless legs syndrome (RLS) symptoms. Other disorders occur during the transition from drowsiness to sleep, for example, rhythmic movement disorder, somniloquy, or propriospinal myoclonus.[2]

It is also possible to find SRMD during sleep-wake patterns, associated with NREM sleep, which predominates during the first 2 hours of the sleep period, such as sleepwalking, sleep terrors, and confusing awakenings. Conversely, REM sleep behavior disorder (RBD) occurs primarily during the second half of the night.[1]

Other disorders can take place at any time of the night, such as nocturnal seizures, or throughout the night, for example, periodic limb movement disorder (PLMD), which consists of repetitive cramping or jerking of the legs during sleep. This disorder is frequently associated with RLS.[1] According to the literature, more than 80% of patients with RLS also have PLMD.[3–5]

Inquiries should also be made on whether involuntary movements are present during the daytime, especially if there is clinical suspicion of epilepsy, as abnormal involuntary movements during sleep could be nocturnal seizures.[1,2]

The duration of the events helps to differentiate whether they occur during REM sleep or NREM sleep. For example, movements associated with RBD usually last a few seconds, rarely exceeding

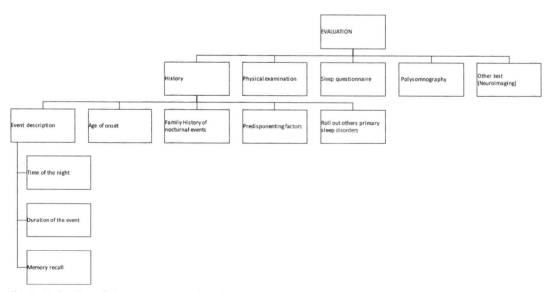

Fig. 1. Evaluation of sleep movements disorders.

1 minute in duration. In contrast, disorders of arousal can last from seconds to several minutes. For epileptic seizures, some can last seconds, whereas others may consist of abnormal behaviors lasting from 30 to 60 seconds. Prolonged events, which last more than 30 minutes, are usually more likely to be of a psychiatric origin.[1,2]

Abnormal movements and behaviors that occur during the first part of sleep, either with partial recall or without recall the next day, suggest an arousal disorder. Motor disorders and complex behaviors that occur from the second half of the night onwards are characteristic of RBD. Patients may remember some dream content that corresponds to the observed behaviors.[1,2]

It is important to ask the patient and their bed partner/caregiver about these behaviors and their level of complexity. Some of the movements that occur during sleep can be violent and cause injuries to the patient or his/her bed partner (this is suggestive of RBD). Patients with seizures of the frontal lobe show chorea-like and stereotyped movements during sleep. Patients with wounds, such as tongue bites or nocturnal enuresis, highly suggest nocturnal seizures. Abnormal movements of abrupt onset and sudden ending, along with subsequent confusion of the event, suggest nocturnal seizures. If abnormal movements have a gradual beginning and ending, if they occur in the middle of the night, or if they are not accompanied by subsequent confusion, they are suggestive of a nonepileptic seizure.[1,2]

The physician needs to make a detailed neurologic history, focusing on abnormal movements and behaviors that occur during sleep at night, because they may precede symptoms of an underlying neurologic disease.[1] For instance, RBD symptoms (abnormal behaviors and complex movements during sleep) may be a precursor of neurodegenerative disease.[1]

If the patient presents with a disorder of arousal, such as sleepwalking, and symptoms of sleep fragmentation, it is essential to rule out another sleep problem that may be causing the awakenings. For example, in patients with symptoms like snoring and cessation of breathing during sleep, a diagnosis of obstructive sleep apnea syndrome (OSAS) should be suspected.[6,7] Other indicators of this disease are elevated blood pressure, increased body mass index, crowded airway, enlarged tonsils, and large neck circumference.[6,7] Likewise, symptoms, such as tiredness and numbness when the patient wakes up in the morning, may suggest that there is a medical cause that is disrupting sleep, such as OSAS. Excessive sleepiness and fatigue throughout the day are additional symptoms of OSAS to bear in mind. If drowsiness

manifests as an irresistible need to fall asleep during the day or by the need to take short naps that make the patient feel refreshed and rested narcolepsy should be suspected.[1,6,7]

There are medical problems that should be questioned that have been reported to initiate sleep-related movements or behaviors, such as chronic obstructive pulmonary disease, hypoglycemia, gastroesophageal reflux, congestive heart failure, or renal disease, as well as neurologic issues.[2]

The physician should pay attention to any signs of a possible psychiatric condition, such as anxiety, depression, life stress, obsessions, personality traits, or even psychosis, because sometimes abnormal movements and behaviors during sleep can be due to a psychiatric illness.[1,2] In most of these patients, however, symptoms are not limited to the sleep period. Most patients with dissociation or panic have diurnal symptoms, a history of traumatic events, or other symptoms of major mood disorders.[2] If abnormal movements or behaviors during sleep are secondary to a psychiatric illness, appropriate treatment will eliminate them in most cases. Otherwise, the physician should suspect a coexisting primary sleep disorder.[1]

Patients should be questioned about drug use that may induce or provoke the symptoms. For example, some sedative-hypnotics, those with short half-lives, such as nonbenzodiazepine or benzodiazepine receptor agonists (eg, zolpidem, zaleplon, eszopiclone), are involved in the development of complex sleep-related behaviors, such as sleep-related eating, sleepwalking, or even driving. Some other medications, such as lithium, triazolam, and other central nervous system depressants, may trigger arousal disorders. Selective serotonin reuptake inhibitors (SSRIs) and tricyclic antidepressants are known for inducing symptoms of RBD. It is also known that RBD symptoms may worsen by the withdrawal of substances like alcohol or barbiturates.[1,2]

Some nocturnal episodes can be triggered or exacerbated by different situations, such as poor sleep, poor sleep hygiene, sleep deprivation, circadian rhythm disturbances, medications, or emotional factors. The anamnesis should include questions about these predisposing factors.[1,2]

Family history can be of great relevance in some cases. Genetic factors play a key role in disorders of arousal from NREM sleep, particularly sleepwalking, as well as in some sleep-related epilepsy syndromes.

Sleep questionnaires are useful tools that can help distinguish types of motor behaviors, predisposing factors, and so forth. They should contain several partially validated questions. Questions must be related to sleep habits, sleep hygiene, medical history, psychiatric history, previous neurologic disorders, and drug or alcohol use. Another supportive tool could be a sleep diary that can be provided to the patient for some time to record data from sleep hygiene, bedtime, nighttime awakenings, motor episodes and their time of appearance, the waking hour, total sleep time, and the feeling upon awaking (refreshed or tired). Other episodes, moods, and naps during daytime should be logged in the diary too.[1]

All of this is important for making a clinical diagnosis of patients with abnormal movements or behavior during sleep.

PHYSICAL EXAMINATION

Patients who present abnormal movements or behaviors during sleep usually have an unaltered physical and neurologic examination. A physical examination should always be performed to detect an underlying cause. The goal is to find out if there are signs of trauma from an event that occurred while the patient was asleep. If any abnormal sign is found during the neurologic examination, then there is a possibility of an underlying neurologic disease that is associated with motor events during sleep.[1,2]

A history of repeated awakening throughout the night, breathing pauses, and snoring is indicative of a sleep fragmentation disorder, such as obstructive sleep apnea (OSA).[1,7]

Individuals with dream enactment behaviors suggestive of RBD or older adults with nighttime confusion should be screened for depression and undergo a comprehensive neurologic examination to look for signs of cognitive impairment, cogwheeling, lack of arm swing, masklike facies, orthostatic hypotension, hypokinesis, or other signs of parkinsonism.[2] If there is a clinical suspicion of epileptic seizures, patients should also be evaluated for focal neurologic findings, suggesting a cerebral hemisphere lesion.[2]

SLEEP QUESTIONNAIRES AND SCALES TO MEASURE SLEEPINESS

A wide variety of scales have been created for assessing drowsiness. Excessive daytime sleepiness is a common complaint raised by patients who present abnormal movements and behaviors during sleep.[1] Symptoms can range from falling asleep while watching television or reading until falling asleep in public places or, in the most extreme cases, while eating or even driving.[1] These patients complain a lot about difficulties

concentrating and low productivity at work or school; they are often involved in traffic or work accidents. Usually, patients present a feeling of daytime fatigue and unrefreshing sleep and often take several naps during the day.[1]

The Stanford Sleepiness Scale is a 1-item self-report questionnaire for measuring levels of sleepiness throughout the day.[1] Another scale used to assess sleepiness is the Visual Analog Scale of Alertness and Well-being, in which the patients indicate their global vigor. This scale has been successfully used in the treatment of circadian rhythm disorders.[1] The Epworth Sleepiness Scale is used to assess daytime sleepiness. This test consists of a list of 8 situations in which patients must rate their tendency to become sleepy in each of them. Patients rate this tendency on a scale from 0 (no chance of dozing) to 3 (high chance of dozing). The maximum score is 24. A score equal to or more than 10 suggests the presence of excessive daytime sleepiness.[1] This scale has been weakly correlated with multiple sleep latency test (MSLT) scores.

LABORATORY ASSESSMENT

Laboratory studies are an essential part of the complete evaluation of these patients. Laboratory studies should be included in the diagnostic evaluation for primary conditions that may suggest movement and behavior disorders during sleep and for the evaluation of sleep complaints that are caused by abnormal movements and behaviors.[1]

Overnight polysomnography (PSG), an essential tool for a sleep center, records overall sleep, determines the percentages of the sleep stages, and records any sleep disorder that may appear during the study.[2] Laboratory tests for patients with a history of parasomnias, nocturnal seizures, or other abnormal movements and behavior during sleep at night should include PSG recording as well as an additional video-PSG with video-electroencephalographic monitoring, and an MSLT. Other possible complementary tests to be carried out are actigraphy, long-term video-electroencephalographic monitoring, basal electroencephalogram (EEG), or a 24-hour video-EEG.[1] To differentiate nocturnal epileptic seizures from episodes of a nonepileptic nature (for example, parasomnias or pseudocrisis), it is necessary to carry out a video-PSG with multichannel EEG. To diagnose OSAS or other primary sleep disorders that can simulate and may be mistaken for abnormal movements and behavior during sleep, a PSG can provide important information in determining the cause of the nocturnal events.

PSG studies are not generally necessary in a typical and uncomplicated parasomnia. Patients with parasomnias are relatively unlikely to have events during the PSG, but it may demonstrate suggestive features, such as a continuation of slowing, or prolonged sleep inertia (partial and prolonged confusion) when arousing from slow-wave sleep.[2] However, PSG is indicated for patients with atypical parasomnias or complex behaviors, such as violent events or potentially dangerous behaviors that may cause injuries to themselves or others. A video-PSG should be performed in such cases to correlate the behavior with the PSG recordings.[1] Some arousal disorders may mimic seizures; consequently, PSG or video-PSG plus multichannel EEG should be carried out to properly characterize the event and make a correct diagnosis.[1] Patients with RBD frequently have events during the sleep study, demonstrating increased muscle activity in isolated muscle groups, often exceeding established norms for REM sleep during the PSG.[2] For suspected RBD patients, multiple muscle electromyogram (EMG) from all 4 limbs is essential.[1] There is often a dissociation of activities between the muscles of the upper and lower limbs in these patients.[2] The presence of wakefulness on PSG before and during the nocturnal events may suggest a dissociative disorder, although panic events may occur out of light sleep.[1,8]

OTHER LABORATORY TEST: NEUROIMAGING

Neuroimaging techniques, like MRI and functional MRI, have always been an important tool for neurologists for the diagnosis of a neurologic disorder. In a sleep unit, this tool is important when there is a suspected neurologic disorder that occurs during the night or is associated with sleep disturbances.[8] Some neurologic disorders that present with abnormal movements and behavior during sleep may show structural brain changes on MRI, which may be responsible for such nocturnal events.[1] A neuroimaging test must be performed in the case of a first seizure, especially if it is of late onset or has atypical characteristics, to rule out any type of brain structural alteration.[1] MRI is more sensitive than computed tomography.[1] PET is a powerful technique for investigating in vivo abnormalities in brain metabolism and receptor distribution. It is performed by injecting a biomolecule into the body and waiting for the expected distribution of the radioligand into the whole body.[8] This technique is very useful for locating the epileptogenic area because the area of the cortex that produces the pathologic electrical discharges usually presents a decrease in glucose uptake compared with the normal cerebral cortex.

When EEG and other sleep examinations have already been performed and further information is still required about the pathogenic mechanism of a major sleep disturbance or the cause of the sleep disorder, additional complementary tests are recommended, such as single-photon emission computed tomography, which may reveal regional patterns of specific sleep disorders.[2]

RBD is known to be associated with neurodegenerative diseases, particularly α-synucleinopathies, such as Parkinson disease (PD), multiple system atrophy (MSA), and dementia with Lewy bodies (DLB). RBD may be a prodromal manifestation of neurodegeneration and can precede the clinical symptoms of a neurodegenerative disease several years before its diagnosis. In most case series, most patients develop a neurologic disease within the next 10 years.[1,8] Neuroimaging studies demonstrate coincident and progressive structural abnormalities in patients with RBD before motor symptoms arise. Follow-up with periodic neurologic examinations and neuroimaging studies should be performed to detect other signs of a degenerative neurologic disease as soon as possible.[8]

Studies exploring structural changes in RLS are limited. None or variable morphologic changes in RLS or microstructural abnormalities have been reported in RLS patients; reports are more consistent concerning levels of white matter atrophy. Iron deficiency has also been repeatedly shown to be associated with RLS, especially given that cerebrospinal fluid (CSF) ferritin levels are low and CSF transferrin levels are higher in RLS patients. MRI and transcranial ultrasound studies can be used to assess the iron concentration in the substantia nigra of patients with RLS. Decreased iron levels in the midbrain have been found to correlate with the severity of RLS.[8]

CLASSIFICATION

A clear and unified classification of SRMD, covering any possible differential diagnosis, is of the utmost importance.

In 2014, the American Academy of Sleep Medicine released its third edition of the *International Classification of Sleep Disorders* (*ICSD-3*). Shortly thereafter, other sleep professionals gave their "highlights and modifications" of that classification, whereby they considered just a small group of diseases in this classification an SRMD.[9]

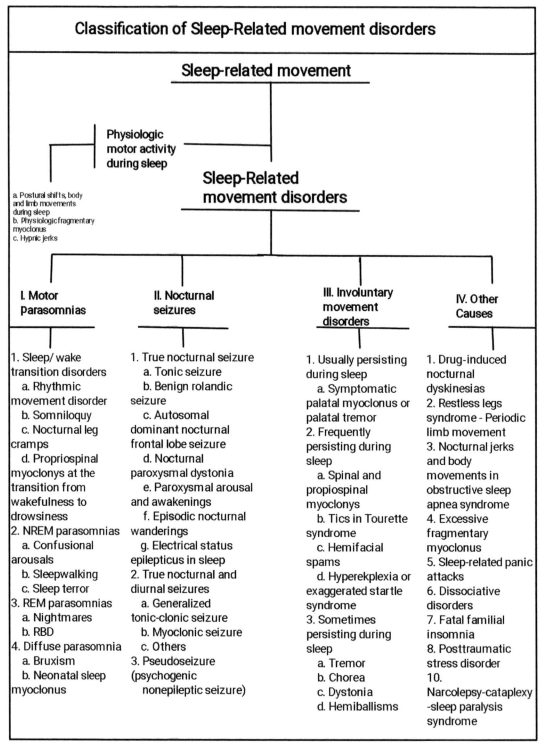

Classification of Sleep-Related movement disorders

Sleep-related movement

Physiologic motor activity during sleep
a. Postural shifts, body and limb movements during sleep
b. Physiologic fragmentary myoclonus
c. Hypnic jerks

Sleep-Related movement disorders

I. Motor Parasomnias

1. Sleep/ wake transition disorders
   a. Rhythmic movement disorder
   b. Somniloquy
   c. Nocturnal leg cramps
   d. Propriospinal myoclonys at the transition from wakefulness to drowsiness
2. NREM parasomnias
   a. Confusional arousals
   b. Sleepwalking
   c. Sleep terror
3. REM parasomnias
   a. Nightmares
   b. RBD
4. Diffuse parasomnia
   a. Bruxism
   b. Neonatal sleep myoclonus

II. Nocturnal seizures

1. True nocturnal seizure
   a. Tonic seizure
   b. Benign rolandic seizure
   c. Autosomal dominant nocturnal frontal lobe seizure
   d. Nocturnal paroxysmal dystonia
   e. Paroxysmal arousal and awakenings
   f. Episodic nocturnal wanderings
   g. Electrical status epilepticus in sleep
2. True nocturnal and diurnal seizures
   a. Generalized tonic-clonic seizure
   b. Myoclonic seizure
   c. Others
3. Pseudoseizure (psychogenic nonepileptic seizure)

III. Involuntary movement disorders

1. Usually persisting during sleep
   a. Symptomatic palatal myoclonus or palatal tremor
2. Frequently persisting during sleep
   a. Spinal and propiospinal myoclonys
   b. Tics in Tourette syndrome
   c. Hemifacial spams
   d. Hyperekplexia or exaggerated startle syndrome
3. Sometimes persisting during sleep
   a. Tremor
   b. Chorea
   c. Dystonia
   d. Hemiballisms

IV. Other Causes

1. Drug-induced nocturnal dyskinesias
2. Restless legs syndrome - Periodic limb movement
3. Nocturnal jerks and body movements in obstructive sleep apnea syndrome
4. Excessive fragmentary myoclonus
5. Sleep-related panic attacks
6. Dissociative disorders
7. Fatal familial insomnia
8. Posttraumatic stress disorder
10. Narcolepsy-cataplexy -sleep paralysis syndrome

Fig. 2. Classification of RMDs. (*Data from* Chokroverty, Sudhansu. Hening, Wayne. Walters Arthur. An approach to a Patient with movement Disorders during Sleep and Classification. In: Sleep and Movement Disorders. 2013:800.)

If the strict meaning of the term "sleep-related movement disorder" is taken, then, is any movement that occurs during sleep considered a part of this group of disorders? In 2013, Chokroverty and colleagues[1] proposed a classification of what one would think as an SRMD, separating it into 2 large groups; the first group consisted of the physiologic movements during sleep, and the second group included pathologic movements. However, the word "disorder" implies the meaning of illness/not-normal, that is why we suggest the term "sleep-related movements" as any movement that occurs during sleep, where there could be physiologic or pathologic movements, and the term "sleep-related movement disorder" only for the pathologic movements (**Fig. 2**).

This classification includes 4 different groups according to the type of activity shown during sleep: motor parasomnias, nocturnal seizures, involuntary movement disorders, and movement disorders owing to other causes, as those syndromes that are unable to fit the characteristics of the previous 3 categories.

Clinical characteristics of some of the most important SRMD are described in later discussion. The other articles in this issue provide more detailed information.

RESTLESS LEGS SYNDROME

RLS, also known as Willis-Ekbom disease, is a common sleep-related disorder characterized by a feeling of discomfort predominantly in the lower limbs, often described as an urge to move the legs. Upper limbs and even the trunk can be affected in the most severe cases. Symptoms appear mainly in the evening and at bedtime when the patient is at rest. As a result, patients with RLS have problems falling and maintaining sleep. Clinical criteria most used goes by the mnemonic URGED:[1,3-5]

- *U*rge or a need to move the limbs, mostly accompanied by dysesthesia.
- *R*est worsens the dysesthesia and the need to move.
- *G*etting up and moving decrease the dysesthesia.
- *E*vening or night worsens symptoms.
- *D*isorders that simulate RLS have been excluded.

Other supportive criteria for RLS are a positive response to dopaminergic therapy, presence of family history, and detection of periodic limb movements (PLMs) in PSG (during sleep) or a pathologic M-SIT (multiple suggested immobilization test) during the late evening.[1,3,4]

NOCTURNAL MOVEMENTS RELATED TO OBSTRUCTIVE SLEEP APNEA SYNDROME

Patients with severe OSAS may have flailing and jerking movements that may resemble PLMS. These movements are associated with repeated apneas, hypopneas, or hypoxemia. Both directed anamnesis and nocturnal PSG help us to correctly differentiate between these different types of movements.[1]

NON–RAPID EYE MOVEMENT PARASOMNIAS

Also known as disorders of arousals, NREM parasomnias take place during NREM sleep, mainly during the first hours of sleep, and include confusional arousals, sleepwalking, and sleep terrors. Most NREM parasomnias begin during childhood. They may overlap sometimes, with patients presenting episodes of sleepwalking and night terrors on different days. All NREM parasomnias have automatic behaviors, lack of interaction with the environment, and amnesia of the episode the next day. Most cases are benign and idiopathic. Family aggregation has been described, but a genetic signature has not yet been found. If these disorders appear during adulthood, they are often caused by medications, such as zolpidem.[1,10]

RAPID EYE MOVEMENT SLEEP BEHAVIOR DISORDER

RBD is probably the first disorder that often comes to mind when talking about REM sleep parasomnia. It is more common in the elderly. The most characteristic feature of RBD is the presence of muscle tone during REM sleep, which allows a dream-enacting behavior, usually violent, that may cause injuries to the patient or their bed partner. RBD is highly associated with neurodegenerative disorders, such as PD, DLB, and MSA. Diagnosis of RBD requires confirmation with video-PSG with EMGs on the upper and lower extremities to record the absence of muscle atonia during REM sleep. RBD is sometimes associated with the withdrawal of REM suppressant medications, barbiturates, or alcohol.[1,10]

NOCTURNAL SEIZURES

Seizures can be classified into 3 groups depending on the moment of the day when they take place. Nocturnal seizures occur predominately during sleep; diurnal seizures appear during the daytime, and diffuse epilepsy is characterized by seizures that can occur throughout the day. Nocturnal seizures may be mistaken for motor and behavioral parasomnias or other movement disorders; for this reason, multichannel EEG must be performed together with the PSG or the previous night under sleep deprivation.[1]

PERIODIC LIMB MOVEMENT DISORDER

Before starting to discuss PLMD, it is important to know what periodic limb movements in sleep (PLMS) are. PLMS are any limb movements recorded in a PSG, that fulfill 2 criteria: they present in series of 4 or more movements separated by more than 5 seconds and less than 90 seconds; after counting how many PLMS there are during the total sleep time, this number should be divided by the number of sleep hours, obtaining then the PLMS index.[11]

In 2005, the *ICSD-2* established the following criteria for diagnosing PLMD: a PSG that demonstrates the presence of PLMS, a PLMS index greater than 15 per hour in adults and greater than 5 per hour in children, presence of sleep disturbance or any other functional impairment, and other sleep disorders must be excluded that may be the cause of the presence of PLMS, like RLS, narcolepsy, RBD, or even an untreated OSA.[9,11,12]

The sleep disturbances seen in PLMD is an impairment to fall asleep and/or problems maintaining sleep. It is also important to keep in mind that excessive daytime sleepiness is most of the time absent in this disorder.[11,12]

It is also important to know that PLMS are not only seen in sleep-related disorders. In recent studies, an elevated PLMS index has been registered in association with other medical conditions, such as essential hypertension, alcohol dependency, and end-stage renal disease. They have also been associated with a higher risk of cardiovascular events, and they are present when medications, such as SSRIs, lithium, or clomipramine, are used.[12,13]

SLEEP BRUXISM

Sleep bruxism is defined as a recurrent contraction of the masseter, temporalis, and other jaw muscles, which is seen as "clenching or grinding of the teeth." This definition was proposed in 2017 in the *ICSD-3*. The diagnosis of this disorder may be made by a proper anamnesis, patient or bed partner report, a clinical examination whereby the loss of tooth surface or masticatory muscle hypertrophy is observed, or it can also be confirmed by performing a PSG or just by recording the muscle activity with an EMG while the patient is asleep.[14,15]

CLINICS CARE POINTS

- Abnormal movements and behaviors during sleep cover a diverse group of conditions that may lead to significant sleep disturbances, from sleep fragmentation or insomnia to sleep-associated injuries, as well as disabling daytime symptoms, such as fatigue and sleepiness.

- Abnormal movements and behaviors during sleep have been linked to some neurodegenerative diseases and epilepsy syndromes, as their first manifestations. These conditions require specific work up and treatment.

- Nocturnal events may occur at any time throughout the night, and movements are rarely witnessed first-hand.

- A good clinical history depends on a reliable witness (or video recording). A detailed anamnesis is important, and it must include a clear description of the events by the patient or their bed partner/caregiver, to establish clues about the underlying cause. Information about personal background, family history, medication or drug use, and other predisposing factors, as well as symptoms that may indicate other neurologic, medical, or psychiatric disorders, must be considered.

- Complementary tests, such as video-polysomnography, are often required to correctly identify abnormal movements and behaviors during sleep. Video-polysomnography provides important information.

- Neuroimaging studies and other more specific complementary tests must be considered in those patients with suspected nocturnal epilepsy or REM sleep behavior disorder because they can identify the underlying cause.

DISCLOSURE

S.S. Anguizola E, L.M. Botta P, and A. Castro-Villacañas have nothing to disclose. D. García-Borreguero has received research funding from Merck, Sharp and Dohme.

REFERENCES

1. Chokroverty S, Allen RP, Walters AS. An approach to a patient with movement disorders during sleep and classification. In: Sleep and Movement Disorders. Oxford University Press; 2013:800.
2. Vaughn B. Approach to abnormal movements and behaviors during sleep. 2018. Available at: https://www.uptodate.com/contents/approach-to-abnormal-

movements-and-behaviors-during-sleep#H2848 205727. Accessed November 2020.

3. Allen RP, Picchietti DL, Garcia-Borreguero D, et al. Restless legs syndrome/Willis-Ekbom disease diagnostic criteria: updated International Restless Legs Syndrome Study Group (IRLSSG) consensus criteria - history, rationale, description, and significance. Sleep Med 2014;15(8):860–73.

4. Allen RP, Picchietti D, Hening WA, et al. Restless legs syndrome: diagnostic criteria, special considerations, and epidemiology. A report from the restless legs syndrome diagnosis and epidemiology workshop at the National Institutes of Health. Sleep Med 2003;4(2):101–19.

5. Trotti LM. Restless legs syndrome and sleep-related movement disorders. Continuum Lifelong Learn Neurol 2017;23(4, SleepNeurology):1005–16.

6. Viola-Saltzman M, Kumar S, Undevia N. The frequency of parasomnia symptoms in patients with obstructive sleep apnea. Sleep 2009;32:A196.

7. Arnold J, Sunilkumar M, Krishna V, et al. Obstructive sleep apnea. J Pharm Bioall Sci 2017;9(Suppl 1):S26.

8. Yousaf T, Pagano G, Wilson H, et al. Neuroimaging of sleep disturbances in movement disorders. Front Neurol 2018;9:1–19.

9. Sateia MJ. International Classification of Sleep Disorders-Third Edition highlights and modifications. Chest 2014;146(5):1387–94.

10. Iranzo A. Parasomnias and sleep-related movement disorders in older adults. Sleep Med Clin 2018; 13(1):51–61.

11. Ferri R, Gschliesser V, Frauscher B, et al. Periodic leg movements during sleep and periodic limb movement disorder in patients presenting with unexplained insomnia. Clin Neurophysiol 2009;120(2): 257–63.

12. Stefani A, Högl B. Diagnostic criteria, differential diagnosis, and treatment of minor motor activity and less well-known movement disorders of sleep. Curr Treat Options Neurol 2019;21(1):1–14.

13. Hornyak M, Feige B, Riemann D, et al. Periodic leg movements in sleep and periodic limb movement disorder: prevalence, clinical significance and treatment. Sleep Med Rev 2006;10(3):169–77.

14. Beddis H, Pemberton M, Davies S. Sleep bruxism: an overview for clinicians. Br Dent J 2018;225(6): 497–501.

15. Wieczorek T, Wieckiewicz M, Smardz J, et al. Sleep structure in sleep bruxism: a polysomnographic study including bruxism activity phenotypes across sleep stages. J Sleep Res 2020;1–12. https://doi.org/10.1111/jsr.13028.

Restless Legs Syndrome - Clinical Features

Celia Garcia-Malo, MD[a,*], Sofia Romero-Peralta, MD[a,b], Irene Cano-Pumarega, MD, PhD[a,c]

KEYWORDS

- Restless legs syndrome • Clinical features • Willis-Ekbom disease • Restless legs mimics
- Complementary tests • Iron replacement therapy • Therapeutic approach

KEY POINTS

- Restless legs syndrome (RLS) is a common neurologic disorder, characterized by the appearance of abnormal sensations, mainly located in the lower limbs accompanied by an uncomfortable urge to move the affected regions, which leads to transitory relief. Symptoms worsen when at rest and during the evening, following a circadian pattern.
- Many conditions, such as iron deficiency (with or without anemia), pregnancy, chronic kidney failure, multiple sclerosis, polyneuropathy, Parkinson disease, major depressive disorder, generalized anxiety disorder, or attention-deficit/hyperactivity disorder, have been associated with RLS. Among them, iron deficiency stands out as the most well-known risk factor for RLS.
- The diagnosis of RLS is clinical. Five clinical criteria must be met to establish the diagnosis. Complementary tests could be useful to support diagnosis, exclude mimics, or for monitoring the response to treatment.
- Nonpharmacologic therapy and iron replacement therapy should be considered as first-line treatment. When necessary, symptomatic treatment of RLS should be started. Although efficacious, the role of dopamine agonists is being reconsidered because of the risk of long-term complications, such as augmentation of symptoms.

DEFINITION

Restless legs syndrome (RLS) is a common neurologic disorder, characterized by the appearance of abnormal sensations, mainly located in the lower limbs, although it can affect other body regions. The patients experience an uncomfortable urge to move the affected limbs/other body regions, which leads to transitory relief. Symptoms frequently appear during the evening or night and worsen when at rest, following a circadian pattern. Many patients with RLS also have insomnia. Overall, RLS has a great negative impact on patients' quality of life.

RLS diagnosis is essentially clinical and is based on the diagnostic criteria proposed by the International Restless Legs Syndrome Study Group (IRLSSG), which were updated in 2014.[1]

EPIDEMIOLOGY AND COMORBID CONDITIONS

RLS prevalence varies greatly, as shown by several epidemiologic studies. A higher prevalence seems to exist among people of European and North American heritage (estimated to be 2%–5%).[2] However, among those of Asian and African heritage, the prevalence seems to be lower (estimated to be 0.6%–0.1% and 0.11%, respectively).[3,4] These results are probably linked to the genetic factors related to this disorder.

[a] Sleep Research Institute, Calle del Padre Damián, 44, Madrid 28036, Spain; [b] Sleep Unit, Respiratory Department, Hospital de Guadalajara, Guadalajara, Spain; [c] Sleep Unit, Respiratory Department, Hospital Ramón y Cajal, IRYCIS, CIBERES, Madrid, Spain
* Corresponding author.
E-mail address: cgarcia@iis.es

Sleep Med Clin 16 (2021) 233–247
https://doi.org/10.1016/j.jsmc.2021.02.002
1556-407X/21/© 2021 Elsevier Inc. All rights reserved.

Both the prevalence and severity of RLS seem to increase with age. The estimated prevalence among children is 2%.[5] Regarding sex, the incidence of RLS is higher among women after the age of 35 years. This finding could probably be explained by the higher rates of iron deficiency occurring among this population, as discussed later.

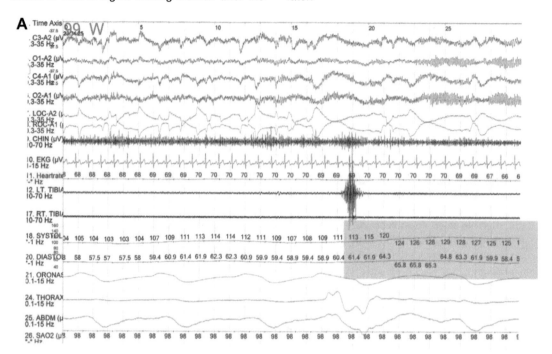

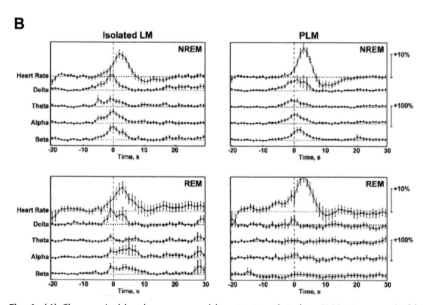

Fig. 1. (A) Changes in blood pressure and heart rate related to PLMs. Increase in blood pressure with PLM in wakefulness in a 30-s epoch. Please find blood pressure values highlighted in violet. (modified From Siddiqui, F., Strus, J., Ming, X., Lee, I. A., Chokroverty, S., & Walters, A. S. (2007). Rise of blood pressure with periodic limb movements in sleep and wakefulness. Clinical Neurophysiology, 118(9), 1923–1930. https://doi.org/10.1016/j.clinph.2007.05.006 with permission.) (B) Leg movements (LMs) during sleep are accompanied by evident changes in heart rate. (From Ferri, R., Zucconi, M., Rundo, F., Spruyt, K., Manconi, M., & Ferini-Strambi, L. (2007). Heart rate and spectral EEG changes accompanying periodic and non-periodic leg movements during sleep. Clinical Neurophysiology, 118(2), 438–448. https://doi.org/10.1016/j.clinph.2006.10.007 with permission.)

Table 1
Drugs that can contribute to the exacerbation of restless legs syndrome symptoms

Prokinetics agents	• Metoclopramide • Cinnarizine
Antipsychotics	More likely with typical antipsychotics
Vestibular sedatives	• Sulpiride • Flunarizine • Triethilperazine
Antihistamines	• Promethazine • Alimemazine
Antidepressants	Tricyclics antidepressants, SSRI, and SNRI Based on its dopaminergic activity, bupropion is the antidepressant that is less likely to worsen RLS

Abbreviations: SNRI, serotonin-norepinephrine reuptake inhibitor; SSRI, selective serotonin reuptake inhibitor.

Medical conditions associated with systemic iron deficiency are related to a greater risk for RLS, including iron deficiency (with or without anemia), pregnancy, and chronic kidney failure. Regarding pregnancy, RLS prevalence has been estimated to be 21%, with percentages of 8%, 16%, and 22% in the first, second, and third trimesters, respectively.[6] Pregnancy is considered to be a risk factor for developing or worsening RLS symptoms, with odds ratios of 1.98, 3.04, and 3.57 for 1, 2, and 3 or more pregnancies.[7]

Other conditions that have been associated with RLS include multiple sclerosis, polyneuropathy, Parkinson disease, major depressive disorder, and generalized anxiety disorder, although their ultimate causal relationship has yet to be elucidated. The relationship between attention-deficit/hyperactivity disorder (ADHD) and RLS has been widely investigated. Sleep disorders are common among patients with ADHD, especially RLS, with an estimated prevalence of 44% in ADHD.[8] Lower serum ferritin levels have also been observed among patients with ADHD.[9] The severity of ADHD has been reported to be significantly higher

Table 2
Diagnostic criteria for restless legs syndrome

Criteria	Notes
1. An urge to move the legs usually but not always accompanied by or caused by unpleasant sensations in the legs	• RLS may also involve the arms or other body parts • The symptoms are frequently bilateral
2. The urge to move the legs and any accompanying unpleasant sensations begin or worsen during periods of rest or inactivity, such as lying down or sitting	• Symptoms in the legs increase with the duration of rest
3. The urge to move the legs and any accompanying unpleasant sensations are partially or totally relieved by movement, such as walking or stretching, at least as long as the activity continues	• When symptoms are severe, relief by activity may not be noticeable but must previously have been present
4. The urge to move the legs and any accompanying unpleasant sensations during rest or inactivity only occur or are worse in the evening or night than during the day	• When symptoms are severe, the worsening in the circadian variation may not be noticeable but must previously have been present
5. The occurrence of the above features is not solely accounted for as symptoms primary to another medical or behavioral condition (mimics of RLS have been excluded: eg, neuropathy, myalgia, venous stasis, leg edema, arthritis, leg cramps, positional discomfort, or habitual foot tapping)	• RLS may also occur with any of these conditions, but the RLS symptoms will then be greater in severity, expression, or character than those usually occurring as part of the other condition

All clinical criteria must be met to establish the diagnosis.
Adapted from Allen, R. P., Picchietti, D., Hening, W. A., Trenkwalder, C., Walters, A. S., Montplaisi, J., ... Zucconi, M. (2003). Restless legs syndrome: Diagnostic criteria, special considerations, and epidemiology. A report from the restless legs syndrome diagnosis and epidemiology workshop at the National Institutes of Health. Sleep Medicine, 4(2), 101–119. https://doi.org/10.1016/S1389-9457(03)00010-8.[1]

in children with iron deficiency than in those without iron deficiency.[10] This finding suggests that iron deficiency and dopaminergic dysfunction link these disorders.

RLS has been investigated as a risk factor for vascular diseases such as coronary heart disease and stroke.[11,12] It has been proposed that the existence of periodic limb movements (PLMs) of sleep, the main motor sign of RLS, leads to more fragmented sleep and also has been associated with an increase in heart rate (of about 10%–20%)[13,14] and increases in blood pressure (10–15 mm Hg for diastolic and 25–30 mm Hg for systolic),[15] contributing to the development of diurnal hypertension among patients with RLS (**Fig. 1**). Greater frequency or severity of RLS symptoms could be related to a higher risk of coronary artery disease and cerebrovascular disease (odds ratio, 2.4; 95% confidence interval, 1.6–3.7) compared with controls.[12]

RLS symptoms can appear or worsen as a consequence of using certain drugs that act as dopamine blockers. Prokinetics, antipsychotics, vestibular sedatives, antihistamines, and antidepressants are the most common. Because they are all commonly used drugs in daily practice, it is important to evaluate current patient medication. Particular attention should be paid to antidepressants because depression often coexists in patients with RLS. **Table 1** summarizes drugs acting as dopamine blockers that could exacerbate RLS symptoms.

DIAGNOSTIC CRITERIA

The diagnosis of RLS is clinical. Five clinical criteria must be met to establish the diagnosis (**Table 2**). The first 4 criteria enable a positive diagnosis to be made and were established by the National Institutes of Health conference and published in 2003.[16] The fifth criterion enables differential diagnosis by excluding conditions that mimic RLS, and was added by the IRLSSG in 2012.[1] Four supportive criteria (not essential) in addition to these 5 essential criteria are useful in equivocal cases (**Box 1**).

At present, the pediatric diagnosis of RLS requires meeting the adult criteria, although children should describe their leg discomfort in their own words. A valid assessment method for the diagnosis of RLS for the cognitively impaired or elderly remains unavailable.[1]

DIFFERENTIAL DIAGNOSIS

Many conditions associated with discomfort or pain in the lower limbs can mimic RLS. As

---

Box 1
Supportive criteria in restless legs syndrome

1. Family history of RLS among first-degree relatives.

2. Presence of PLMs of sleep or resting wake at rates or intensity greater than expected for age or medical status.

3. Lack of profound daytime sleepiness.

4. Symptoms improvement with dopaminergic treatment.

These criteria are not essential for diagnosis but should be noted when present because they are useful in equivocal cases.
Adapted from Allen, R. P., Picchietti, D. L., Garcia-Borreguero, D., Ondo, W. G., Walters, A. S., Winkelman, J. W., ... Lee, H. B. (2014). Restless legs syndrome/Willis-Ekbom disease diagnostic criteria: Updated International Restless Legs Syndrome Study Group (IRLSSG) consensus criteria - history, rationale, description, and significance. Sleep Medicine, 15(8), 860–873. https://doi.org/10.1016/j.sleep.2014.03.025.

---

discussed later, some of them can even get worse during the afternoon or appear during sleep, making differential diagnosis more difficult. Because RLS diagnosis is essentially

---

Box 2
Secondary sleep-related leg cramps causes

- Metabolic alterations (eg, hypokalemia, hypocalcemia, hypomagnesemia)
- Dehydration
- Neurologic alterations (eg, spinal stenosis, peripheral neuropathy)
- Peripheral vascular disease
- Cirrhosis
- Drugs
  - Oral contraceptives
  - Diuretics
  - Intravenous iron sucrose
  - Raloxifene
  - Teriparatide
  - Pyrazinamide
  - Long-acting β-agonists
  - Statins

Adapted from Brown, T. (2015). Sleep-Related Leg Cramps: A Review and Suggestions for Future Research. Sleep Medicine Clinics, 10(3), 385–392. https://doi.org/10.1016/j.jsmc.2015.05.002.

Table 3
clinical features of the main restless legs syndrome mimics

	Location and Character of the Distress	Maneuvers Causing Relief	Circadian Pattern	Response to Dopaminergic Agonists	Neurologic Evaluation	Electromyography	Additional Features
RLS	Diffuse, usually in calf, unpleasant sensations	While walking or changing position	Yes	Yes	Normal	Normal	Frequent family history Association with iron deficiency Insomnia
Sleep-related leg cramps	Painful involuntary muscle contractions, preferably affecting muscles in the calf or foot, often visible	Stretching or massaging affected muscles	No	No	Normal	Normal	Muscular contraction can be palpable or even visible Secondary causes (see **Box 2**) must be evaluated
Positional leg discomfort	Unpleasant sensations in the legs that are caused after sitting or lying in the same position for a long time	Changing position	No	No	Normal	Normal	No other symptoms are associated, and it does not affect patient's quality of life
Venous disorder	Sensory discomfort in legs when standing	At rest or while elevating legs	No	No	Normal	Normal	Sometimes skin alterations can be observed
Akathisia	Feeling of inner restlessness not exclusively located in legs	Movement	No	No	Normal	Normal	History of exposure to neuroleptic medications or associated extrapyramidal symptoms
Polyneuropathy	Painful burning sensations in the upper and lower extremities (sometimes glove-and-sock distribution)	Inactivity can worsen symptoms	No or weak	No	Altered (except sometimes if small-fiber polyneuropathy)	Altered (except sometimes if small-fiber polyneuropathy)	The urge to move the legs does not exist or is less than RLS/WED Familiar history could be present

Abbreviation: WED, Willis-Ekbom disease.

From: Garcia-Malo, C., Romero Peralta, S., & Garcia-Borreguero, D. (2020). Restless Legs Syndrome and Other Common Sleep-Related Movement Disorders. Continuum (Minneapolis, Minn.), 26(4), 963–987. https://doi.org/10.1212/CON.0000000000000886; with permission.

clinical, a careful and systematic evaluation is mandatory to exclude these mimics. The main conditions that should be considered are the following:

- Sleep-related leg cramps: leg cramps are painful involuntary muscle contractions that generally affect calf or foot muscles. Muscular contraction can be palpable or even visible. Sixty-percent of adults report that they have had nocturnal leg cramps. The symptoms are usually relieved with stretching or massaging affected muscles, which is what patients do intuitively.[17] Leg cramps are mostly defined as idiopathic, although they can be secondary to other disorders such as metabolic alterations or related to the use of certain drugs (**Box 2**). Most of the secondary causes are related to changes in the permeability of the cell membrane. Neurologic evaluation and electromyography are normal. There is limited evidence on the efficacy of stretching or exercise. Several medications have been tested for treating leg cramps, such as magnesium and calcium channel blockers, all with poor evidence. Quinine is no longer recommended because of its known side effects.[18,19] Unlike RLS, no response to dopamine agonists is observed.
- Venous disorder: venous peripheral vascular disease can lead to sensory discomfort mainly affecting the lower limbs. Sometimes, the symptoms worsen at the end of the day, not because of a pure circadian pattern but because of having spent most of the day standing or walking, which usually aggravates symptoms. When experiencing discomfort, some relief can be obtained through rest or by elevating the limbs, the opposite of what occurs in RLS, where rest worsens symptoms.
- Polyneuropathy: sensory polyneuropathy can provoke painful burning sensations. In most cases, the pattern of length-dependent involvement occurs, initially affecting the lower limbs and extending over time to the upper limbs, with a glove-and-stocking distribution. Sometimes the symptoms can worsen when at rest; however, the urge to move is usually absent. Neurologic evaluation and electromyography are usually altered, except in the case of some small-fiber polyneuropathies.
- Akathisia: akathisia is described as the feeling of inner restlessness that can affect any part of the body but can be more intense in the lower limbs. History of exposure to neuroleptic medications or associated extrapyramidal symptoms can help with diagnosis. Unlike RLS, no circadian pattern or response to dopaminergic agents are observed.
- Positional leg discomfort: this entity cannot be defined as a disorder, but some individuals describe having unpleasant sensations in the legs after sitting or lying in the same position for a long time, obtaining relief by changing position. However, no other symptoms are present, and it does not affect the individual's quality of life.

Box 3
Laboratory test recommended in patients with restless legs syndrome

Complete blood cell count

Iron parameters

- Serum iron
- Serum ferritin
- Serum transferrin
- TSAT
- TIBC

Acute phase reactants

- C-reactive protein
- Erythrocyte sedimentation rate

Serum levels of electrolytes

- Potassium
- Calcium
- Sodium

Kidney function markers

- Creatinine
- Urea

Liver function markers

- Alanine aminotransferase
- Aspartate aminotransferase
- Serum bilirubin
- Serum albumin
- International Normalized Ratio

Vitamins

- Vitamin B_{12}
- Folic acid
- Vitamin D

Thyroid hormones

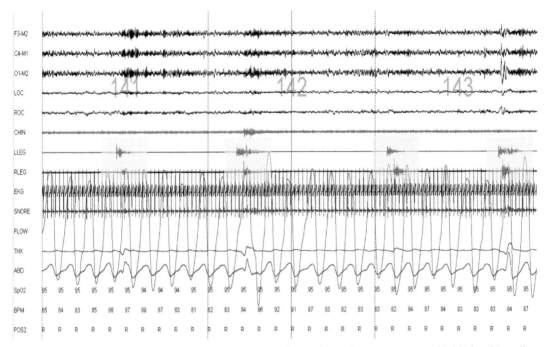

Fig. 2. Example of PLMs of sleep during a polysomnography study. Limb movements are highlighted in yellow.

Careful evaluation of the symptoms (including location and maneuvers that provide symptom relief), evaluating the circadian pattern of symptoms, response to dopaminergic agonists, and neurologic examination are all mandatory for RLS differential diagnosis. **Table 3** summarizes the clinical features of the main RLS mimics.

COMPLEMENTARY TESTS IN RESTLESS LEGS SYNDROME

Diagnosis of RLS can be challenging in some cases, mainly because of the presence of mimics and other confounders. Although the diagnosis of RLS is clinical, complementary tests can be useful to support diagnosis, exclude mimics, or for monitoring the response to treatment. The main complementary tests that could be useful are discussed here.

The International Restless Legs Syndrome Study Group Rating Scale

The International Restless Legs Syndrome Study Group Rating Scale (IRLS) can be used to assess RLS severity, reflecting the intensity and frequency of RLS symptoms and associated sleep problems. It also includes questions that probe the impact of this disorder on the patient's mood and daily functioning.[20] The scale consists of 10 questions with 5 possible responses, each scored between 0 and 4. Higher scores indicate more severe disease.

The severity of RLS symptoms is scored as mild (total score of 1–10), moderate,[11–20] severe,[21–30] or very severe.[31–40] The scale is validated as a satisfactory instrument for use without contribution from an expert clinical interview and offers the possibility of being easy to use in clinical practice. The scale is also useful for evaluating the clinical benefit of any treatment.

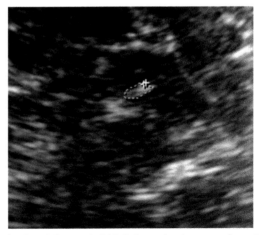

Fig. 3. TCS image in RLS. Substantia nigra area from 1 side is encircled. Left and right areas must be summed to obtain a value called substantia nigra echogenicity index, a direct marker of iron deposits in the substantia nigra. In RLS, because there is lower iron content in the substantia nigra, hypoechogenicity is observed compared with healthy controls.

Laboratory

Every patient with RLS should have a complete blood test, including every systemic iron parameter: serum iron, serum ferritin, serum transferrin, transferrin saturation index (TSAT), and total iron-binding capacity (TIBC). It is recommended to also include C-reactive protein and erythrocyte sedimentation rate, because serum ferritin can be falsely increased like an acute phase reactant in the presence of inflammation. Blood samples should be obtained in the fasted state in the morning, because circadian changes can affect ferritin levels. It is also recommended to perform a complete blood cell count and obtain information regarding liver and kidney function markers, among others (**Box 3**).

Polysomnography

Polysomnography is not required for the diagnosis of RLS. However, it can be useful, because it enables the objectification and quantification of PLMs (a motor sign of this disorder), and to assess the quality of sleep in patients with RLS. During a polysomnography study, PLMs can be quantified by using tibialis anterior surface electromyography (EMG) electrodes. A leg movement (LM) is defined as any anterior tibialis EMG event that increases to greater than or equal to 8 µV and decreases to less than 2 µV above resting baseline. The duration of the LM must be 0.5 to 10 seconds. The period length for 2 consecutive movements to be considered PLMs must be at least 10 seconds and no more than 90 seconds. PLMs are defined as at least 4 limb movements in a row.[21] **Fig. 2** shows PLMs in a real polysomnography study.

The PLM index (PLMI) obtained by the polysomnography is calculated by dividing the total number of PLMs by sleep time in hours. PLMs have been reported to occur in 80% to 89% of patients with RLS.[22] The PLMI reflects the degree of motor symptoms, giving an indirect index of RLS severity. A PLMI greater than 15/h can support the diagnosis of RLS in doubtful cases.[23] PLMs are not specific and are also present in healthy controls[24] and patients with other sleep disorders with or without RLS, such as narcolepsy, REM behavior disorder, and sleep apnea.[25–27]

The Multiple Suggested Immobilization Test

The Multiple Suggested Immobilization Test (m-SIT) provides a standardized testing condition to evaluate RLS severity. This test measures the number of PLMs during relaxed wakefulness preceding sleep onset (PLMW). The PLMW during the m-SIT are objectively measured using the

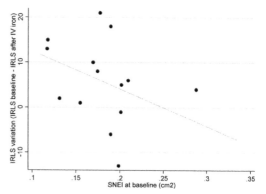

Fig. 4. Variation in severity of symptoms (assessed by IRLS) depending on the baseline Substantia Nigra Echogenicity Index (SNEI). SNEI is directly related to substantia nigra iron content. Variation in IRLS is represented on the y axis, obtained as IRLS value baseline minus IRLS value after intravenous (IV) iron. The baseline SNEI value is represented on x axis. Note the negative relation between IRLS and SNEI (the lower the baseline SNEI, the greater the clinical improvement after IV iron, represented as a change in IRLS). IRLS, The International Restless Legs Syndrome Study Group Rating Scale. (*From*: Garcia-Malo C, Wanner V, Miranda C, Romero Peralta S, Agudelo L, Cano-Pumarega I, Granizo JJ, Garcia-Borreguero D, (2019). Quantitative transcranial sonography of the substantia nigra as a predictor of therapeutic response to intravenous iron therapy in restless legs syndrome. Sleep Medicine, 66, 123–129. https://doi.org/10.1016/j.sleep.2019.09.020, with permission.)

same criteria for measuring PLM of sleep during a polysomnography study. This test has been proposed as a standardized laboratory test for diagnosis and evaluation of the severity of RLS.[22] Values of PLMW greater than 50/h are highly suggestive of RLS.[28] The patient reclines quietly and is told to keep the voluntary movements to a minimum for the entire test. The patient is also asked to indicate the urge to move and leg discomfort on a visual analog scale.[29] During the test, both motor and sensory symptoms frequently worsen, following a circadian pattern.[30]

Electromyography and Nerve Conduction Studies

EMG and nerve conduction studies should be considered if polyneuropathy or radiculopathy is suspected on clinical grounds.

Neuroimaging Studies

Different neuroimaging techniques can be useful to support the diagnosis of RLS.[31] Most of these studies have been investigational and are not currently part of the standard assessment. These studies are based on the fact that central iron deficiency present in most patients seems to be critical in the pathogenesis of RLS.[32] Central iron deficiency can occur despite normal systemic iron parameters, so the direct quantification of iron into the regions of interest inside the central nervous system is becoming more important.[33]

Transcranial sonography (TCS) is one of the most accessible neuroimaging techniques in daily practice. Patients with RLS showed a significant hypoechogenicity of the substantia nigra compared with healthy controls.[34] TCS has shown its usefulness in quantifying midbrain iron deposits (**Fig. 3**). Recent studies have shown that TCS could be a predictor of therapeutic response to intravenous iron in RLS and could enable the selection of candidates for this treatment to be improved[35] (**Fig. 4**). Reduction in brain iron content in the substantia nigra in patients with RLS was also confirmed using functional MRI.

Box 4
General recommendations on oral iron treatment

Recommendations to optimize oral iron treatment absorption

- Iron generally should not be given with food.
- Iron should especially be taken separately from calcium-containing foods and beverages (milk), calcium supplements, cereals, dietary fiber, tea, coffee, and eggs.
- Iron should be given 2 hours before, or 4 hours after, ingestion of antacids.
- Coadministration of 250 mg of ascorbic acid or a half-glass of orange juice with iron to enhance its absorption.
- Once-a-day could be as effective as twice-a-day administration, because oral iron increases serum hepcidin and absorption can be reduced. Compliance may also be higher with this posology.

Recommendations to minimize adverse effects derived from oral iron treatment

- Change from every-day administration to every other day.
- Take oral iron with food or milk, although this may lead to a reduction in its absorption.
- Switch to a lower elemental iron presentation.

From: Garcia-Malo, C., Miranda, C., Romero Peralta, S., Cano-Pumarega, I., Novo Ponte, S., & Garcia-Borreguero, D. (2020). Iron Replacement Therapy in Restless Legs Syndrome. Current Treatment Options in Neurology, 22(11), 1–16. https://doi.org/10.1007/s11940-020-0617-7. With permission.

TREATMENT

At present, the decision about whether or not to treat RLS is determined by how the disorder affects the patient's life. This approach may change in the future because RLS has been related to an increase in vascular risk (discussed earlier in relation to epidemiology and comorbid conditions").

Because many drugs can trigger or worsen RLS symptoms (see **Table 1**), it is important to evaluate which medications a patient is being treated with, and, where possible, their withdrawal considered in the first instance.

The therapeutic options for RLS can be divided into 3 groups: (1) nonpharmacologic therapy, (2) iron replacement therapy, and (3) symptomatic treatments.

Nonpharmacologic Therapy

There are behavioral strategies that can provide a relief of RLS symptoms. It is important that patients have proper sleep hygiene, avoid sleep deprivation and caffeine and other stimulants, and implement moderate regular exercise.[36]

Iron Replacement Therapy

Because of the essential role of iron in RLS pathophysiology, iron replacement therapy should always be considered as first-line treatment. To date, iron replacement is indicated if transferrin

---

Box 5
Recommended questions for the detection of augmentation phenomena

- Do RLS symptoms appear earlier than when the drug was first started?
- Are higher doses of the drug now needed or do you need to take the medicine earlier to control the RLS symptoms compared with the original effective dose?
- Has the intensity of symptoms worsened since starting the medication?
- Have symptoms spread to other parts of the body (eg, arms) since starting the medication?

When any answer is yes, augmentation should be considered. See Laura M. Botta P's article, "Restless Legs Syndrome: Challenges to Treatment," in this issue, for further information regarding how to manage augmentation.
Adapted from: Garcia-Borreguero, D., Silber, M. H., Winkelman, J. W., Högl, B., Bainbridge, J., Buchfuhrer, M., ... Allen, R. P. (2016). Guidelines for the first-line treatment of restless legs syndrome/Willis-Ekbom disease, prevention and treatment of dopaminergic augmentation: A combined task force of the IRLSSG, EURLSSG, and the RLS-foundation. Sleep Medicine, 21, 1–11. https://doi.org/10.1016/j.sleep.2016.01.017.

Table 4
Summary of dosage, administration, pharmacokinetic details, and common side effects of the dopaminergic agonists and $\alpha 2\delta$-ligands for restless legs syndrome

Therapeutic Group	Preparation	Initial Dosage (mg/d)	Titration	Maximum Recommended Dosage (mg/d)	Usual Effective Daily Dose (mg)	Time to Peak (h)	Half-lives (h)	Recommended Time of Administration	Common Side Effects
Dopaminergic agonists	Pramipexole immediate release	0.125	The dose may be doubled every 4–7 d	0.75	0.18–0.54	~2	~8.5	2–3 h before bedtime	• Nausea, headache, sleepiness, and impulse control disorders (reported to develop in 6% to 17%). The patient must be specifically questioned about this complication)
	Ropinirole immediate release	0.25	The dose may be doubled after 2 d and titrated upward in increments of 0.5 mg every week	4	2	~1–2	~6	1–3 h before bedtime	• Augmentation phenomena (for more information, see Laura M. Botta P's article,
	Rotigotine (Transdermal patch)	1	1 mg every day; dose may be increased by 1 mg/24 h every week	3	2	15–18; can occur 4–27 after application	After removal of the patch: ~5–7	Replace it every day, preferably at the same time	

α2δ Ligands								("Restless Legs Syndrome: Challenges to Treatment," in this issue)
Gabapentin	300	Increase 300 mg/d every 2 or 3 d	2400	900–2400	2–4	5–7	2 h before bedtime	Somnolence, dizziness, fatigue, weight gain, and headache
Pregabalin	75	Increase 75 mg/d every 2 or 3 d	450	150–450	1.5	6.3	2 h before bedtime	
Gabapentin enacarbil	600	The dose may be doubled after 1 wk	1200	600–1200	5–7.3	5–6	5:00–7:00 PM	

Adapted from: Garcia-Borreguero, D., Silber, M. H., Winkelman, J. W., Högl, B., Bainbridge, J., Buchfuhrer, M., … Allen, R. P. (2016). Guidelines for the first-line treatment of restless legs syndrome/Willis-Ekbom disease, prevention and treatment of dopaminergic augmentation: A combined task force of the IRLSSG, EURLSSG, and the RLS-foundation. Sleep Medicine, 21, 1–11. https://doi.org/10.1016/j.sleep.2016.01.01.

saturation is less than 45% and the serum ferritin level is less than 300 ng/mL.[37] When these cutoff points are respected, the risk of causing iron overload is very unlikely.[38] The decision about when to indicate iron replacement therapy currently depends only on the evaluation of systemic iron parameters, although it is known that having normal peripheral iron measures does not exclude having central iron deficiency.[32]

It is recommended to check systemic iron parameters with a blood test together with other parameters (see **Box 3**), both at the moment of diagnosis and during follow-up.

Both oral and intravenous routes can be useful for RLS; however, the intravenous route is preferred when any of the answers to the following questions is yes:

- Is there any contraindication for the use of the oral route?
- Has intestinal iron malabsorption or previous failure with oral treatment been reported?
- Is a more rapid response needed?
- Is the serum ferritin level less than 100 ng/mL?

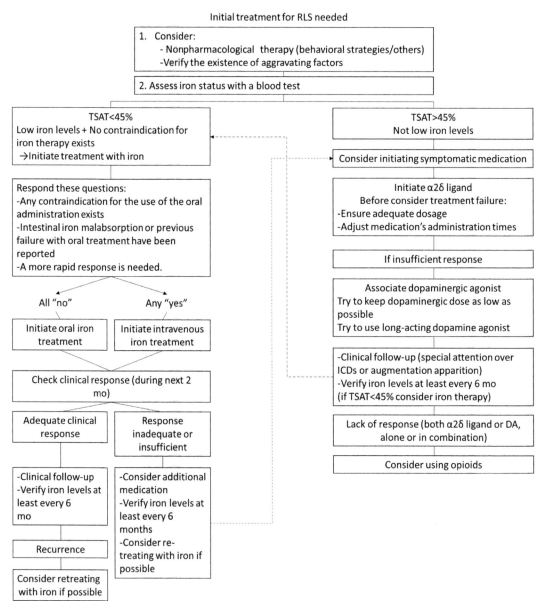

Fig. 5. General approach algorithm for initial treatment of RLS. DA, dopaminergic agonists; ICD, impulse control disorder. (*From*: Garcia-Malo, C., Peralta, S. R., & Garcia-Borreguero, D. (2020). Restless Legs Syndrome and Other Common Sleep-Related Movement Disorders. Continuum (Minneapolis, Minn.), 26(4), 963–987. https://doi.org/10.1212/CON.0000000000000886 with permission.)

Among the different formulations of intravenous iron that are available, the most compelling evidence for treating RLS is ferric carboxymaltose, using a total dose of 1000 mg.[37]

Among oral preparations, ferrous sulfate is the one that has been specifically investigated for RLS.[39–41] The main disadvantage of using the oral route is that up to 70% of patients report gastrointestinal side effects, resulting in low compliance.[42] **Box 4** summarizes general recommendations on oral iron treatment[43]

Symptomatic Treatments

When no response is obtained with nonpharmacologic therapy or correction of iron deficiency, symptomatic treatment should be considered. Classically, the treatment of choice has been dopamine agonists; however, their relation to long-term complications, such as augmentation of symptoms, is leading to changes in their role when initiating symptomatic treatment.[44] **Box 5** summarizes the questions that should alert physicians to the presence of augmentation. Although the effectiveness of dopamine agonists for the treatment of RLS is well documented, the risk of developing long-term complications has led to investigations of other therapeutic targets.

$\alpha 2\delta$-Ligands (gabapentin, pregabalin, and gabapentin enacarbil) were initially approved as anticonvulsants and later for neuropathic pain. When used in RLS, $\alpha 2\delta$-ligands have been shown to be both effective and safe in the long term.[44] Compared with dopaminergic therapy, $\alpha 2\delta$-ligands are more effective in consolidating sleep.[45]

Table 4 summarizes dosage, administration, pharmacokinetic details, and common side effects of the dopaminergic agonists and $\alpha 2\delta$-ligands for RLS.

Other therapeutic options include benzodiazepines; however, although used historically for RLS, there is no evidence for their efficacy in treating RLS. Opioids are now considered a second-line treatment of RLS (when refractory symptoms or complications derived from the treatment exist). Both methadone and oxycodone have been shown to be efficacious for RLS.[45,46] These drugs should only be prescribed by a trained physician and the patient must be closely monitored because of the potential risk of side effects such as sedation, constipation, depression, anxiety, altered consciousness, increased risk for opioid-induced respiratory depression, and substance use.[47]

Emerging treatments for RLS include perampanel, which acts on the glutamate route as a selective α-amino-3-hydroxy-5-methyl-4-isoxazolepropionic acid (AMPA) receptor antagonist,[48] and dipyridamole, which acts on the adenosine route.[49]

RLS treatment can be challenging and the decision of whether to initiate RLS treatment should be based on a risk-benefit assessment. Iron replacement therapy should be considered as a first-line treatment. Symptomatic treatment should be tailored to the patient's needs. **Fig. 5** includes an algorithm for the initial treatment of RLS.

CLINICS CARE POINTS

- RLS should be considered in every patient complaining of abnormal sensations located in the lower limbs. Patients should be asked about the urge to move the affected region and whether movement leads to a transitory relief. A circadian pattern is also observed in RLS.

- The diagnosis of RLS is clinical and is based on meeting the clinical criteria. A careful evaluation and the exclusion of other conditions producing abnormal sensations in the lower limbs are essential, such as sleep-related leg cramps, venous disorder, polyneuropathy, or akathisia.

- Every condition associated with systemic iron deficiency (with or without anemia) is related to a greater risk of RLS.

- Systemic iron parameters should be evaluated both at the beginning and periodically during the follow-up of these patients, because the choice of first-line treatment greatly depends on iron status.

- Although a clinical evaluation is essential, some complementary tests can be useful both to support RLS diagnosis and to exclude mimics. Among these, polysomnography studies, the m-SIT, and some neuroimaging techniques can be helpful in equivocal cases.

- The decision about whether to initiate RLS treatment should be based on a risk-benefit assessment. Both nonpharmacologic therapy and iron replacement therapy should be considered as first-line treatment. When necessary, symptomatic treatments should be recommended.

- The therapeutic role of dopamine agonists as the first-line treatment of RLS is undergoing reconsideration because of long-term complications (eg, augmentation phenomena). For this reason, $\alpha 2\delta$-ligands are preferred for symptomatic treatment.

- Other therapeutic options include opioids as a second-line treatment and emerging treatments acting on glutamate and adenosine receptors.

DISCLOSURE

C. Garcia-Malo reports grants from IRLSSG, outside the submitted work. The other authors have nothing to disclose.

REFERENCES

1. Allen RP, Picchietti DL, Garcia-Borreguero D, et al. Restless legs syndrome/Willis-Ekbom disease diagnostic criteria: updated International Restless Legs Syndrome Study Group (IRLSSG) consensus criteria - history, rationale, description, and significance. Sleep Med 2014;15(8):860–73.
2. Ohayon MM, O'Hara R, Vitiello MV. Epidemiology of restless legs syndrome: a synthesis of the literature. Sleep Med Rev 2012;16(4):283–95.
3. Tan EK1, Seah A, See SJ, et al. Restless legs syndrome in an Asian population: a study in Singapore. Mov Disord 2001;16(3):577–9.
4. Winkler AS, Trendafilova A, Meindl M, et al. Restless legs syndrome in a population of northern Tanzania: a community-based study. Mov Disord 2010;25(5):596–601.
5. Picchietti D, Allen RP, Walters AS, et al. Restless legs syndrome: prevalence and impact in children and adolescents - the peds REST study. Pediatrics 2007;120(2):253–66.
6. Chen SJ, Shi L, Bao YP, et al. Prevalence of restless legs syndrome during pregnancy: a systematic review and meta-analysis. Sleep Med Rev 2018;40:43–54.
7. Pantaleo NP, Hening WA, Allen RP, et al. Pregnancy accounts for most of the gender difference in prevalence of familial RLS. Sleep Med 2010;11(3):310–3.
8. Cortese S, Konofal E, Lecendreux M, et al. Restless legs syndrome and attention-deficit/hyperactivity disorder: a review of the literature. Sleep 2005;28(8):1007–13.
9. Wang Y, Huang L, Zhang L, et al. Iron status in attention-deficit/hyperactivity disorder: a systematic review and meta-analysis. PLoS One 2017;12(1):e0169145.
10. Tseng PT, Cheng YS, Yen CF, et al. Peripheral iron levels in children with attention-deficit hyperactivity disorder: a systematic review and meta-analysis. Sci Rep 2018;8(1):788.
11. Ferri R, Koo BB, Picchietti DLFS. Periodic leg movements during sleep: phenotype, neurophysiology, and clinical significance. Sleep Med 2017;31:29–38.
12. Winkelman JW, Shahar E, Sharief IGD. Association of restless legs syndrome and cardiovascular disease in the Sleep Heart Health Study. Neurology 2008;70(1):35–42.
13. Winkelman JW. The evoked heart rate response to periodic leg movements of sleep. Sleep 1999;22(5):575–80.
14. Ferri R, Zucconi M, Rundo F, et al. Heart rate and spectral EEG changes accompanying periodic and non-periodic leg movements during sleep. Clin Neurophysiol 2007;118(2):438–48.
15. Siddiqui F, Strus J, Ming X, et al. Rise of blood pressure with periodic limb movements in sleep and wakefulness. Clin Neurophysiol 2007;118(9):1923–30.
16. Allen RP, Picchietti D, Hening WA, et al. Restless legs syndrome: diagnostic criteria, special considerations, and epidemiology. A report from the restless legs syndrome diagnosis and epidemiology workshop at the National Institutes of Health. Sleep Med 2003;4(2):101–19.
17. Hallegraeff J, de Greef M, Krijnen W, et al. Criteria in diagnosing nocturnal leg cramps: a systematic review. BMC Fam Pract 2017;18(1):29.
18. Allen RE, Kirby KA. Nocturnal leg cramps. Am Fam Physician 2012;86(4):350–5.
19. Brown T. Sleep-related leg cramps: a review and Suggestions for future research. Sleep Med Clin 2015;10(3):385–92.
20. Walters AS, LeBrocq C, Dhar A, et al. Validation of the International restless legs syndrome study group rating scale for restless legs syndrome. Sleep Med 2003;4(2):121–32.
21. Ferri R, Fulda S, Manconi M, et al. World Association of Sleep Medicine (WASM) 2016 standards for recording and scoring leg movements in polysomnograms developed by a joint task force from the International and the European Restless Legs Syndrome Study Groups (IRLSSG and EURLSSG). Sleep Med 2016;26:86–95.
22. Montplaisir J, Boucher S, Nicolas A, et al. Immobilization tests and periodic leg movements in sleep for the diagnosis of restless leg syndrome. Mov Disord 1998;13(2):324–9.
23. Ferri R, Rundo F, Zucconi M, et al. Diagnostic accuracy of the standard and alternative periodic leg movement during sleep indices for restless legs syndrome. Sleep Med 2016;22:97–9.
24. Pennestri MH, Whittom S, Adam B, et al. PLMS and PLMW in healthy subjects as a function of age: prevalence and interval distribution. Sleep 2006;29(9):1183–7.
25. Mattarozzi K, Bellucci C, Campi C, et al. Clinical, behavioural and polysomnographic correlates of cataplexy in patients with narcolepsy/cataplexy. Sleep Med 2008;9(4):425–33.
26. Manconi M, Ferri R, Zucconi M, et al. Time structure analysis of leg movements during sleep in REM sleep behavior disorder. Sleep 2007;30(12):1779–85.
27. Al-Alawi A, Mulgrew A, Tench ERC. Prevalence, risk factors and impact on daytime sleepiness and hypertension of periodic leg movements with arousals in patients with obstructive sleep apnea. J Clin Sleep Med 2006;15(2):281–7.

28. Garcia-Borreguero D, Kohnen R, Boothby L, et al. Validation of the multiple suggested immobilization test: a test for the assessment of severity of restless legs syndrome (Willis-Ekbom disease). Sleep 2013; 36(7):1101–9.

29. Michaud M, Paquet J, Lavigne G, et al. Sleep laboratory diagnosis of restless legs syndrome. European Neurology 2002;48(2):108–13.

30. Trenkwalder C, Hening WA, Walters AS, et al. Circadian rhythm of periodic limb movements and sensory symptoms of restless legs syndrome. Mov Disord 1999;14(1):102–10.

31. Provini F, Chiaro G. Neuroimaging in restless legs syndrome. Sleep Med Clin 2015;10(3):215–26.

32. Earley CJ, Connor J, Garcia-Borreguero D, et al. Altered brain iron homeostasis and dopaminergic function in restless legs syndrome (Willis-Ekbom disease). Sleep Med 2014;15(11):1288–301.

33. Godau J, Schweitzer KJ, Liepelt I, et al. Substantia nigra hypoechogenicity: Definition and findings in restless legs syndrome. Mov Disord 2007;22(2): 187–92.

34. Schmidauer C, Sojer M, Seppi K, et al. Transcranial ultrasound shows nigral hypoechogenicity in restless legs syndrome. Ann Neurol 2005;54(4):630–4.

35. Garcia-Malo C, Wanner V, Miranda C, et al. Quantitative transcranial sonography of the substantia nigra as a predictor of therapeutic response to intravenous iron therapy in restless legs syndrome. Sleep Med 2019;66:123–9.

36. Aukerman MM, Aukerman D, Bayard M, et al. Exercise and restless legs syndrome: a randomized controlled trial. J Am Board Fam Med 2006;19(5):487–93. Available at: http://www.embase.com/search/results? subaction=viewrecord&from=export&id=L4457720 7%5Cnhttp://www.jabfm.org/cgi/reprint/19/5/487% 5Cnhttp://rd8hp6du2b.search.serialssolutions.com? sid=EMBASE&issn=15572625&id=doi:&atitle= Exercise+and+restless+legs+syndrome:+A.

37. Allen RP, Picchietti DL, Auerbach M, et al. Evidence-based and consensus clinical practice guidelines for the iron treatment of restless legs syndrome/Willis-Ekbom disease in adults and children: an IRLSSG task force report. Sleep Med 2018;41: 27–44.

38. Garcia-Malo C, Miranda C, Novo Ponte S, et al. Low risk of iron overload or anaphylaxis during treatment of restless legs syndrome with intravenous iron: a consecutive case series in a regular clinical setting. Sleep Med 2020;74:48–55.

39. Davis BJ, Rajput A, Rajput ML, et al. A randomized, double-blind placebo-controlled trial of iron in restless legs syndrome. Eur Neurol 2000;43(2):70–5.

40. Wang J, O'Reilly B, Venkataraman R, et al. Efficacy of oral iron in patients with restless legs syndrome and a low-normal ferritin: a randomized, double-blind, placebo-controlled study. Sleep Med 2009; 10(9):973–5.

41. Lee CS, Lee SD, Kang SH, et al. Comparison of the efficacies of oral iron and pramipexole for the treatment of restless legs syndrome patients with low serum ferritin. Eur J Neurol 2014;21(2):260–6.

42. Tolkien Z, Stecher L, Mander AP, et al. Ferrous sulfate supplementation causes significant gastrointestinal side-effects in adults: a systematic review and meta-analysis. PLoS One 2015;10(2):e0117383.

43. Garcia-Malo C, Miranda C, Romero Peralta S, et al. Iron replacement therapy in restless legs syndrome. Curr Treat Options Neurol 2020;22(11):1–16.

44. Garcia-Borreguero D, Silber MH, Winkelman JW, et al. Guidelines for the first-line treatment of restless legs syndrome/Willis-Ekbom disease, prevention and treatment of dopaminergic augmentation: a combined task force of the IRLSSG, EURLSSG, and the RLS-foundation. Sleep Med 2016;21:1–11.

45. Silver N, Allen RP, Senerth J, et al. A 10-year, longitudinal assessment of dopamine agonists and methadone in the treatment of restless legs syndrome. Sleep Med 2011;12(5):440–4.

46. Silber MH, Becker PM, Buchfuhrer MJ, et al. The appropriate use of opioids in the treatment of refractory restless legs syndrome. Mayo Clin Proc 2018; 93(1):59–67.

47. Wanner V, Garcia Malo C, Romero S, et al. Non-dopaminergic vs. dopaminergic treatment options in restless legs syndrome. Adv Pharmacol 2019; 84:187–205.

48. Garcia-Borreguero D, Cano I, Granizo JJ. Treatment of restless legs syndrome with the selective AMPA receptor antagonist perampanel. Sleep Med 2017; 34:105–8.

49. Garcia-Borreguero D, Guitart X, Garcia Malo C, et al. Treatment of restless legs syndrome/Willis-Ekbom disease with the non-selective ENT1/ENT2 inhibitor dipyridamole: testing the adenosine hypothesis. Sleep Med 2018;45:94–7.

Akathisia and Restless Legs Syndrome
Solving the Dopaminergic Paradox

Sergi Ferré, MD, PhD[a,*], Xavier Guitart, PhD[a], César Quiroz, PhD[a], William Rea, MA[a], Celia García-Malo, MD[b], Diego Garcia-Borreguero, MD[b], Richard P. Allen, PhD[c], Christopher J. Earley, MBBCh, PhD[c]

KEYWORDS

- Akathisia • Restless legs syndrome • Striatum • Dopamine • Glutamate • Adenosine
- Receptor heteromers

KEY POINTS

- Akathisia is associated with the treatment with dopamine receptor blocking agents (DRBAs) and with restless legs syndrome (RLS).
- It is proposed that akathisia depends on the alteration of specific presynaptic and postsynaptic mechanisms in the ventral striatum.
- Presynaptically, there is an increase in dopamine neurotransmission secondary to autoreceptor inactivation (with DRBA) or to a brain iron deficiency–induced increase in glutamate release (in RLS).
- Postsynaptically, there is an increased activation of dopamine D_1 receptors, which form complexes (heteromers) with dopamine D_3 and adenosine A_1 receptors.
- Adenosine and dopamine receptor heteromers localized in the ventral striatum provide potential targets for the treatment of akathisia.

INTRODUCTION: THE CLINICAL COMPLEXITY OF RESTLESS LEGS SYNDROME

Restless legs syndrome (RLS), also known as Willis-Ekbom disease, is a sensorimotor disorder characterized by an urge to move the legs, usually accompanied by or felt to be caused by uncomfortable or unpleasant sensations in the legs. Its diagnosis requires the following subjective clinical criteria: (1) urgency to move the legs, usually with unpleasant sensations; (2) appearance of symptoms during inactivity or rest; (3) relief with movement; (4) a worsening condition in the evening or at night; and (5) such features not solely accounted for as symptoms primary to another medical or a behavioral condition.[1] The latest updated consensus includes the following 4 clinical features supporting the diagnosis of RLS: (1) periodic limb movements (PLMs) during sleep (PLMS) or resting wakefulness at rates or intensity greater than expected for age or medical/medication status; (2) positive response to the treatment with dopamine receptor agonists; (3) family history of RLS among first-degree relatives; and (4) lack of profound daytime sleepiness.[1]

The term, akathisia, is used to define a feeling of restlessness, an urgent need to move— objectively perceived as psychomotor agitation, an inability to stay still. Therefore, akathisia is implicit in the description of the symptoms of RLS, which add a significant unpleasant sensory component in the legs. Pathophysiologically, RLS can be separated into 2 clinical phenomena, deficits of sensorimotor integration that produce akathisia

[a] Integrative Neurobiology Section, Intramural Research Program, National Institute on Drug Abuse, National Institutes of Health, Triad Building, 333 Cassell Drive, Baltimore, MD 21224, USA; [b] Sleep Research Institute, Paseo de la Habana 151, Madrid 28036, Spain; [c] Department of Neurology, Johns Hopkins University, Johns Hopkins Bayview Medical Center, 5501 Hopkins Bayview Circle, Baltimore, MD 21224, USA
* Corresponding author.
E-mail address: sferre@intra.nida.nih.gov

Sleep Med Clin 16 (2021) 249–267
https://doi.org/10.1016/j.jsmc.2021.02.012
1556-407X/21/Published by Elsevier Inc.

and PLMs, both more pronounced at the end of the day and beginning of the sleep period, and an enhanced arousal state or hyperarousal.[2] When studying the underlying neuropathologic mechanisms of akathisia, it is important to underscore its occurrence outside the frame of RLS. Thus, akathisia is considered as the most frequent movement disorder that develops as a complication of the exposure to dopamine receptor blocking agents (DRBAs), with a reported incidence of 21% to 75% and a prevalence of 20% to 35%.[3,4] There are 2 main distinctive forms of DRBA-induced akathisia, acute and tardive. Tardive akathisia is included in the tardive syndrome, a broad spectrum of DRBA-induced abnormal movements, which include tardive dyskinesia among other manifestations.[5–7] The tardive syndrome has 2 main characteristics: it appears late after prolonged exposure to the DRBA, and it persists and continues, and often worsens, after the offending drug is withdrawn.[6,7] Acute akathisia, on the other hand, is a condition with identical symptoms that tardive akathisia that occurs fairly early after the DRBA is introduced and dissipates upon its withdrawal.[7] Apart from the more focal predominant need to move the legs, usually associated with unpleasant sensations of the legs, akathisia of RLS differs from DRBA-induced akathisia in its predominant occurrence in the evening and at night, whereas DRBA-induced akathisia occurs mostly at daytime.[1–4]

PLMs are more pronounced in the legs, are more frequent during sleep (PLMS), and have very specific characteristics: (1) they involve the extension of the big toe and dorsiflexion of the ankle, the knee, and occasionally with flexion of the hip, and (2) they are grouped as repetitive runs of movements of a duration of 0.5 to 10 seconds, with at least 4 movements in a row, with an intermovement interval of 10 to 90 seconds.[8,9] PLMS do not only occur in RLS, where they represent a supportive diagnostic criterion, because they do not occur in all but in approximately 90% of the patients,[10] and they also occur in other sleep disorders, such as narcolepsy, rapid eye movement sleep behavior disorder, and obstructive sleep apnea syndrome.[8,9] But they also occur with high prevalence that increases with age in the general healthy population.[11] PLMS by themselves can be considered a sleep disorder when associated with clinical sleep disturbance or daytime fatigue that cannot be attributed to another sleep disorder or condition and when the PLMS index (runs of PLMS per hour) is greater than 15 in adults and 5 in children.[8,9] As first stated by Moore and colleagues,[12] the demonstration of the same gene polymorphisms being associated with an increased risk of RLS and an increased risk of PLMS without RLS strongly suggests that RLS and PLMS form part of a spectrum disorder.[11,12] It could be said that akathisia and PLMS are pathophysiologically linked clinical features of a spectrum disorder that include the PLMS disorder, RLS with PLMS, and RLS without PLMS.

Hyperarousal in RLS manifests, first, as a short sleep time (4.0–5.5 h)[13] with episodes of arousal (awakening) during sleep, related but not caused by the PLMs. Thus, in approximately half of all cases, the onset of the episodes of arousal precedes the onset of the leg movements.[14] Second, as part of the clinical features supporting the diagnosis of RLS, there often is a lack of profound sleepiness during the day, which would be expected given the significant total sleep loss at night.[15] The mechanisms of the 3 separate pathophysiologic phenomena, akathisia, PLMS, and hyperarousal still need to be determined. An additional challenge is the pathophysiologic integration of these apparently disconnected phenomena. This article focuses on akathisia and its main mechanisms but also reviews a recently proposed heuristic hypothesis for a specific integrative pathophysiologic mechanism in RLS, an alteration of the adenosinergic system secondary to brain iron deficiency (BID).[2,16]

THE DOPAMINERGIC PARADOX OF AKATHISIA

The neural mechanisms of akathisia have been difficult to dissect because of the apparent conundrum of a syndrome that seems to result from a hyperdopaminergic state and yet, in case of DRBA-induced akathisia, it is associated with a high occupancy of striatal D_2 receptors (here abbreviated D2R).[17] Adding to the apparent conundrum, akathisia of RLS also is associated with a neurochemical hyperdopaminergic state (discussed later) and yet dopamine receptor agonists provide an initial significant relief. To explain the akathisia paradox, in 1980, Marsden and Jenner invoked the autoreceptor hypothesis,[18] based on an ample experimental evidence indicating the existence of dopamine autoreceptors and their role in locomotor depression induced by low doses of dopamine receptor agonists. Thus, ex vivo and in vitro experiments in rodents showed that small doses or concentrations of the nonselective dopamine receptor agonist apomorphine reduced tyrosine hydroxylase (TH) activity (dopamine synthesis), dopamine release, and dopamine neuronal impulse flow.[19–22]

Subsequent studies clearly establish the existence of autoreceptors both in the terminals and somatodendritic region of the midbrain dopaminergic neurons of the substantia nigra pars compacta and in the ventral tegmental area (VTA).[23–25] There has been a long debate about which are the dopamine receptor subtypes that function as autoreceptors. Dopamine receptors are classified in Gs protein–coupled dopamine D_1–like receptors, with dopamine D_1 and D_5 receptor subtypes (here abbreviated D1R and D5R, respectively), and Gi-coupled dopamine D_2–like receptors, with D2R and dopamine D_3 and D_4 receptor subtypes (here abbreviated D3R and D4R, respectively).[26] Some studies indicate that dopamine autoreceptors are predominantly of the D2R subtype with a predominant contribution of its short isoform (D2SR) versus its long isoform (D2L). These studies used different genetic approaches, with selective genetic inactivation of different D_2-like receptor subtypes (D2R vs D3R subtypes),[27] of the 2 different D2R isoforms (D2SR vs D2LR isoforms)[28] or of D2R in the dopaminergic cells.[29] Nevertheless, D3R and D3R mRNA clearly also have been identified in the rodent and human midbrain dopaminergic cells, albeit with lower density than D2R.[30–33] In addition, recent studies using highly selective D3R antagonists strongly support their additional role as autoreceptors, with a possible preferential inhibitory effect on dopamine uptake and with less influence than the D2R on dopamine synthesis and release.[34–36]

The autoreceptor hypothesis of DRBA-induced akathisia then would imply that a preferential blockade of presynaptic versus postsynaptic D2R or D3R could lead to a presynaptic hyperdopaminergic state by disinhibition of dopamine synthesis and release or by decrease in the dopamine uptake. This would lead to an increase in the extracellular concentration of dopamine that still could promote a significant activation of postsynaptic dopamine receptors, at least of the nonblocked D1R. Following a similar rationale, the clinical efficacy of D_2-like receptor agonists in RLS would depend on a presynaptic effect, on their ability to preferentially block the dopamine autoreceptors and counteract the associated presynaptic hyperdopaminergic state (discussed later). But, 3 more considerations need to be reviewed in order to understand the behavioral effects of D_2-like receptor ligands and the possible contribution of autoreceptors and postsynaptic dopamine receptors to the akathisia induced by DRBAs or akathisia in RLS: (1) the existence of different functional striatal compartments in the striatum, mostly the dorsal and ventral striatum, innervated by the dopaminergic cells of the substantia nigra pars compacta and the VTA, respectively; (2) the differential expression and role of dopamine receptor subtypes in different striatal neuronal populations; and (3) the existence of indirect interactions at the circuit level between specific dopamine receptor subtypes and the existence of direct intermolecular interactions (heteromerization) within the same neuron.

INDIRECT INTERACTIONS BETWEEN DOPAMINE RECEPTORS SUBTYPES: THE D1R-D2R COOPERATION AT THE CIRCUIT LEVEL

The dorsal striatum corresponds to the anatomically defined caudate-putamen and the ventral striatum corresponds to the nucleus accumbens with its 2 subcompartments, shell and core, and the olfactory tubercle. A main role of the ventral striatum, labeled by Mogenson[37] as an interface between motivation and action, can be synthesized as determining "whether to respond" whereas that of the dorsal striatum determines "how to respond" to reward-associated stimuli.[38,39] In rodents, systemic administration of psychostimulants produces psychomotor activation, manifested as locomotor activation and orofacial stereotypies,[40] which classically has been associated with the respective dopaminergic activation of the ventral and dorsal striatum. Thus, locomotor activation can be produced by the intracranial infusion in the ventral but not the dorsal striatum of psychostimulants, such as amphetamine or cocaine, drugs that increase the extracellular concentration of dopamine, or the infusion of nonselective dopamine receptor agonists, such as apomorphine.[41–47] Also, the selective lesion of the dopaminergic nerve terminals in the ventral striatum markedly reduces locomotion induced by the systemic administration of amphetamine or cocaine.[48] On the other hand, the infusion in the dorsal but not the ventral striatum of psychostimulants or dopamine led to orofacial stereotypies.[44,49] The ventral striatal–dependent locomotor activation induced by psychostimulants and dopamine receptor agonists, therefore, seems to represent an experimental animal counterpart of the akathisia induced by psychostimulants, whereas the dorsal striatal–dependent stereotypies represents the associated stereotypies and dyskinesias.[50,51]

Apart from their localization in dopaminergic neurons as autoreceptors, striatal D2R also are localized postsynaptically in the GABAergic striatopallidal neuron, which is in 1 of the 2 main striatal neuronal populations.[52] The other main population is represented by the GABAergic striatonigral neuron, which connects the striatum with the substantia nigra pars reticulata and substantia nigra pars compacta, the VTA, and the internal segment of the globus pallidus (the entopeduncular nucleus in rodents).[52] The striatonigral neurons constitute the direct striatal efferent pathway, which directly connect the input structure of the basal ganglia, the striatum, with the output structures of the basal ganglia, which are the substantia nigra pars reticulata and the internal segment of the globus pallidus (**Fig. 1**). The striatopallidal neurons, on the other hand, give rise to the indirect striatal efferent pathway, which indirectly connects the striatum with the output structures through the external segment of the globus pallidus (globus pallidus in rodents), ventral pallidum, and subthalamic nucleus (see **Fig. 1**).[52] A segregation of dopamine receptor subtypes exists in the 2 striatal GABAergic efferent neurons, with striatopallidal neurons expressing D2R and the striatonigral neurons expressing D1R (see **Fig. 1**).[52]

The same dichotomic classification of D1R striatonigral and D2R striatopallidal GABAergic neurons applies to the dorsal and ventral striatum and activation of the ventral striatonigral and ventral striatopallidal neurons leads to psychomotor activation and inactivation, respectively.[38] Dopamine promotes psychomotor activation by activating stimulatory D1R in the striatonigral and inhibitory D2R in the striatopallidal neurons. This has been long advocated as the mechanism responsible for the well-established cooperative effect of the activation of dopamine D1R and D2R receptors in the ventral and dorsal striatum in the elicitation of locomotor activity and orofacial stereotypies in rodents, respectively.[45–47,53–56]

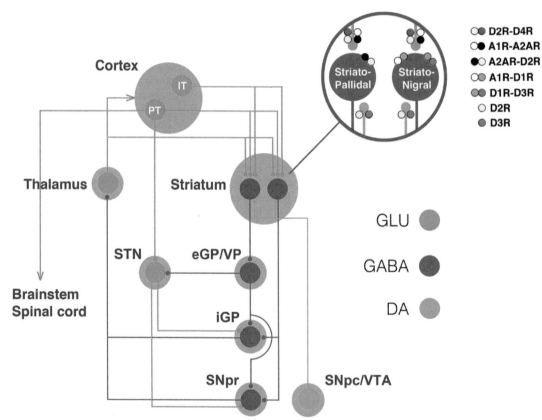

Fig. 1. Scheme of the corticostriatal-thalamic-cortical circuits and the localization of striatal presynaptic and postsynaptic adenosine and dopamine receptors. Presynaptic D2R and D3R localized in striatal dopaminergic terminals and A1R-A2AR and D2R-D4R heteromers localized in corticostriatal glutamate terminals modulate dopamine and glutamate release, respectively. Postsynaptic A2AR-D2R heteromers control the function of striatopallidal neurons and postsynaptic A1R-D1R and D1R-D3R heteromers control the function of striatonigral neurons. DA, dopamine neurons; eGP/VP, external segment of the globus pallidus/ventral pallidum; GABA, γaminobutyric acid; GLU, glutamate; iGP, internal segment of the globus pallidus; IT, intratelencephalic neurons; PT, pyramidal tract neurons; SNpc, substantia nigra pars compacta; SNpr, substantia nigra pars reticulata; STN, subthalamic nucleus.

Results of the locomotor activating effects of single and combined systemic administration of D1R and D2R agonists then can be explained in the frame of 3 main populations of dopamine receptors: postsynaptic D1R, localized in the ventral striatonigral neurons, presynaptic D2R, localized in the somatodendritic region and terminals of VTA dopaminergic cells (autoreceptors), and postsynaptic D2R, localized in the ventral striatopallidal neurons.

An illustrative experiment was performed by Jackson and colleagues in 1988.[57] They showed that the systemic administration of the D2R-D3R agonists bromocriptine and quinpirole produce a dose-dependent locomotor depression in naïve mice, which apparently was counteracted by coadministrations of D1R agonists. The investigators concluded that the D2R agonist–induced locomotor depression is mediated via D2R autoreceptors (the identity of D3R had not been established yet), which mediate an inhibition of dopamine release onto postsynaptic DA receptors, depriving postsynaptic D1R and D2R from dopamine. Nevertheless, postsynaptic D2R still were activated by the experimenter-administered D2R agonists, indicating that activation of postsynaptic D2R promotes little behavioral activation effect and that the concomitant D1R activation, that is, the activation of the ventral striatonigral neuron, is critical for promoting locomotor activation.

From these considerations, speculations about D2R antagonists can be made. D2R antagonists, at specific doses, should be able to promote dopamine release by blocking a tonic activation of autoreceptors by endogenous dopamine, which should promote the activation of D1R in the ventral striatonigral neurons. It then could be surmised that, unless completely blocked by the D2R antagonist, the remaining activation of postsynaptic D2R in the ventral striatopallidal neurons is sufficient to allow cooperation with the activation of the ventral striatonigral neurons. This interpretation would be based on the assumption that synergistic interactions of D1R and D2R agonists is established at the circuit level, by the simultaneous activation of the ventral striatonigral and inactivation of the ventral striatopallidal neuron. An additional significant factor, direct interactions between D1R and D3R at the neuronal level, is discussed later.

It is well established that locomotor activity induced by dopamine receptor agonists in reserpinized mice represents activation of striatal postsynaptic dopamine receptors, without the confounding effect of endogenous dopamine or any influence of exogenous D2R-D3R agonists on dopamine release. Systemic administration of reserpine produces a pronounced depletion of catecholamines,[58] which produces an almost complete immobility that can be reversed partially by D1R or D2R agonists and largely reversed by concomitant administration of both D1R and D2R agonists.[58–60] Experiments in reserpinized mice would support the D1R-D2R cooperation model not only of locomotor activation but also of segregated striatal D1R and D2R and, therefore, of an integration of D1R-mediated and D2R-mediated signaling at the circuit level. For instance, a differential effect of adenosine receptor agonists with different selectivity for the adenosine receptor subtypes A_1 (A1R) and A_{2A} (A2AR) could be demonstrated in their respective abilities to counteract the locomotor activation in reserpinized mice induced by D1R and D2R agonists.[60] These experiments led to the discovery of a respective segregation of A1R and A2AR in the striatonigral and striatopallidal neurons and to specific molecular interactions, heteromerization, between A1R and D1R and between A2A and D2R (see Fig. 1).[39,61–63] The A2AR-D2R heteromers have been the focus of extensive research and found to be main targets for the psychostimulant effects of caffeine.[62,64] As discussed later, A1R-D1R heteromers also are localized in the spinal motoneurons[65] and both striatal and spinal A1R-D1R heteromers might play a significant role in the pathogenesis of RLS.

DIRECT INTERACTIONS BETWEEN DOPAMINE RECEPTORS SUBTYPES: THE D1R-D3R HETEROMER

Several experiments indicated, however, that D1R-D2R cooperation also can take place within the striatum, probably at the cellular level. Thus, in ex vivo experiments, D1R and D2R agonists showed a synergistic effect on neuronal activation (c-fos expression) that was insensitive to tetrodotoxin, which implied being independent of action potentials and, therefore, circuit independent.[66] D1R-D2R cooperation could be demonstrated at the cellular level, in striatal GABAergic efferent neurons, with electrophysiologic experiments in slice preparations of the nucleus accumbens.[67] Those results then would be in conflict with the predominant striatal segregation of D1R and D2R in different neuronal populations. An answer to this problem was found by investigating the localization and functional role of the different striatal D_2-like receptor subtypes, which had been hampered by the lack of sensitive techniques and selective ligands. A seminal experiment by Surmeier and colleagues,[68] using a method of amplification of mRNA sequences from individual striatal neurons in rats, confirmed the predominant segregation of D1R and D2R subtypes in different striatal efferent neurons but also demonstrated an additional significant expression of the D3R subtype in the D1R-expressing neurons. Some other studies would demonstrate that this colocalization preferentially occur in the ventral striatum (discussed later), the brain area with maximal expression of D3R in rodents.[30,31] In the human brain, a higher expression of D3R also was found in the ventral striatum but with less pronounced higher expression than in the dorsal striatum compared with rodents.[33] Also, in humans, D3R were highly expressed in the internal segment of the globus pallidus and substantia nigra pars reticulata, localization of the nerve terminals of striatonigral neurons. In these areas, the expression of D2R was significantly lower and the opposite pattern of expression, a significantly higher expression of D2R versus D3R, also was observed in the substantia nigra pars compacta,[33] in agreement with the predominant role of D2R as autoreceptors.

In 1998, Schwartz and colleagues[69] put forward the hypothesis of the D1R-D3R coexistence. Based on their results from in vitro and ex vivo experiments in rodents, they suggested that D3R activation can sometimes promote inhibition of adenylyl cyclase (AC) signaling and sometimes promote activation of mitogenesis, most probably by activation of the mitogen-activated protein kinase (MAPK) signaling pathway, which could respectively inhibit or potentiate D1R-mediated activation of AC or MAPK signaling. They then suggested that "the two receptor subtypes may affect neurons in either synergy or opposition according to the cell or signal generated."[69] More recently, using ligands with different selectivity for D2R and D3R and genetic blockade of D3R in reserpinized mice, the authors obtained results that suggested that the indirect D1R-D2R cooperation model of psychomotor activation should be revisited and put forward the direct D1R-D3R cooperation model. In reserpinized mice, isolated activation of postsynaptic striatal D3R did not produce any behavioral effect, but it significantly potentiated the locomotor activity induced by D1R agonists.[70,71] Coexpression of D1R and D3R and their cooperation subsequently has been demonstrated in the rat substantia nigra pars reticulata, in the terminals of the GABAergic striatonigral neurons, providing a significant amplification of the same mechanism at the neuronal terminal level.[72]

Several in vitro experiments in mammalian transfected cells and parallel ex vivo experiments in reserpinized mice provide the molecular and signaling mechanisms responsible for the D1R-D3R cooperation, which depend on the ability of D1R and D3R to form complexes, D1R-D3R heteromers.[70,71,73,74] G protein–coupled receptors (GPCRs) form precoupled functional complexes that include the same or other receptors making receptor oligomers. A receptor oligomer is defined as a "macromolecular complex composed of at least 2 (functional) receptor units (protomers) with biochemical properties that are demonstrably different from those of its individual components."[75] The pentameric structure constituted by 1 GPCR homodimer and 1 heterotrimeric G protein provides a main functional unit and GPCR heteromers often have a tetrameric structure, constituted by 2 homodimers coupled to their preferred G protein.[76,77] This is of particular functional importance with heteromers that include a GPCR homodimer coupling to a Gs protein, like the D1R or the A2AR, and another homodimer coupling to a Gi protein, like the D2R or the A1R. Such a GPCR heterotetramer provides a functional precoupled macromolecular complex that includes 2 molecularly different GPCRs, their cognate G proteins, and the plasma membrane effector AC, which provides the frame for the canonical antagonistic interaction at the AC level, the ability of a Gi-coupled GPCR to counteract AC activation induced by a Gs-coupled GPCR.[77] That this canonical interaction at the AC level depends on the integrity of the heterotetramer and its precoupling to AC was demonstrated by using specific synthetic peptides that disrupt their intermolecular interactions and, simultaneously, disrupt the canonical interaction.[63]

The D1R-D3R heteromer was the first GPCR heterotetramer described, constituted by a D1R homomer coupled to Gs (or to the Golf subtype in the striatum)[78] and a D3R homomer coupled to Gi (or Go subtype) (**Fig. 2**).[71] Initially demonstrated In cells in culture, the D1R-D3R heteromer provided the frame for a canonical interaction at the AC level, with the ability of D3R agonists to counteract D1R agonist–induced AC activation, which leads to cyclic adenosine monophosphate (cAMP) formation and protein kinase A (PKA) activation (see **Fig. 2**).[71,74] That the canonical antagonistic interaction at the AC level is a property of the D1R-D3R heteromer was demonstrated with synthetic peptides that specifically disrupted the quaternary structure of the heteromer.[74] This canonical interaction could explain some results of interactions between D1R and D3R ligands in the nucleus accumbens, particularly those of D3R antagonists,[36] because the much higher affinity of D3R for dopamine than the D1R implies that endogenous dopamine is occupying a significant proportion of D3R under basal conditions, which

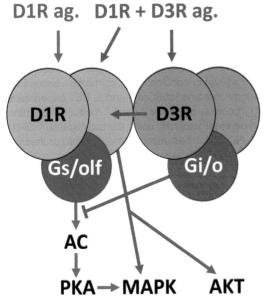

D1R ag.   D1R + D3R ag.

Fig. 2. Scheme of the molecular mechanism of the cellular D1R-D3R cooperation in the striatal D1R-D3R heterotetramer. Selective activation of the D1R in the D1R-D3R heterotetramer leads to a Gs/olf protein–dependent AC–PKA-MAPK signaling (*blue arrows*). Coactivation of D1R and D3R in the D1R-D3R heterotetramer leads to a Gi/o-Gs/olf canonical antagonistic interaction and AC inhibition and to a synergistic G protein–independent and ß-arrestin–dependent MAPK and AKT activation (*red arrows*). The G protein–independent signaling by the D1R-D3R heteromer explains the D1R-D3R cooperation, such as the synergistic locomotor activation of D1R and D3R agonists (ag.) in reserpinized mice.

tonically counteracts a D1R-mediated AC activation (discussed later). This would predict that D3R agonists are mainly pharmacologically silent under conditions of physiologic dopamine release, whereas D3R antagonists should significantly potentiate D1R-mediated AC signaling. Recent electrophysiologic experiments in slices of the mouse nucleus accumbens found that a selective D3R antagonist significantly potentiated a D1R-mediated increase in the neural activity of the D1R-expressing neurons.[36] These experiments also suggested that a significant population of D1R in the nucleus accumbens are forming D1R-D3R heteromers.

If that is the case and D3R are constantly suppressing the ability of D1R to signal the AC-PKA pathway in the nucleus accumbens, what is the function of the D1R in the D1R-D3R heteromer in vivo? Furthermore, can D1R-D3R heteromerization simultaneously mediate the canonical antagonistic interaction and the D1R-D3R cooperation demonstrated in reserpinized mice? First in mammalian transfected cells, it could be

demonstrated that although D1R and D3R agonists interact antagonistically at the G protein-dependent AC-PKA-MAPK signaling, they interact synergistically at the G protein–independent ß-arrestin/ MAPK/AKT signaling (see **Fig. 2**).[71,74] Again, D1R-D3R heteromer-disrupting peptides disrupted the G protein–independent synergistic interaction between D1R and D3R agonists.[71] More specifically, these studies indicate that D3R activation promotes a change in the D1R signaling from a G protein–dependent to a G protein–independent mechanism (see **Fig. 2**).[74] This switch also could be observed by analyzing D1R agonist–mediated MAPK activation in ex vivo experiments in reserpinized mice. A D1R agonist alone or coadministered with a D3R agonist promoted a selective striatal MAPK activation in the nucleus accumbens, which was respectively and selectively inhibited by an inhibitor of PKA activation or by the D1R-D3R heteromer-disrupting peptide.[74] Finally, the synergistic locomotor activation of D1R and D3R agonists in reserpinized mice correlated with a synergistic AKT activation in the ventral striatum.[74] In summary, the D1R-D3R cooperation responsible for the synergistic locomotor activation of D1R and D3R agonists is mediated by the G protein–independent signaling of the D1R-D3R heteromer localized in the striatonigral neurons of the nucleus accumbens (see **Fig. 2**).

DOPAMINERGIC MECHANISMS IN ACUTE DOPAMINE RECEPTOR BLOCKING AGENT–INDUCED AKATHISIA

Putting together the significant role of particularly D2R, but also D3R, as autoreceptors and the significant role of the D1R-D3R heteromer localized in the ventral striatonigral neuron in locomotor activation, a mechanism for DRBA-induced akathisia could be proposed with 1 final consideration, which is the different affinity of dopamine and DRBAs for the different dopamine receptor subtypes. Dopamine has the highest affinity for D3R compared with the other D2R subtypes. Thus, dopamine has twice more affinity for the D3R than for D4R and between 4 times and 5 times more affinity for D3R than for the D2R (both isoforms, D2SR and D2LR).[79] In addition, dopamine has significantly higher affinity for D2R than for D1R. Therefore, D2R are more activated than D1R by basal dopamine levels and are more sensitive to the effects of dopamine pauses, whereas D1R are more sensitive to dopamine bursts.[80] Bursts of dopamine neurons produce conditions of high dopamine release, which activate stimulatory D1R in the striatonigral neurons, activating the direct striatal efferent pathway (also called the Go pathway), to promote reward-associated movements, whereas dopamine pauses produce conditions of low dopamine release, which remove the activation of inhibitory D2R in the striatopallidal neurons, activating the indirect pathway (also called the NoGo pathway), to suppress non–reward-and-punishment–associated movements.[81,82]

On the other hand, in general, DRBAs (first or second generation) have higher affinities for D2R than for not only D1R but also for D3R or D4R.[83] Following the autoreceptor hypothesis, at doses that promote high occupancy of postsynaptic D2R in the ventral striatopallidal neuron, most DRBAs should be associated with a significant autoreceptor blockade and, therefore, increased extracellular concentrations of dopamine, which could be sufficient to activate postsynaptic D1R in the ventral striatonigral neuron. Because dopamine can compete better for the binding of DRBA to the D3R than to the D2R (because of the relative differences in the affinities of dopamine and the DRBAs for the 2 receptor subtypes), a predominant occupation of the postsynaptic D3R by dopamine should promote the D1R-D3R cooperation in the D1R-D3R heteromer and promote akathisia.

This mechanism could be sufficient to explain the high incidence of acute DRBA-induced akathisia and predicts that an increased sensitivity of D3R should increase the susceptibility to develop akathisia. This is the case and a significant association has been demonstrated for a D3R gene (DRD3) polymorphism and an increased susceptibility of akathisia and tardive dyskinesia.[84–87] The polymorphism occurs in the coding sequence and gives rise to a serine to glycine substitution in the N terminus of the receptor (Ser9Gly), which determines a significant increase in the affinity of dopamine.[88]

DOPAMINERGIC MECHANISMS IN THE TARDIVE SYNDROME

Another mechanism that could result in increased sensitivity to develop akathisia is an increase in the number of D3R, a D3R up-regulation. The sustained treatment with L-dopa or a D1R agonist in rodents with unilateral dopamine denervation leads to a behavioral sensitization (increase in the asymmetric locomotor activation or turning behavior) that is associated with a selective and pronounced up-regulation of striatal D3R.[89] D3R up-regulation with a concomitant increase in its synergistic interactions with D1R was then suggested to provide a mechanism for the behavioral sensitization to psychostimulants, which would probably involve the ventral striatum, and a mechanism for a major complication

of the long-term treatment of Parkinson disease with levodopa (L-dopa), L-dopa–induced dyskinesia (LID), which would depend on D3R up-regulation in the dorsal striatum.[89] D3R up-regulation in the ventral striatum has been demonstrated in rats self-administering cocaine,[90] in postmortem tissue from human cocaine fatalities[91] and in PET experiments in cocaine-dependent and methamphetamine-dependent subjects, using the radioligand [^{11}C]-(1)-PHNO, which has approximately 20-fold preferential affinity for D3R versus D2R.[92,93]

Dopamine denervation and sustained activation of postsynaptic striatal receptors, therefore, seem to be the 2 main factors that promote D3R up-regulation, which here is hypothesized that implies an increase in D1R-DR3 heteromerization and a consequent increased ability of D1R to signal through a G protein–independent mechanism. D3R up-regulation in the ventral striatum then could represent a key mechanism involved in tardive akathisia. But there also is experimental evidence indicating that D3R up-regulation potentially can extend to the dorsal striatum. The same discrete ventral striatal MAPK activation obtained in reserpinized mice upon administration of a D1R agonist also was reported previously in naïve rats upon systemic administration of D1R agonists or upon endogenous dopamine release (by electrical activation of midbrain striatal dopaminergic afferents).[71] In the same study, it also was demonstrated that the pattern of D1R agonist–mediated MAPK activation extended to the whole striatum upon 6-hydroxydopamine–induced striatal dopamine denervation.[94] The investigators concluded that D1R supersensitivity induced by prolonged dopamine denervation is related to a switch in MAPK signaling, with an extension of D1R agonist–induced MAPK activation from the ventral to the dorsal striatum.[94] Selective D3R up-regulation (with a concomitant increase in D1R-D3R heteromerization) provides the most plausible mechanistic explanation, as supported by electrophysiologic studies in acutely dissociated striatal neurons obtained from rodents with unilateral 6-hydroxydopamine–induced striatal dopamine denervation.[95]

D3R up-regulation in the dorsal striatum then could be a main pathogenetic mechanism involved in LID and tardive dyskinesia. Selective D3R up-regulation was demonstrated in the dorsal striatum of rodent models of LID[96–98] and also in nonhuman primates and human subjects with LID.[99,100] In MPTP-induced parkinsonian nonhuman primates showing dyskinesia after treatment with L-dopa, there was a selective increase in D3R versus D1R or D2R density in the dorsal striatum as well as in the D3R-rich section of the globus pallidus, its internal segment.[99] A recent PET study also could demonstrate a significant heightened binding in the D3R-rich section of the globus pallidus compared to nondyskinetic patients.[100]

Finally, apart from homozygosity for the Ser9Gly variant (allele 2) of the DRD3 gene, experimental evidence indicates that D3R up-regulation also is involved in tardive dyskinesia. Thus, in a nonhuman primate model of tardive dyskinesia, chronic treatment with haloperidol produced a selective increase in D3R density in both the dorsal and ventral striatum and internal segment of the globus pallidus.[101] It also was shown that the D3R up-regulation was selective for the GABAergic striatal neurons of the direct efferent pathway, the D1R-expressing striatal neurons.[101] Finally, a more recent study by the same research group found an increase in AKT activation (phosphorylated AKT) in the putamen of monkeys chronically treated with haloperidol that develop dyskinesia, which correlated with dyskinetic scores.[102] The study also showed up-regulated levels of D3R and that colocalization of D3R and phosphorylated AKT was enriched in haloperidol-treated animals displaying tardive dyskinesia.[102]

DOPAMINERGIC MECHANISMS IN RESTLESS LEGS SYNDROME: DEPENDENCE ON BRAIN IRON DEFICIENCY

Different to DRBA-induced akathisia, in RLS. clinical data clearly indicate the presence of a presynaptic hyperdopaminergic state. In this case, as discussed previously, the dopaminergic paradox is related to the very effective initial treatment with D_2-like receptor agonists, such as pramipexole and ropinirole. Importantly, however, long-term treatment with dopamine receptor agonists leads to a reversal of their therapeutic effect and to augmentation of RLS symptomatology.[103] Unfortunately, there is no clue as to the mechanisms involved in the augmentation phenomenon, which is leading to a revision of the guidelines for the pharmacologic treatment of RLS.[103] Nevertheless, there are compelling experimental data about the main factor that leads to the hyperdopaminergic state in RLS. This is BID, which now is well recognized as a main initial pathogenetic mechanism in the development of RLS. The role of BID is based on the results from studies analyzing cerebrospinal fluid (CSF) samples and autopsy material and from brain imaging studies, which consistently indicate a reduction of brain iron in RLS patients.[104] This is without a concomitant iron deficient anemia, although peripheral iron deficiency (with or without anemia) predisposes to BID and RLS.[105,106]

The cause of BID is still not well determined, but several experimental, clinical, and postmortem studies indicate that it is associated with alterations in the expression or function of iron management proteins involved in the acquisition or export of iron by the brain.[107–111] The results of these studies are not discussed in detail, and interested readers are referred to the references herein and to additional reviews.[104,112,113] Nevertheless, there is evidence for the involvement of genetic factors. This is indirectly supported by the experimental evidence of a differential susceptibility to BID in recombinant inbred mouse strains and of alterations in iron homeostasis associated with RLS-risk gene polymorphisms, such as MEIS1 and BTB9.[112,114–117] It also should be underlined that the involvement of BID in RLS is promoting the use of iron therapy, not only in refractory RLS but also as a first-line treatment.[118]

The alterations of the dopaminergic system in RLS that imply a hyperdopaminergic state are based on analysis of CSF samples and postmortem material, which reflect an increase in dopamine synthesis, secondary to an increase in TH activity. Thus, TH is a critical enzyme in dopamine synthesis that utilizes iron and tetrahydrobiopterin as cofactors.[119] CSF in RLS patients showed an increase in tetrahydrobiopterin and 3-ortho-methyldopa and homovanillic acid, which together indicate an increase in dopamine synthesis.[104,120] In addition, the neurochemical dopaminergic profile in postmortem tissue from RLS patients includes an increase in the density of phosphorylated TH in the substantia nigra and in the striatum as well as a decreased density of striatal D2R.[110] Because phosphorylated TH is the active form of the enzyme, its up-regulation can explain the increased dopamine synthesis, whereas the decrease in D2R density most probably represents an adaptation, down-regulation, secondary to an increased dopamine release. An in vivo decrease in D2R radioligand binding potential also has been shown in the striatum of RLS patients with PET and single-photon emission computed tomography techniques (reviewed by Earley and colleagues).[104] Nevertheless, the most recent interpretation is that the significant decrease in D2R radioligand binding potential mostly reflects an increased extracellular concentration of endogenous dopamine displacing the D2R radiogand,[121] again indicating the existence of a presynaptic hyperdopaminergic state.

Support for the assumption that these dopaminergic alterations are BID-dependent comes from the repeated demonstration of a preferential decrease in iron content in the substantia nigra, as measured by magnetic resonance imaging (MRI) and transcranial sonography and in postmortem studies (reviewed by Earley and colleagues).[104] It is difficult, however, to directly link a reduction in neuronal iron content with an increased activity of the nonheme iron protein TH. In addition, most iron in the substantia nigra is localized in oligodendrocytes and it is very low, histochemicaly undetectable, in the dopaminergic (neuromelanin-containing) neurons.[109] Furthermore, in rodents and nonhuman primates, iron content is much higher in the substantia nigra pars reticulata than the substantia nigra pars compacta.[122,123] Other brain areas with maximal content of iron included the other target areas of the striatonigral and striatopallidal neurons: the globus pallidus (external segment of the globus pallidus in primates), the ventral pallidum, and the interpeduncular nucleus (internal segment of the globus pallidus in primates) and their myelinated tracts.[122,123] Consequently, the values of nigral iron content as measured with different techniques in humans most probably represent values from the oligodendrocytes of the substantia nigra pars reticulata and, therefore, the significant reduction of nigral iron content in RLS should not represent, after all, an iron deficiency of the dopaminergic neurons. Nevertheless, alterations in the expression of transferrin and transferrin receptors that support a specific impairment of iron acquisition could be specifically demonstrated in the neuromelanin-containing cells of the substantia nigra pars compacta of RLS patients.[109]

The question remains about if BID is directly and predominantly affecting the dopaminergic neurons of the substantia nigra, which, if anything, should result in a dorsal striatal clinical symptomatology. According to this review, akathisia in RLS should depend on a hyperdopaminergic state in the ventral striatum, whereas other components of the syndrome, mainly PLMS, still could involve the dorsal striatum. The complete picture also would require a mechanism behind the circadian-dependent expression of akinesia and PLMS in RLS. There are, in fact, results that imply a more generalized BID in RLS, including the striatum and thalamus.[124,125] It also could be expected that the functional abnormalities in the dopaminergic system be secondary to BID-dependent alterations in other functionally connected brain areas or neurotransmitter systems. This new mechanistic explanation comes from results obtained in animal models.

It could be argued that the best demonstration of the dependence on BID for the development of the dopaminergic alterations in RLS is their recapitulation in rodents with BID. BID is difficult to study in adult rodents, because of the very efficient capacity of the adult rodent brain to keep normal iron stores, even with severe anemia. Nevertheless, BID in rodents can be optimally induced by providing an iron deficiency diet during the postweaning period.[104] BID in weanling rodents constitutes an animal model of RLS with construct and face validity. Thus, weanling rodents with BID consistently have shown correlational neurochemical changes in the dopaminergic system as those found in RLS, mainly the increased TH activity in the substantia nigra and in the striatum and the reduced striatal density of D2R.[2,104,110,126] In addition, several studies have shown that rodents with an iron-deficient diet during the postweaning period develop an RLS-like clinical phenotype, with akathisia-like behavior (locomotor activation) and leg movements with practically the same characteristic to those of PLMS. This RLS-like phenotype demonstrates the same circadian variation than RLS symptoms, with their maximal expression at the end of the active period and beginning of the active period (for most recent studies, see Lai and colleagues[127] and Allen and colleagues[128]). In addition, the BID-induced RLS-like phenotype in rodents can be counteracted by clinically effective dopamine receptor agonists,[127,128] which is 1 of the 4 clinical features supporting the diagnosis of RLS (discussed previously).

Of particular construct validity is the BXD40 mouse strain, selected from BXD strains derived from the C57BL/6J and DBA/2J progenitor strains. Evaluation of more than 20 BXD strains, including BXD40, demonstrated a differential effect of an iron-deficient diet during the postweaning period on peripheral and brain iron levels, indicating different genetic regulation of peripheral and brain iron.[115] Upon the iron-deficient diet during the postweaning period, BXD40 female mice (BXD40f) showed an increased locomotor activation with the circadian characteristics of RLS.[128] More importantly, BXD40f were identified as having an RLS iron biological pattern of significant BID. BXD40f mice with BID initially were shown to display a significant decrease in iron content in the ventral midbrain (which includes the substantia nigra and VTA) and striatum.[115] In a subsequent study in BXD40f mice, BID was shown to be significantly more pronounced in the ventral than the dorsal striatum.[129] In addition, alterations of striatal dopaminergic neurotransmission in the ventral striatum, including an increased concentration of dopamine and a decrease in D2R density already had been described in rats after an iron-deficient diet during the postweaning period.[130,131] Altogether, these studies in animal models provide evidence for the ability of BID to promote alterations in the VTA/ventral striatal dopaminergic system, which, if also present in RLS, would provide a neurochemical correlate of akathisia.

GLUTAMATERGIC MECHANISMS IN RESTLESS LEGS SYNDROME: HYPERSENSITIVITY OF STRIATAL GLUTAMATERGIC TERMINALS

The rodent with BID also has been used to study if alterations in neurotransmitter systems other than the dopaminergic system can be involved in the pathophysiology of RLS. Those alterations could be either secondary or represent primary alterations in a chain of events leading to the hyperdopaminergic state an akathisia. A magnetic resonance spectroscopy study in subjects with RLS compared with controls showed results compatible with an increased thalamic concentration of glutamate, which correlated with the time spent awake during the sleep period.[132] These findings suggested the presence of a presynaptic hyperglutamatergic state, which would be involved in the hyperarousal component of RLS and would agree with the therapeutic efficacy of $\alpha_2\delta$ ligands (such as gabapentin) in RLS.[103] Hence, the main mechanism of action of $\alpha_2\delta$ ligands is binding to the $\alpha_2\delta$-subunits of the voltage-dependent calcium channels localized in glutamatergic terminals and promote an inhibition of glutamate release (Fig. 3).[133] Importantly, $\alpha_2\delta$ ligands are effective not only for the hyperarousal but also for the sensorimotor symptoms, akathisia, and PLMs.[103]

An increased glutamate release could promote a local increase in dopamine and be involved in the hyperdopaminergic state of RLS. Striatal dopamine release is known to be triggered by 2 main mechanisms. One mechanism involves action potential firing initiated in the somatodendritic region of the midbrain dopaminergic neurons, which propagates through dense axonal arborizations to reach active zone–like release sites of the striatal dopaminergic terminals.[134,135] The other mechanism takes place in the dopaminergic terminals, which are locally activated by an action potential–independent mechanism. This intrastriatal mechanism of dopamine signal generation is just beginning to be understood and depends on the following sequence of events: glutamate release from striatal glutamatergic inputs, activation of glutamate ionotropic N-methyl-D-aspartate (NMDA) receptors in cholinergic interneurons, which promotes acetylcholine release and activation of ionotropic nicotinic acetylcholine receptors (of the $\alpha_4\beta_2$ subtype) localized in the dopaminergic terminals, which leads to dopamine release (see Fig. 3).[136–138]

Evidence for a BID-dependent increase in presynaptic glutamatergic transmission in the dorsal striatum could be recently demonstrated in the BID rat model of RLS, using an optogenetic-microdialysis method.[139] This method allowed

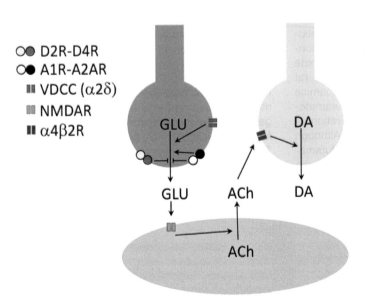

- ◯● D2R-D4R
- ◯● A1R-A2AR
- ▮▮ VDCC ($\alpha_2\delta$)
- ▮▮ NMDAR
- ▮▮ $\alpha_4\beta_2$R

Fig. 3. Action potential–independent and glutamate-dependent mechanism of striatal dopamine release. Glutamate release from striatal glutamatergic terminals is under the control of $\alpha_2\delta$ subunit-containing voltage-dependent calcium channels (VDCC-$\alpha_2\delta$), which are targets of gabapentin, D2R-D4R heteromers, which are targets of D_2-like receptor agonists like pramipexole, and A1R-A2AR heteromers, which are indirect targets of inhibitors of adenosine transporters like dipyridamole. Apart from the striatal dopamine release induced by the propagation of action potentials initiated in the somatodendritic region of the midbrain dopaminergic neurons, there is a local striatal mechanism of dopamine release that involves glutamate and acetylcholine. Glutamate release from striatal glutamatergic terminals leads to activation of NMDA of cholinergic interneurons, which promotes acetylcholine release and activation of nicotinic acetylcholine receptors (of the $\alpha_4\beta_2$ subtype) localized in the dopaminergic terminals, which leads to dopamine release.

the measurement of light-induced glutamate release by corticostriatal glutamatergic terminals and the ability of locally perfused drugs to modulate this glutamate release. It first was shown that BID in rats produces hypersensitivity of corticostriatal glutamatergic terminals in the dorsal striatum, by which glutamate release can be induced by a lower frequency of optogenetic stimulation.[139] In addition, application of clinically effective drugs, either the $\alpha_2\delta$ ligand gabapentin or the dopamine receptor agonists pramipexole or ropinirole, completely blocked glutamate release induced by optogenetic stimulation, both in controls and in animals with BID. This would strongly suggest that inhibitory dopamine receptors and voltage-dependent calcium channels expressing $\alpha_2\delta$ units localized in striatal glutamatergic terminals might represent key targets for the therapeutic effects of both dopamine receptor agonists and $\alpha_2\delta$ ligands in RLS.[139] The differential effect of several dopamine receptor antagonists with different selectivity for the different dopamine receptor subtypes in counteracting the effect of pramipexole indicated the involvement of D2R and D4R but not D3R.[139] These results agree with previous studies indicating that D2R and D4R localized in glutamatergic terminals and forming D2R-D4R heteromers mediate the inhibitory control of dopamine on glutamate release in the rodent dorsal and ventral striatum (see Fig. 3).[140,141]

Using the same methodology, the optogenetic-microdialysis method, it recently has been demonstrated that optogenetically induced glutamate release from corticostriatal terminals in the rat ventral striatum locally induces striatal dopamine release secondary to a concomitant glutamate-induced acetylcholine release and activation of nicotinic acetylcholine receptors.[138] Although BID-induced hypersensitivity of striatal glutamatergic terminals still needs to be replicated in the ventral striatum, these results strongly support that BID-induced striatal presynaptic hyperdopaminergic state is secondary to a striatal presynaptic hyperglutamatergic state. The increased glutamate and concomitant dopamine release should lead to an increased activation of the D1R forming heteromers with D3R (discussed previously) and with A1R (discussed later) localized in the striatonigral neuron. This provides a very plausible mechanism for akathisia in RLS and a very plausible target for the therapeutic effects of the D$_2$-like receptor agonists for akathisia in RLS, the ventral striatal glutamatergic terminals.

The results of the BID rodent model of RLS, therefore, implies considering the striatum as a more relevant brain area involved in the pathogenesis of RLS than the ventral midbrain (substantia nigra or VTA). A glutamate-dependent locally generated increase in presynaptic dopaminergic transmission in the ventral and dorsal striatum could be mainly responsible for akathisia and PLMS, respectively. More accurately, the alterations in glutamatergic and dopaminergic neurotransmission in different striatal compartments should result in dysfunction of their corresponding corticostriatal-thalamic-cortical (C-S-T-C) circuits (see Fig. 1). Clinical and human genetic studies support this hypothesis. A functional MRI study found particularly significant changes in regional spontaneous activity of RLS patients in the striatum and thalamus and also significant but less pronounced changes in frontal cortical areas.[142] These findings, therefore, indicate the existence of predominant alterations in C-S-T-C circuits in the pathogenesis of RLS.[2] A more recent MRI study showed a significant decrease in cortical thickness in the somatosensory cortex of RLS patients.[143] It is well established that corticostriatal projections from reciprocally connected cortical regions often converge in the striatum. In particular, motor and somatosensory cortical areas are heavily interconnected, directly, by cortical reciprocal projections, and indirectly, by convergent projections to even the same striatal neurons.[144,145] This provides the framework for a dysfunction of the C-S-T-C circuits that include the motor and somatosensory cortices and dorsal striatum, which could be particularly involved in the PLMS component of RLS.

Genetic factors play a significant role in RLS and family and twin studies have estimated that RLS heritability is 50% to 60%.[146] In fact, several RLS risk gene polymorphisms have been identified by genome-wide association studies, which include MEIS1, BTBD9, PTPRD, MAP2K5, and TOX3.[147] These genetic findings provided a new pathogenetic clue based on the relation of these genes with neurodevelopment. For instance, MEIS1 polymorphism has been confirmed as the strongest genetic risk factor. A risk allele polymorphism in the cis-regulatory locus of the MEIS1 gene specifically reduces its enhancer activity in the mouse embryonic ganglionic eminences.[148] Significantly, the ganglionic eminences develop into the basal striatum and the other basal ganglia in the adult brain. In fact, also the transcripts of BTBD9, PTPRD, MAP2K5, and TOX3 all are expressed during development in the ganglionic eminences.[148] It is out of the scope of this review to analyze all the epidemiologic and experimental studies involving RLS risk polymorphisms, but it can be underlined that most of these studies point to a significant neurodevelopmental component in the pathogenesis of RLS that leads to an increased vulnerability to dysfunction of C-S-T-C circuits. The recent experimental work on *BTBD9* is discussed as one the clearest examples of a connection between an RLS risk gene polymorphism and dysfunction of C-S-T-C circuits. These studies used behavioral, electrophysiologic, and imaging techniques in global *BTBD9* knockout mice and conditional knockout mice with selective blockade of the expression of *BTBD9* in the GABAergic striatal efferent neurons.[149] The results showed a specific increase in neuronal activity in the striatum of *BTBD9* knockout mice, more specifically in striatal GABAergic efferent neurons, with an increase in the amplitude of excitatory postsynaptic currents indicative of an enhanced striatal glutamatergic transmission.[149] Behaviorally, *BTBD9* knockout mice showed akathisia-like behavior with the circadian characteristics of RLS, which was reproduced in the conditional *BTBD9* knockout of striatal GABAergic efferent neurons.[149]

ADENOSINERGIC MECHANISMS IN RESTLESS LEGS SYNDROME: DOWN-REGULATION OF A1R

An important question is what determines the hyperglutamatergic state, the hypersensitivity of striatal glutamatergic terminals upon BID. The authors hypothesized that BID-induced alterations in the adenosinergic system, a hypoadenosinergic state, might represent an initial pathogenetic step leading to the hyperglutamatergic state.[2,16] The assumption was based on the well-established modulatory role of adenosine on glutamatergic and dopaminergic transmission and its role in homeostatic sleep. Thus, adenosine is a universal inhibitor of glutamate release by acting on presynaptic A1R.[150] In the striatal glutamatergic terminals, A1R form heteromers with A2AR, providing a mechanism for a fine-tune modulation of glutamate release (see **Fig. 3**).[151] In addition, also in the striatum, adenosine exerts an inhibitory control of dopaminergic transmission by acting on the A2AR-D2R and A1R-D1R heteromers respectively localized in the striatopallidal and striatonigral neurons (see **Fig. 1**).[39,60–63] In both heteromers, activation of the adenosine receptor leads to a decrease in the signaling of the dopamine receptor. Apart from the striatonigral neuron, A1R-D1R heteromers also recently have been demonstrated in the spinal motoneuron, where they exert a significant functional control.[65] Importantly, A1R also are localized in the cells of origin and terminals of the multiple interconnected ascending arousal systems and are directly involved in the role of adenosine on homeostatic sleep, mediating the sleepiness

induced by prolonged wakefulness.[2,152] A recent study, using a genetically encoded adenosine sensor and selective neuronal-type specific ablation and optogenetic activation techniques, demonstrated a particularly salient role of the basal forebrain ascending glutamatergic neurons in the adenosine-mediated control of homeostatic sleep.[153]

A BID-induced hypoadenosinergic state then could explain the clinical complexity of RLS and link its apparently disconnected symptomatology with its circadian expression. RLS symptoms then could result from a reduced adenosine tone in the ventral striatum (akathisia), in the dorsal striatum or spinal cord (PLMS) and in the basal forebrain (hyperarousal). The alteration in the adenosinergic system could also explain the circadian expression of RLS symptoms.[2] A significant down-regulation of A1R could be demonstrated in different brain areas (cortex and whole striatum) from mice and rats with BID.[126] Additional BID-induced neurochemical alterations included the expected down-regulation of striatal D2R and an up-regulation of striatal A2AR. Striatal A1R and D2R down-regulation, however, were correlated and were observed with mild and severe BID, whereas A2AR up-regulation would occur only with severe BID.[126] It, therefore, would be possible that BID-induced down-regulation of A1R in striatal glutamatergic terminals, by decreasing the A1R-mediated inhibition of glutamate release (associated with a reduced number of A1R-A2AR heteromers), would lead to the hypersensitivity of striatal glutamatergic terminals, to the locally induced increase in dopamine release and a secondary down-regulation of postsynaptic D2R. In addition, down-regulation of postsynaptic A1R should result in a decrease in the population of D1R forming heteromers with A1R and, therefore, an increase in the effect of dopamine on D1R-mediated signaling by the striatonigral GABAergic neurons. In agreement with the involvement of A1R in the hypersensitivity of striatal glutamatergic terminals induced by BID, using the optogenetic-microdialysis technique, it recently could be demonstrated that local striatal application of an A1R antagonist significantly decreases the minimal frequency of optogenetic stimulation promoting corticostriatal glutamate release.[154] In the same study, BID-induced hypersensitivity of striatal glutamatergic terminals could be counteracted by the local application of dipyridamole, an inhibitor of the equilibrative adenosine transporters ENT1 and ENT2.[154]

Support for the hypoadenosinergic hypothesis recently has been obtained from 2 clinical studies: First, a prospective, 2-month, open-label, non–placebo-controlled clinical trial, with 13 untreated patients with idiopathic RLS[155]; second, a double-blind, crossover, placebo-controlled study, with 28 untreated patients with idiopathic RLS, treated for 2 weeks with either dipyridamole or placebo (García-Borreguero et al., submitted). In both cases, the inhibitor of adenosine transporters proved to be significantly effective in all major RLS rating scales.

SUMMARY

This article proposes that the main common mechanism of akathisia involves an increase in presynaptic dopaminergic transmission in the ventral striatum and a concomitant strong activation of D1R localized in the ventral GABAergic striatonigral neurons, which form heteromers with D3R and A1R (see **Fig. 1**). The authors hypothesize that in DRBA-induced akathisia, ventral striatal dopamine release is promoted by inactivation of autoreceptors and D1R activation is facilitated by up-regulation of D3R (in tardive syndrome). In akathisia of RLS, ventral striatal dopamine release would be dependent on a BID-induced increase in striatal glutamate release, which would depend on down-regulation of A1R localized in the striatal glutamatergic terminals. D1R activation then would be facilitated by a concomitant down-regulation of postsynaptic A1R, which form heteromers with D1R. The hypotheses provide a mechanism for understanding the dopamine paradox: the hyperdopaminergic state associated with DRBA treatment and the clinical response to D_2-like receptor agonists in the akathisia of RLS, were the D_2-like receptor localized in the dopaminergic and glutamatergic terminals play a significant role, respectively. It also is proposed that the phenomenon of augmentation could be understood in the frame of changes in the sensitivity of postsynaptic D1R localized in the ventral striatonigral neuron, possibly secondary to changes in the expression of D3R upon chronic agonist treatment. A corollary of these hypotheses is that A1R-D1R and D1R-D3R heteromers localized in the ventral striatonigral neurons provide potential targets for the treatment of akathisia and augmentation.

IN MEMORIAM

Professor Richard Allen was at the center of most of the advances in RLS research over the last 25 years and sadly passed away on 12/09/2020.

ACKNOWLEDGMENTS

S. Ferré, X. Guitart, C. Quiroz, and W. Rea are supported by the intramural funds of the National Institute on Drug Abuse.

DISCLOSURE

The authors have nothing to disclose.

REFERENCES

1. Allen RP, Picchietti DL, Garcia-Borreguero D, et al. Restless legs syndrome/Willis-Ekbom disease diagnostic criteria: updated International Restless Legs Syndrome Study Group (IRLSSG) consensus criteria–history, rationale, description, and significance. Sleep Med 2014;15(11):860–73.
2. Ferré S, García-Borreguero D, Allen RP, et al. New insights into the neurobiology of restless legs syndrome. Neuroscientist 2019;25(2):113–25.
3. Braude WM, Barnes TR, Gore SM. Clinical characteristics of akathisia. A systematic investigation of acute psychiatric inpatient admissions. Br J Psychiatry 1983;143:139–50.
4. Halstead SM, Barnes TR, Speller JC. Akathisia: prevalence and associated dysphoria in an inpatient population with chronic schizophrenia. Br J Psychiatry 1994;164(2):177–83.
5. Kane JM, Fleischhacker WW, Hansen L, et al. Akathisia: an updated review focusing on second-generation antipsychotics. J Clin Psychiatry 2009; 70(5):627–43.
6. Aquino CC, Lang AE. Tardive dyskinesia syndromes: current concepts. Parkinsonism Relat Disord 2014;20(Suppl 1):S113–7.
7. Frei K, Truong DD, Fahn S, et al. The nosology of tardive syndromes. J Neurol Sci 2018;389:10–6.
8. Ferri R, Rundo F, Zucconi M, et al. Diagnostic accuracy of the standard and alternative periodic leg movement during sleep indices for restless legs syndrome. Sleep Med 2016;22:97–9.
9. Figorilli M, Puligheddu M, Congiu P, et al. The clinical importance of periodic leg movements in sleep. Curr Treat Options Neurol 2017;19(3):10.
10. Rye DB, Trotti LM. Restless legs syndrome and periodic leg movements of sleep. Neurol Clin 2012; 30(4):1137–66.
11. Haba-Rubio J, Marti-Soler H, Marques-Vidal P, et al. Prevalence and determinants of periodic limb movements in the general population. Ann Neurol 2016;79(3):464–74.
12. Moore H 4th, Winkelmann J, Lin L, et al. Periodic leg movements during sleep are associated with polymorphisms in BTBD9, TOX3/BC034767, MEIS1, MAP2K5/SKOR1, and PTPRD. Sleep 2014;37(9):1535–42.
13. Saletu B, Gruber G, Saletu M, et al. Sleep laboratory studies in restless legs syndrome patients as compared with normals and acute effects of ropinirole. 1. Findings on objective and subjective sleep and awakening quality. Neuropsychobiology 2000;41(4):181–9.

14. Ferri R, Rundo F, Zucconi M, et al. An evidence-based analysis of the association between periodic leg movements during sleep and arousals in restless legs syndrome. Sleep 2015;38(6):919–24.

15. Gamaldo C, Benbrook AR, Allen RP, et al. Evaluating daytime alertness in individuals with Restless Legs Syndrome (RLS) compared to sleep restricted controls. Sleep Med 2009;10(1):134–8.

16. Ferré S, Quiroz C, Guitart X, et al. Pivotal role of adenosine neurotransmission in restless legs syndrome. Front Neurosci 2018;11:722.

17. Farde L, Nordström AL, Wiesel FA, et al. Positron emission tomographic analysis of central D1 and D2 dopamine receptor occupancy in patients treated with classical neuroleptics and clozapine. Relation to extrapyramidal side effects. Arch Gen Psychiatry 1992;49(7):538–44.

18. Marsden CD, Jenner P. The pathophysiology of extrapyramidal side-effects of neuroleptic drugs. Psychol Med 1980;10(1):55–72.

19. Carlsson A. Receptor-mediated control of dopamine metabolism. In: Udsin E, Bunney WE Jr, editors. Pre- and postsynaptic receptors. New York: Marcel Dekker; 1975. p. 49–66.

20. Farnebo LO, Hamberger B. Drug-induced changes in the release of 3 H-monoamines from field stimulated rat brain slices. Acta Physiol Scand Suppl 1971;371:35–44.

21. Aghajanian GK, Bunney BS. Central dopaminergic neurons: neurophysiological identification and responses to drugs. In: Snyder SH, Usdin E, editors. Frontiers in catecholamine research. New York: Pergamon Press; 1973. p. 643.

22. Aghajanian GK, Bunney BS. Dopamine"autoreceptors": pharmacological characterization by microiontophoretic single cell recording studies. Naunyn Schmiedebergs Arch Pharmacol 1977;297(1):1–7.

23. Adell A, Artigas F. The somatodendritic release of dopamine in the ventral tegmental area and its regulation by afferent transmitter systems. Neurosci Biobehav Rev 2004;28(4):415–31.

24. Ford CP. The role of D2-autoreceptors in regulating dopamine neuron activity and transmission. Neuroscience 2014;282:13–22.

25. Rice ME, Patel JC. Somatodendritic dopamine release: recent mechanistic insights. Philos Trans R Soc Lond B Biol Sci 2015;370(1672):20140185.

26. Missale C, Nash SR, Robinson SW, et al. Dopamine receptors: from structure to function. Physiol Rev 1998;78(1):189–225.

27. Li SM, Collins GT, Paul NM, et al. Yawning and locomotor behavior induced by dopamine receptor agonists in mice and rats. Behav Pharmacol 2010;21(3):171–81.

28. Radl D, Chiacchiaretta M, Lewis RG, et al. Differential regulation of striatal motor behavior and related cellular responses by dopamine D2L and D2S isoforms. Proc Natl Acad Sci U S A 2018;115(1):198–203.

29. Bello EP, Mateo Y, Gelman DM, et al. Cocaine supersensitivity and enhanced motivation for reward in mice lacking dopamine D2 autoreceptors. Nat Neurosci 2011;14(8):1033–8.

30. Bouthenet ML, Souil E, Martres MP, et al. Localization of dopamine D3 receptor mRNA in the rat brain using in situ hybridization histochemistry: comparison with dopamine D2 receptor mRNA. Brain Res 1991;564(2):203–19.

31. Diaz J, Lévesque D, Lammers CH, et al. Phenotypical characterization of neurons expressing the dopamine D3 receptor in the rat brain. Neuroscience 1995;65(3):731–45.

32. Diaz J, Pilon C, Le Foll B, et al. Dopamine D3 receptors expressed by all mesencephalic dopamine neurons. J Neurosci 2000;20(23):8677–84.

33. Gurevich EV, Joyce JN. Distribution of dopamine D3 receptor expressing neurons in the human forebrain: comparison with D2 receptor expressing neurons. Neuropsychopharmacology 1999;20(1):60–80.

34. Castro-Hernández J, Afonso-Oramas D, Cruz-Muros I, et al. Prolonged treatment with pramipexole promotes physical interaction of striatal dopamine D3 autoreceptors with dopamine transporters to reduce dopamine uptake. Neurobiol Dis 2015;74:325–35.

35. McGinnis MM, Siciliano CA, Jones SR. Dopamine D3 autoreceptor inhibition enhances cocaine potency at the dopamine transporter. J Neurochem 2016;138(6):821–9.

36. Manvich DF, Petko AK, Branco RC, et al. Selective D_2 and D_3 receptor antagonists oppositely modulate cocaine responses in mice via distinct postsynaptic mechanisms in nucleus accumbens. Neuropsychopharmacology 2019;44(8):1445–55.

37. Mogenson GJ, Jones DL, Yim CY. From motivation to action: functional interface between the limbic system and the motor system. Prog Neurobiol 1980;14(2–3):69–97.

38. Ferré S. Adenosine control of striatal Function. Implications for the treatment of apathy in basal ganglia disorders. In: Blum D, Lopes LV, editors. Adenosine receptors in neurodegenerative diseases. Amsterdam: Academic Press; 2017. p. 231–55.

39. Ferré S, Bonaventura J, Zhu W, et al. Essential control of the function of the striatopallidal neuron by pre-coupled complexes of adenosine a_{2a}-dopamine d_2 receptor heterotetramers and adenylyl cyclase. Front Pharmacol 2018;9:243.

40. Wise RA, Bozarth MA. A psychomotor stimulant theory of addiction. Psychol Rev 1987;94(4):469–92.

41. Kelly PH, Seviour PW, Iversen SD. Amphetamine and apomorphine responses in the rat following 6-OHDA lesions of the nucleus accumbens septi and corpus striatum. Brain Res 1975;94(3):507–22.

42. Staton DM, Solomon PR. Microinjections of d-amphetamine into the nucleus accumbens and

caudate-putamen differentially affect stereotypy and locomotion in the rat. Physiol Psycol 1984;12: 159–62.

43. Carr GD, White NM. Effects of systemic and intra-cranial amphetamine injections on behavior in the open field: a detailed analysis. Pharmacol Biochem Behav 1987;27(1):113–22.

44. Kelley AE, Gauthier AM, Lang CG. Amphetamine microinjections into distinct striatal subregions cause dissociable effects on motor and ingestive behavior. Behav Brain Res 1989;35(1):27–39.

45. Plaznik A, Stefanski R, Kostowski W. Interaction between accumbens D1 and D2 receptors regulating rat locomotor activity. Psychopharmacology 1989; 99(4):558–62.

46. Delfs JM, Schreiber L, Kelley AE. Microinjection of cocaine into the nucleus accumbens elicits locomotor activation in the rat. J Neurosci 1990;10:303–10.

47. Ikemoto S. Ventral striatal anatomy of locomotor activity induced by cocaine, D-amphetamine, dopamine and D1/D2 agonists. Neuroscience 2002; 113(4):939–55.

48. Kelly PH, Iversen SD. Selective 6OHDA-induced destruction of mesolimbic dopamine neurons: abolition of psychostimulant-induced locomotor activity in rats. Eur J Pharmacol 1976;40(1):45–56.

49. Delfs JM, Kelley AE. The role of D1 and D2 dopamine receptors in oral stereotypy induced by dopaminergic stimulation of the ventrolateral striatum. Neuroscience 1990;39(1):59–67.

50. Brust JC. Substance abuse and movement disorders. Mov Disord 2010;25(13):2010–20.

51. Asser A, Taba P. Psychostimulants and movement disorders. Front Neurol 2015;6:75.

52. Gerfen CR. Basal ganglia. In: Paxinos G, editor. The rat nervous system. Amsterdam: Academic Press; 2004. p. 445–508.

53. Braun AR, Chase TN. Obligatory D-1/D-2 receptor interaction in the generation of dopamine agonist related behaviors. Eur J Pharmacol 1986;131(2–3):301–6.

54. Arnt J, Hyttel J, Perregaard J. Dopamine D-1 receptor agonists combined with the selective D-2 agonist quinpirole facilitate the expression of oral stereotyped behaviour in rats. Eur J Pharmacol 1987;133(2):137–45.

55. Dreher JK, Jackson DM. Role of D1 and D2 dopamine receptors in mediating locomotor activity elicited from the nucleus accumbens of rats. Brain Res 1989;487(2):267–77.

56. Bordi F, Meller E. Enhanced behavioral stereotypies elicited by intrastriatal injection D1 and D2 dopamine agonists in intact rats. Brain Res 1989; 504(2):276–83.

57. Jackson DM, Ross SB, Hashizume M. Dopamine-mediated behaviours produced in naive mice by bromocriptine plus SKF 38393. J Pharm Pharmacol 1988;40(3):221–3.

58. Starr BS, Starr MS, Kilpatrick IC. Behavioural role of dopamine D1 receptors in the reserpine-treated mouse. Neuroscience 1987;22(1):179–88.

59. Ferré S, Giménez-Llort L, Artigas F, et al. Motor activation in short- and long-term reserpinized mice: role of N-methyl-D-aspartate, dopamine D1 and dopamine D2 receptors. Eur J Pharmacol 1994;255(1–3):203–13.

60. Ferré S, Popoli P, Giménez-Llort L, et al. Postsynaptic antagonistic interaction between adenosine A1 and dopamine D1 receptors. Neuroreport 1994;6(1):73–6.

61. Ginés S, Hillion J, Torvinen M, et al. Dopamine D1 and adenosine A1 receptors form functionally interacting heteromeric complexes. Proc Natl Acad Sci U S A 2000;97(15):8606–11.

62. Ferré S. An update on the mechanisms of the psychostimulant effects of caffeine. J Neurochem 2008;105(4):1067–79.

63. Navarro G, Cordomí A, Casadó-Anguera V, et al. Evidence for functional pre-coupled complexes of receptor heteromers and adenylyl cyclase. Nat Commun 2018;9(1):1242.

64. Ferré S. Mechanisms of the psychostimulant effects of caffeine: implications for substance use disorders. Psychopharmacology 2016;233(10): 1963–79.

65. Rivera-Oliver M, Moreno E, Álvarez-Bagnarol Y, et al. Adenosine A_1-Dopamine D_1 receptor heteromers control the excitability of the spinal motoneuron. Mol Neurobiol 2019;56(2):797–811.

66. LaHoste GJ, Henry BL, Marshall JF. Dopamine D1 receptors synergize with D2, but not D3 or D4, receptors in the striatum without the involvement of action potentials. J Neurosci 2000;20(17): 6666–71.

67. Hopf FW, Cascini MG, Gordon AS, et al. Cooperative activation of dopamine D1 and D2 receptors increases spike firing of nucleus accumbens neurons via G-protein betagamma subunits. J Neurosci 2003;23(12):5079–87.

68. Surmeier DJ, Song WJ, Yan Z. Coordinated expression of dopamine receptors in neostriatal medium spiny neurons. J Neurosci 1996;16(20): 6579–91.

69. Schwartz JC, Diaz J, Bordet R, et al. Functional implications of multiple dopamine receptor subtypes: the D1/D3 receptor coexistence. Brain Res Rev 1998;26(2–3):236–42.

70. Marcellino D, Ferré S, Casadó V, et al. Identification of dopamine D1-D3 receptor heteromers. Indications for a role of synergistic D1-D3 receptor interactions in the striatum. J Biol Chem 2008;283(38): 26016–25.

71. Guitart X, Navarro G, Moreno E, et al. Functional selectivity of allosteric interactions within G protein-coupled receptor oligomers: the dopamine

D1-D3 receptor heterotetramer. Mol Pharmacol 2014;86(4):417–29.

72. Cruz-Trujillo R, Avalos-Fuentes A, Rangel-Barajas C, et al. D3 dopamine receptors interact with dopamine D1 but not D4 receptors in the GABAergic terminals of the SNr of the rat. Neuropharmacology 2013;67:370–8.

73. Fiorentini C, Busi C, Gorruso E, et al. Reciprocal regulation of dopamine D1 and D3 receptor function and trafficking by heterodimerization. Mol Pharmacol 2008;74(1):59–69.

74. Guitart X, Moreno E, Rea W, et al. Biased G protein-independent signaling of dopamine D_1-D_3 receptor heteromers in the nucleus accumbens. Mol Neurobiol 2019;56(10):6756–69.

75. Ferré S, Baler R, Bouvier M, et al. Building a new conceptual framework for receptor heteromers. Nat Chem Biol 2009;5(3):131–4.

76. Ferré S, Casadó V, Devi LA, et al. G protein-coupled receptor oligomerization revisited: functional and pharmacological perspectives. Pharmacol Rev 2014;66(2):413–34.

77. Ferré S. The GPCR heterotetramer: challenging classical pharmacology. Trends Pharmacol Sci 2015;36(3):145–52.

78. Yano H, Cai NS, Xu M, et al. Gs- versus Golf-dependent functional selectivity mediated by the dopamine D_1 receptor. Nat Commun 2018;9(1):486.

79. Sánchez-Soto M, Bonifazi A, Cai NS, et al. Evidence for noncanonical neurotransmitter activation: norepinephrine as a dopamine D2-like receptor agonist. Mol Pharmacol 2016;89(4):457–66.

80. Dreyer JK, Herrik KF, Berg RW, et al. Influence of phasic and tonic dopamine release on receptor activation. J Neurosci 2010;30(42):14273–83.

81. Bromberg-Martin ES, Matsumoto M, Hikosaka O. Dopamine in motivational control: rewarding, aversive, and alerting. Neuron 2010;68(5):815–34.

82. Macpherson T, Morita M, Hikida T. Striatal direct and indirect pathways control decision-making behavior. Front Psychol 2014;5:1301.

83. Li P, Snyder GL, Vanover KE. Dopamine targeting drugs for the treatment of schizophrenia: past, present and future. Curr Top Med Chem 2016;16(29):3385–403.

84. Steen VM, Løvlie R, MacEwan T, et al. Dopamine D3-receptor gene variant and susceptibility to tardive dyskinesia in schizophrenic patients. Mol Psychiatry 1997;2(2):139–45.

85. Eichhammer P, Albus M, Borrmann-Hassenbach M, et al. Association of dopamine D3-receptor gene variants with neuroleptic induced akathisia in schizophrenic patients: a generalization of Steen's study on DRD3 and tardive dyskinesia. Am J Med Genet 2000;96(2):187–91.

86. Lerer B, Segman RH, Fangerau H, et al. Pharmacogenetics of tardive dyskinesia: combined analysis of 780 patients supports association with dopamine D3 receptor gene Ser9Gly polymorphism. Neuropsychopharmacology 2002;27(1):105–19.

87. Bakker PR, van Harten PN, van Os J. Antipsychotic-induced tardive dyskinesia and the Ser9Gly polymorphism in the DRD3 gene: a meta analysis. Schizophr Res 2006;83(2–3):185–92.

88. Lundstrom K, Turpin MP. Proposed schizophrenia-related gene polymorphism: expression of the Ser9Gly mutant human dopamine D3 receptor with the Semliki Forest virus system. Biochem Biophys Res Commun 1996;225(3):1068–72.

89. Bordet R, Ridray S, Carboni S, et al. Induction of dopamine D3 receptor expression as a mechanism of behavioral sensitization to levodopa. Proc Natl Acad Sci U S A 1997;94(7):3363–7.

90. Neisewander JL, Fuchs RA, Tran-Nguyen LT, et al. Increases in dopamine D3 receptor binding in rats receiving a cocaine challenge at various time points after cocaine self-administration: implications for cocaine-seeking behavior. Neuropsychopharmacology 2004;29(8):1479–87.

91. Staley JK, Mash DC. Adaptive increase in D3 dopamine receptors in the brain reward circuits of human cocaine fatalities. J Neurosci 1996;16(19):6100–6.

92. Boileau I, Payer D, Houle S, et al. Higher binding of the dopamine D3 receptor-preferring ligand [11C]-(+)-propyl-hexahydro-naphtho-oxazin in methamphetamine polydrug users: a positron emission tomography study. J Neurosci 2012;32(4):1353–9.

93. Payer DE, Behzadi A, Kish SJ, et al. Heightened D3 dopamine receptor levels in cocaine dependence and contributions to the addiction behavioral phenotype: a positron emission tomography study with [11C]-+-PHNO. Neuropsychopharmacology 2014;39(2):311–8.

94. Gerfen CR, Miyachi S, Paletzki R, et al. D1 dopamine receptor supersensitivity in the dopamine-depleted striatum results from a switch in the regulation of ERK1/2/MAP kinase. J Neurosci 2002;22(12):5042–54.

95. Prieto GA, Perez-Burgos A, Palomero-Rivero M, et al. Upregulation of D2-class signaling in dopamine-denervated striatum is in part mediated by D3 receptors acting on Ca V 2.1 channels via PIP2 depletion. J Neurophysiol 2011;105(5):2260–74.

96. Visanji NP, Fox SH, Johnston T, et al. Dopamine D3 receptor stimulation underlies the development of L-DOPA-induced dyskinesia in animal models of Parkinson's disease. Neurobiol Dis 2009;35(2):184–92.

97. Farré D, Muñoz A, Moreno E, et al. Stronger dopamine D1 receptor-mediated neurotransmission in dyskinesia. Mol Neurobiol 2015;52(3):1408–20.

98. Solís O, Garcia-Montes JR, González-Granillo A, et al. Dopamine D3 Receptor Modulates l-DOPA-

induced dyskinesia by targeting D1 receptor-mediated striatal signaling. Cereb Cortex 2017; 27(1):435–46.

99. Guigoni C, Aubert I, Li Q, et al. Pathogenesis of levodopa-induced dyskinesia: focus on D1 and D3 dopamine receptors. Parkinsonism Relat Disord 2005;11(Suppl 1):S25–9.

100. Payer DE, Guttman M, Kish SJ, et al. D3 dopamine receptor-preferring [11C]PHNO PET imaging in Parkinson patients with dyskinesia. Neurology 2016;86(3):224–30.

101. Mahmoudi S, Lévesque D, Blanchet PJ. Upregulation of dopamine D3, not D2, receptors correlates with tardive dyskinesia in a primate model. Mov Disord 2014;29(9):1125–33.

102. Hernandez G, Mahmoudi S, Cyr M, et al. Tardive dyskinesia is associated with altered putamen Akt/GSK-3β signaling in nonhuman primates. Mov Disord 2019;34(5):717–26.

103. Garcia-Borreguero D, Silber MH, Winkelman JW, et al. Guidelines for the first-line treatment of restless legs syndrome/Willis-Ekbom disease, prevention and treatment of dopaminergic augmentation: a combined task force of the IRLSSG, EURLSSG, and the RLS-foundation. Sleep Med 2016;21:1–11.

104. Earley CJ, Connor J, Garcia-Borreguero D, et al. Altered brain iron homeostasis and dopaminergic function in restless legs syndrome (Willis-Ekbom disease). Sleep Med 2014;15(8):1288–301.

105. Allen RP, Auerbach S, Bahrain H, et al. The prevalence and impact of restless legs syndrome on patients with iron deficiency anemia. Am J Hematol 2013;88(4):261–4.

106. Zhu XY, Wu TT, Wang HM, et al. Correlates of non-anemic iron deficiency in restless legs syndrome. Front Neurol 2020;11:298.

107. Clardy SL, Wang X, Boyer PJ, et al. Is ferroportin-hepcidin signaling altered in restless legs syndrome? J Neurol Sci 2006;247(2):173–9.

108. Earley CJ, Ponnuru P, Wang X, et al. Altered iron metabolism in lymphocytes from subjects with restless legs syndrome. Sleep 2008;31(6):847–52.

109. Connor JR, Boyer PJ, Menzies SL, et al. Neuropathological examination suggests impaired brain iron acquisition in restless legs syndrome. Neurology 2003;61(3):304–9.

110. Connor JR, Wang XS, Allen RP, et al. Altered dopaminergic profile in the putamen and substantia nigra in restless leg syndrome. Brain 2009;132(9): 2403–12.

111. Chawla S, Gulyani S, Allen RP, et al. Extracellular vesicles reveal abnormalities in neuronal iron metabolism in restless legs syndrome. Sleep 2019; 42(7):zsz079.

112. Connor JR, Patton SM, Oexle K, et al. Iron and restless legs syndrome: treatment, genetics and pathophysiology. Sleep Med 2017;31:61–70.

113. Wade QW, Chiou B, Connor JR. Iron uptake at the blood-brain barrier is influenced by sex and genotype. Adv Pharmacol 2019;84:123–45.

114. Jellen LC, Beard JL, Jones BC. Systems genetics analysis of iron regulation in the brain. Biochimie 2009;91(10):1255–9.

115. Jellen LC, Unger EL, Lu L, et al. Systems genetic analysis of the effects of iron deficiency in mouse brain. Neurogenetics 2012;13(2):147–57.

116. Catoire H, Dion PA, Xiong L, et al. Restless legs syndrome-associated MEIS1 risk variant influences iron homeostasis. Ann Neurol 2011;70(1):170–5.

117. DeAndrade MP, Johnson RL Jr, Unger EL, et al. Motor restlessness, sleep disturbances, thermal sensory alterations and elevated serum iron levels in Btbd9 mutant mice. Hum Mol Genet 2012; 21(18):3984–92.

118. Allen RP, Picchietti DL, Auerbach M, et al. International Restless Legs Syndrome Study Group (IRLSSG). Evidence-based and consensus clinical practice guidelines for the iron treatment of restless legs syndrome/Willis-Ekbom disease in adults and children: an IRLSSG task force report. Sleep Med 2018;41:27–44.

119. Goodwill KE, Sabatier C, Stevens RC. Crystal structure of tyrosine hydroxylase with bound cofactor analogue and iron at 2.3 A resolution: self-hydroxylation of Phe300 and the pterin-binding site. Biochemistry 1998;37(39):13437–45.

120. Allen RP, Connor JR, Hyland K, et al. Abnormally increased CSF 3-Ortho-methyldopa (3-OMD) in untreated restless legs syndrome (RLS) patients indicates more severe disease and possibly abnormally increased dopamine synthesis. Sleep Med 2009;10(1):123–8.

121. Earley CJ, Kuwabara H, Wong DF, et al. Increased synaptic dopamine in the putamen in restless legs syndrome. Sleep 2013;36(1):51–7.

122. Francois C, Nguyen-Legros J, Percheron G. Topographical and cytological localization of iron in rat and monkey brains. Brain Res 1981;215(1–2):317–22.

123. Hill JM, Switzer RC 3rd. The regional distribution and cellular localization of iron in the rat brain. Neuroscience 1984;11(3):595–603.

124. Godau J, Klose U, Di Santo A, et al. Multiregional brain iron deficiency in restless legs syndrome. Mov Disord 2008;23(8):1184–7.

125. Rizzo G, Manners D, Testa C, et al. Low brain iron content in idiopathic restless legs syndrome patients detected by phase imaging. Mov Disord 2013;28(13):1886–90.

126. Quiroz C, Gulyani S, Ruiqian W, et al. Adenosine receptors as markers of brain iron deficiency: implications for Restless Legs Syndrome. Neuropharmacology 2016;111:160–8.

127. Lai YY, Cheng YH, Hsieh KC, et al. Motor hyperactivity of the iron-deficient rat - an animal model of

restless legs syndrome. Mov Disord 2017;32(12): 1687–93.

128. Allen RP, Earley CJ, Jones BC, et al. Iron-deficiency and dopaminergic treatment effects on RLS-Like behaviors of an animal model with the brain iron deficiency pattern of the restless legs syndrome. Sleep Med 2020;71:141–8.

129. Unger EL, Bianco LE, Jones BC, et al. Low brain iron effects and reversibility on striatal dopamine dynamics. Exp Neurol 2014;261:462–8.

130. Nelson C, Erikson K, Piñero DJ, et al. In vivo dopamine metabolism is altered in iron-deficient anemic rats. J Nutr 1997;127(12):2282–8.

131. Beard J, Erikson KM, Jones BC. Neonatal iron deficiency results in irreversible changes in dopamine function in rats. J Nutr 2003;133(4):1174–9.

132. Allen RP, Barker PB, Horská A, et al. Thalamic glutamate/glutamine in restless legs syndrome: increased and related to disturbed sleep. Neurology 2013;80(22):2028–34.

133. Dooley DJ, Taylor CP, Donevan S, et al. Ca2+ channel alpha2delta ligands: novel modulators of neurotransmission. Trends Pharmacol Sci 2007; 28(2):75–82.

134. Matsuda W, Furuta T, Nakamura KC, et al. Single nigrostriatal dopaminergic neurons form widely spread and highly dense axonal arborizations in the neostriatum. J Neurosci 2009;29(2):444–53.

135. Liu C, Kershberg L, Wang J, et al. Dopamine secretion is mediated by sparse active zone-like release sites. Cell 2018;172(4):706–18.e15.

136. Threlfell S, Lalic T, Platt NJ, et al. Striatal dopamine release is triggered by synchronized activity in cholinergic interneurons. Neuron 2012;75(1): 58–64.

137. Kosillo P, Zhang YF, Threlfell S, et al. Cortical control of striatal dopamine transmission via striatal cholinergic interneurons. Cereb Cortex 2016; 26(11):4160–9.

138. Adrover MF, Shin JH, Quiroz C, et al. Prefrontal cortex-driven dopamine signals in the striatum show unique spatial and pharmacological properties. J Neurosci 2020;40(39):7510–22.

139. Yepes G, Guitart X, Rea W, et al. Targeting hypersensitive corticostriatal terminals in restless legs syndrome. Ann Neurol 2017;82(6):951–60.

140. González S, Rangel-Barajas C, Peper M, et al. Dopamine D4 receptor, but not the ADHD-associated D4.7 variant, forms functional heteromers with the dopamine D2S receptor in the brain. Mol Psychiatry 2012;17(6):650–62.

141. Bonaventura J, Quiroz C, Cai NS, et al. Key role of the dopamine D$_4$ receptor in the modulation of corticostriatal glutamatergic neurotransmission. Sci Adv 2017;3(1):e1601631.

142. Zhuo Y, Wu Y, Xu Y, et al. Combined resting state functional magnetic resonance imaging and diffusion tensor imaging study in patients with idiopathic restless legs syndrome. Sleep Med 2017;38: 96–103.

143. Lee BY, Kim J, Connor JR, et al. Involvement of the central somatosensory system in restless legs syndrome: a neuroimaging study. Neurology 2018; 90(21):e1834–41.

144. Hoffer ZS, Alloway KD. Organization of corticostriatal projections from the vibrissal representations in the primary motor and somatosensory cortical areas of rodents. J Comp Neurol 2001;439(1): 87–103.

145. Kress GJ, Yamawaki N, Wokosin DL, et al. Convergent cortical innervation of striatal projection neurons. Nat Neurosci 2013;16(6):665–7.

146. Schormair B, Winkelmann J. Genetics of restless legs syndrome: mendelian, complex, and everything in between. Sleep Med Clin 2011;6(2): 203–15.

147. Schormair B, Zhao C, Bell S, et al. Identification of novel risk loci for restless legs syndrome in genome-wide association studies in individuals of European ancestry: a meta-analysis. Lancet Neurol 2017;16(11):898–907.

148. Spieler D, Kaffe M, Knauf F, et al. Restless legs syndrome-associated intronic common variant in Meis1 alters enhancer function in the developing telencephalon. Genome Res 2014;24(4): 592–603.

149. Lyu S, Xing H, DeAndrade MP, et al. The role of BTBD9 in striatum and restless legs syndrome. eNeuro 2019;6(5). ENEURO.0277-19.

150. Dunwiddie TV, Masino SA. The role and regulation of adenosine in the central nervous system. Annu Rev Neurosci 2001;24:31–55.

151. Ciruela F, Casadó V, Rodrigues RJ, et al. Presynaptic control of striatal glutamatergic neurotransmission by adenosine A1-A2A receptor heteromers. J Neurosci 2006;26(7):2080–7.

152. Ferré S. Role of the central ascending neurotransmitter systems in the psychostimulant effects of caffeine. J Alzheimers Dis 2010;20(Suppl 1): S35–49.

153. Peng W, Wu Z, Song K, et al. Regulation of sleep homeostasis mediator adenosine by basal forebrain glutamatergic neurons. Science 2020; 369(6508):eabb0556.

154. Ferré S, Quiroz C, Rea W, et al. Adenosine mechanisms and hypersensitive corticostriatal terminals in restless legs syndrome. Rationale for the use of inhibitors of adenosine transport. Adv Pharmacol 2019;84:3–19.

155. Garcia-Borreguero D, Guitart X, Garcia Malo C, et al. Treatment of restless legs syndrome/Willis-Ekbom disease with the non-selective ENT1/ENT2 inhibitor dipyridamole: testing the adenosine hypothesis. Sleep Med 2018;45:94–7.

Restless Legs Syndrome: Challenges to Treatment

Laura M. Botta P, MD[a], Samantha S. Anguizola E, MD[b], Andrea Castro-Villacañas, MD[c], Diego Garcia-Borreguero, MD[c],*

KEYWORDS

- Restless legs syndrome • Dopamine agonists • $\alpha 2\delta$ ligands • Gabapentinoids • Opioids
- Glutamate • Adenosine • Dipyridamole

KEY POINTS

- Restless legs syndrome (RLS) patients treated over the long term with dopamine agonists are exposed to an increased risk of loss of efficacy and augmentation.
- Current treatment guidelines recommend initiating treatment with $\alpha 2\delta$ ligands.
- Opioids are used as a second-line option for treatment-resistant cases of RLS/Willis-Ekbom disease.
- Patients with low iron stores should be given iron replacement therapy.
- New therapeutic options are emerging based on current knowledge of glutamatergic and adenosinergic dysfunction.

INTRODUCTION

Over the past decades, dopaminergic agents were the main therapeutic agent for the first-line treatment of restless legs syndrome (RLS). Initially, the first dopaminergic drug to be used was levodopa.[1] Although the first studies were promising, showing a pronounced short-term efficacy, over the long term, levodopa caused early morning rebound of symptoms[2] due to its short half-life and high rates of augmentation of symptoms. This led to the study of dopamine agonists with longer half-lives, and these became the first-line treatment options for RLS.

Different classes of drugs have also undergone clinical development for the treatment of RLS over the past decade. Among the α-2δ ligands, gabapentin enacarbil has been approved by the Food and Drug Administration (FDA), whereas among the opioids, oxycodone extended-release in combination with naloxone has been approved as a second-line treatment in Europe.

The following sections review the main complications arising during long-term treatment and perform a critical analysis of the different types of agents.

DOPAMINE AGONISTS
Dopamine Agonists in Restless Legs Syndrome

Three different non-ergot dopamine agonists have been studied extensively for the short-term treatment of RLS. These drugs are ropinirole, pramipexole, and rotigotine. All are effective in alleviating RLS-specific sensory symptoms, reducing periodic limb movements (PLMs), and improving sleep.[3,4] Based on their therapeutic efficacy over periods of 3 months to 6 months, these 2 agents have been approved by the FDA and the European Medicines Agency for the treatment of idiopathic RLS. Placebo-controlled studies have been performed for a maximal period of 6 months and showed a mild decrease in therapeutic efficacy compared with placebo.[5,6]

[a] European Sleep Institute, Luis Pasteur 5607 Vitacura, Santiago, Chile; [b] European Sleep Institute, Edif. Habitats Plaza, Calle 51, Distr, Panamá; [c] Sleep Research Institute, Calle Padre Damián 44 Madrid 28036, Spain
* Corresponding author.
E-mail address: dgb@iis.es

Sleep Med Clin 16 (2021) 269–277
https://doi.org/10.1016/j.jsmc.2021.02.003

Treatment Failure in Restless Legs Syndrome/ Willis-Ekbom Disease

Over the long term, however, the percentage of patients whose symptoms do not improve or even worsen despite treatment is high, as shown by several long-term retrospective evaluations.[7] A European retrospective evaluation of 160 patients undergoing dopaminergic treatment, over a mean period of 8.1 years ± 2.9 years, found that following the initial stabilization of symptoms, there was a need to repeatedly increase or switch the medication in 59% of these patients. Furthermore, symptoms worsened or remained unchanged in 45% of the patients despite treatment. In another study, Silver and colleagues[8] evaluated the medical records of patients who had been treated for at least 10 years with the dopamine agonists pramipexole and pergolide. The annual rates for discontinuing treatment were constant over the period, with a yearly discontinuation rate of 9% for pramipexole and 8% for pergolide. During follow-up, only 58% persisted for over 5 years with pramipexole and 35% with pergolide.

Lipford and colleagues[9] performed a retrospective long-term analysis on a group of 50 RLS/ Willis-Ekbom disease (WED) patients treated with pramipexole followed for a mean duration of 8 years (range 0.6–12 years). Pramipexole was reported to be partially effective or even ineffective in 60% of the sample. Over the years, the median daily dose was increased from 0.38 mg after initial stabilization, to 1 mg at the end of the study. Additional nondopaminergic medications were needed by 28% of patients.[9]

These studies were performed in tertiary-care centers and hence are at high risk of bias by having included a higher than usual proportion of treatment-resistant cases. Several studies performed in the community, however, have shown fairly similar results:

- Allen and colleagues[10] performed an online survey of more than 266 RLS/WED patients being treated with dopamine agonists by their primary care practitioner/neurologist across the United States. Signs of poor clinical outcome and augmentation were found in 75% of the sample.[10]
- Tzonova and colleagues[11] performed a survey on 224 RLS/WED patients who had been undergoing treatment for a mean duration of 5.9 (± 4.5) years; despite treatment, 68.6% reported RLS/WED symptoms during the daytime.[11]
- Godau and colleagues[12] reported a lack of statistically significant improvement in

International Restless Legs Syndrome (IRLS) rating score and Restless Legs Syndrome Quality-of-Life Questionnaire scores in patients who had been treated in the community for 12 months mostly with dopaminergic agents.

In summary, it seems that both retrospective long-term evaluations performed in specialized centers and cross-sectional studies in the community suggest that partial or total treatment failure is common among patients being treated with dopamine agonists, leading to dose increases and combination treatments with nondopaminergic agents.

Augmentation

Augmentation is defined as an increase in symptom severity despite (mostly dopaminergic) treatment.[13] This worsening of symptoms occurs after an initial positive response to treatment and in the absence of factors, such as changes in medical status, reduced mobility, or the natural progression of the disorder should have been ruled out. The increase in symptom severity should be greater than that seen before treatment initiation. Alternatively, there can be an earlier onset of symptoms in the afternoon by at least 4 hours, and/or a shorter latency of symptoms at rest, a spread of symptoms to previously unaffected body parts, a greater intensity of symptoms, and/ or a shorter duration of relief from symptoms.[13]

Current augmentation treatment guidelines suggest that to facilitate the identification of augmentation in clinical practice the evaluation should be considered anytime a patient who has been on stable treatment for at least 6 months requests more medication.[14] The International Restless Legs Syndrome Study Group (IRLSSG) has outlined 4 screening questions that may be used in clinical practice in patients treated with dopaminergic agents (**Box 1**). An affirmative answer to any of these should lead a physician to suspect the presence of augmentation.

Augmentation can progress over time with a fluctuating course and should be differentiated from the natural progression of RLS/WED, fluctuations in disease severity, tolerance, end-of-dose rebound, and worsening of symptoms due to extrinsic factors (**Table 1**).[14]

- Although RLS/WED might progressively worsen over time, improve with each dose increase, and worsen with each dose decrease,[15] during augmentation, symptoms get better after a reduction in dose.

- Tolerance is a decrease in medication efficacy over time and requires medication dosage to be increased to maintain the initial symptom relief. As discussed below, during tolerance, symptoms do not appear earlier in the day and are not worse than at baseline. Tolerance, however, likely precedes augmentation.[16]

- End-of-dose rebound, which is the reappearance of symptoms in the early morning, has been reported in up to 35% of RLS/WED patients and corresponds to the fall in medication plasma concentration. It, therefore, is more common with drugs with shorter half-lives, such as levodopa.[2] Similarly to augmentation, symptoms of rebound are worse than at baseline, but there is neither a spread of symptoms to the arms nor a worsening with increased dose/improvement with decreased dose.

Several factors have been identified that possibly exacerbate RLS/WED symptoms[14,17]: iron deficiency, poor medication adherence, sleep deprivation, lifestyle changes (eg, more sedentary lifestyle), the appearance of other physiologic or pathologic conditions known to trigger or exacerbate RLS/WED (pregnancy, renal insufficiency, and other sleep disorders, in particular sleep-disordered breathing), and medications, such as antihistamines, dopamine-receptor blockers, and serotonergic antidepressants.

Do all dopaminergic agents cause augmentation?

A comparative evaluation of augmentation across different drugs remains difficult given the variations according to drug, dose, duration, and type of study; criteria used to evaluate augmentation; and number of participants. Nevertheless, the prevalence rates reported increase with the length of the studies: in short-term studies, augmentation

Table 1
Differential diagnosis of augmentation

	Augmentation	End-of-Dose Rebound	Tolerance	Natural Progression	Exacerbating Factors[a]
Worse than before treatment	Yes	Yes, in early morning	No	Yes	Yes
Earlier onset	Yes	Yes, in early morning	No	Yes	Yes
Spread to arms	Yes	No	No	Yes	Yes
Breakthrough at night	Yes	Yes, in early morning	Yes	Yes	Yes
Worse with increased dose	Yes, but not immediately	No	No	No	No
Improved with decreased dose	Yes, but not always[b]	No	No	No	No

[a] For example, low serum ferritin, medications, increased immobility.
[b] Eventually augmentation is overcome when the dose is decreased; and although augmentation symptoms can improve within 72 h on levodopa, it can take several weeks to several months to see an improvement with dopamine agonists.

Reprinted from Garcia-Borreguero D, Silber MH, Winkelman JW, et al. Guidelines for the first-line treatment of restless legs syndrome/Willis-Ekbom disease, prevention and treatment of dopaminergic augmentation: a combined task force of the IRLSSG, EURLSSG, and the RLS-foundation. Sleep Med 2016;21:1-11. Under the Creative Commons license https://creativecommons.org/licenses/by-nc-nd/4.0/.

rates of less than 10% have been reported,[5,6,18–20] whereas in studies lasting 2 to 3 years, augmentation rates are higher at 30%,[10,16,21–23] and in 2 very long-term studies (approximately 10 years) augmentation has been reported to be 42% to 68%.[8,14]

Prevention of augmentation
Reduction of risk factors The use of dopaminergic agents is the main risk for augmentation, and augmentation is likely to be exclusively related to their specific effects on the dopaminergic system. Furthermore, such a risk is strongly associated with the dose and duration of treatment.[14]

According to current guidelines, the most effective preventive strategy is to not use dopaminergic agents unless necessary. Nevertheless, should dopaminergic treatment be necessary to effectively alleviate symptoms or due to side-effects from other therapeutic options, then the guidelines recommend that the dopaminergic load be reduced by using the lowest effective dose for the shortest possible time.[14] Other factors to be considered as potentially contributing to an increased risk of augmentation are

- Lower iron stores[24,25]
- Greater severity of RLS/WED symptoms before the initiation of treatment[10,26]

Starting treatment with a nondopaminergic agent The fact that augmentation tends to develop very slowly after the initial response to treatment makes it harder to differentiate it from the natural progression of the disease, especially in the early stages, before it becomes a significant problem. For these reasons, the current IRLSSG guidelines identified preventive strategies to minimize the dopaminergic load in every de novo patient:

- The physician should consider using medications with little or no risk of augmentation for initial treatment of RLS, such as the $\alpha 2\delta$ ligands.[14,27]

If dopaminergic agents already are being used, then

- Ensure that the lowest possible cumulative daily dopaminergic dose is used and that the total daily dose does not exceed maximum recommended levels by the IRLSSG task force.[14]
- Intermittent dosing can be pursued if symptoms are infrequent (<1–2/wk) or as a preventive measure before situations where the patient knows he/she will be immobile (eg, long car or plane trips or medical procedures).

Daily RLS/WED treatment should be delayed as long as possible.

Loss of Efficacy

Loss of efficacy is a potentially major problem during the long-term treatment of RLS/WED (**Box 2**). One retrospective study reported 46% of patients treated with the dopamine agonist pramipexole experienced a reduction in efficacy over time.[16] There are 2 main reasons why during the long-term treatment of RLS/WED, a reduction of efficacy can occur due to either loss of response or augmentation.

- Loss of response, unlike augmentation, does not require RLS/WED symptoms to become worse than before treatment had been initiated. Neither is the development of additional new RLS/WED symptoms needed.[13]
- A reduction in the therapeutic response of RLS/WED treatment requires medical attention. It might not just be a problem per se but may be an early indicator for RLS/WED augmentation. Such a progressive loss of therapeutic response in the absence of any change in the metabolism of the drug could reflect a process exacerbating the underlying disease process, eventually leading to augmentation (see **Box 2**).

Impulse Control Disorders

Impulse control disorders (ICDs) develop in up to 39% of patients with RLS/WED who are taking dopamine-receptor agonists.[3,28,29] ICDs may occur more often with higher doses of drugs and may be more likely to occur in women.[30] Patients should be questioned about ICDs at each visit. If a significant ICD is present, the drug should be discontinued or at least the dose decreased to a level at which ICDs cease. Other nondopaminergic drugs should be substituted or added.

General side effects
The main side effects of dopamine agonists are nausea (>41%), vomiting, headache, abdominal pain, and daytime somnolence.[3] When rotigotine patches are used, skin reactions also can occur. The nonapproved ergoline derivatives pergolide and cabergoline cause more nausea and vomiting and potentially also can lead to pleuropulmonary fibrosis and valvulopathy over the long term.[3]

Iron loss
Serum iron loss not only can occur long before the initiation of RLS/WED symptoms but also can recur in the course of the disorder and lead to worsening of symptoms.[25,31] Thus, iron

Box 2
Current diagnostic criteria for loss of efficacy

Definition of loss of clinically relevant response for clinical trials—a loss of response occurs when the patient meets both of the following 2 criteria:

Criterion A (defines initial clinically relevant response)—during the first 3 months of treatment, on any 2 consecutive evaluations, at least 1 week apart:

1. There is a reduction in the IRLS scale total score by ≥40% from the baseline value (ie, IRLS ≤60% of the baseline value). Example 1: a baseline IRLS scale score of 25 with decreases after treatment to ≤15

or

2. The IRLS scale score ≤10. Example 2: regardless of the initial score, there is an improvement to ≤10

Criterion B (defines clinically relevant loss of initial response)—once clinically relevant response is established according to criterion A, loss of response is defined as follows:

1. On any 2 consecutive evaluations at least 1 month apart, there is an increase of the IRLS scale score to >70% of the baseline score (example 1: baseline IRLS scale score of 25, treatment response of IRLS scale score ≤15 followed by worsening with IRLS scale score increased on 2 visits to ≥ 18) and there is no re-establishment of response (defined as criterion A) afterwards without a dose increase.

or

2. A dose increase occurring

- After the first 3 months of treatment

   or

- Within the first 3 months of treatment and preceded by 1 evaluation with IRLS scale score >70% of baseline

3. The patient drops out due to loss of response as determined by the investigator

If the patient meets both criteria A and B, indicating loss of response, the investigator should determine the presence of augmentation. The patient should be classified as

- Loss of response with augmentation
- Loss of response without augmentation
- Loss of response—augmentation state not assessed

From Garcia-Borreguero D, Silber MH, Winkelman JW, et al. Guidelines for the first-line treatment of restless legs syndrome/Willis-Ekbom disease, prevention and treatment of dopaminergic augmentation: a combined task force of the IRLSSG, EURLSSG, and the RLS-foundation. Sleep Med 2016;21:1-11.

parameters should be checked regularly, particularly when patients present with a worsening of symptoms (**Box 3**). For example, if serum ferritin levels fall lower than 75 μg/mL or if transferrin saturation is less than 20%, iron stores should be replenished with orally administered iron, unless poorly tolerated or contraindicated, in which case intravenous (IV) iron also can be considered.[32]

$\alpha2\delta$ LIGANDS

Three different $\alpha2\delta$ ligands have undergone controlled trials for RLS/WED: gabapentin, gabapentin enacarbil, and pregabalin. Although the first has hardly been investigated, the other 2 have undergone extensive clinical evaluation.[33] α-2δ ligands are effective agents to alleviate RLS/WED symptoms. Furthermore, these agents improve sleep (increasing thereby slow-wave sleep) and reduce PLMs of sleep.

Two studies have compared the short-term efficacy of $\alpha2\delta$ ligands with dopamine agonists. A first study compared 85 idiopathic RLS/WED patients with sleep disturbance, randomized to treatment with pregabalin, 300 mg/d (n = 75); pramipexole, 0.5 mg/d (n = 76); or placebo (n = 73). RLS/WED severity was not a primary endpoint but the study showed a noninferiority of pregabalin, 300 mg/d, compared with pramipexole, 0.5 mg/d.[34]

In the other study,[18] 719 patients were randomized to receive pregabalin, 300 mg/d; pramipexole, 0.25 mg/d; pramipexole, 0.5 mg/d; or placebo. Over 12 weeks, the improvement (reduction) in the mean score on the IRLS scale score was greater, by 4.5 points, among individuals receiving pregabalin than among those receiving placebo, and the proportion of patients with symptoms that were "very much improved" or "much

Box 3
Parameters that must be evaluated in restless leges syndrome/Willis-Ekbom disease (initially and periodically) including every systemic iron parameter

Hemoglobin

Serum ferritin

Serum iron

Serum transferrin

Total iron-binding capacity

Transferrin saturation

C-reactive protein and erythrocyte sedimentation rate also should be included for the proper interpretation of the results.

improved" also was greater with pregabalin than with placebo: pregabalin, 300 mg, and pramipexole, 0.5 mg, both were superior to placebo but not pramipexole, 0.25 mg. No differences existed between the therapeutic effects of pregabalin and either of the 2 doses of pramipexole. Moreover, the rate of augmentation for pregabalin was not different from the 1 obtained in similar studies for placebo and was lower than the 1 obtained for either of the 2 doses of pramipexole.[18]

In the 52-week double-blind comparative study between pregabalin and pramipexole, discussed previously, the overall rate of occurrence of adverse reactions for patients undergoing treatment with pregabalin was 85.2%, and 27.5% of these patients had to discontinue due to adverse effects. In the group of patients treated with the lower dose (0.25 mg) of pramipexole, adverse effects were reported by 79.8% of them, and 18.5 had to discontinue for that reason. Dizziness and somnolence were far more common during treatment with pregabalin, whereas headache and nausea were more common under the lower dose of pramipexole.[18]

Moreover, in a comprehensive meta-analysis, comprising 58 placebo-controlled and 4 active-controlled clinical trials, Hornyak and colleagues[35] found that changes in the IRLS scale score were comparable ($P<.78$) across dopaminergic and nondopaminergic medications, with a mean reduction in the IRLS scale score of -5.47 points for dopamine agonists and -5.12 points for anticonvulsants ($\alpha 2\delta$ ligands). Taken together, both comparative studies and the meta-analysis suggest that the therapeutic efficacy of pregabalin, 300 mg/d, and pramipexole, 0.5 mg/d, are similar.

However, 1 study[36] found that the efficacy of gabapentin enacarbil, 600 mg/d, was greater in treatment-naive patients than in patients who previously had been treated with dopamine agonists for longer than 5 years, as shown in a placebo-controlled, crossover design that compared 2 groups of closely matched patients. This further supports the IRLSSG recommendations to initiate first-line treatment with nondopaminergic agents.[14]

OPIOIDS

Opioids are used as a second-line treatment of treatment-resistant cases of RLS/WED.

Several reports have been published on different opioids.[33] However, 2 of these drugs, namely methadone and oxycodone, have been investigated with more detail:

- One class III study and another class IV study have evaluated the use of methadone in the treatment of idiopathic and secondary RLS/

WED, and both studies showed sustained therapeutic benefit over a prolonged period, from 2 years to 10 years, in patients who had failed treatment with other agents largely due to augmentation. Dropout rates ranged from 13% to 30% and were due to lack of efficacy and side effects (sedation, depression/anxiety, and altered consciousness).[37]

- A class I double-blind study on 276 RLS patients who had not responded to dopamine agonists showed that oxycodone extended-release with naloxone was efficacious for the short-term treatment of patients with severe RLS/WED inadequately controlled with previous treatment.[38] The study also provided evidence of the long-term efficacy of this treatment. Oxycodone extended-release with naloxone is approved in Europe for the treatment of patients with severe RLS/WED who have had no benefit with first-line drugs.

No comparative studies exist between opioids and any of the other classes of drugs (dopaminergics or $\alpha 2\delta$ ligands).

IRON REPLACEMENT THERAPY

The relation between iron deficiency and RLS/WED is well known. As physicians are more aware of the long-term complications that could occur with the use of symptomatic drugs, the role of iron is gaining ground. The option of initiating iron replacement therapy is, for the moment, the safest and probably the only disease-modifying strategy that currently exists for RLS/WED.

Obtaining a complete blood test and evaluating every systemic iron parameter is mandatory in every patient diagnosed with RLS/WED. It is useful to include C-reactive protein and erythrocyte sedimentation rate as long as isolated high serum ferritin levels could occur as a consequence of inflammatory conditions. **Box 3** summarizes parameters that must be evaluated.

Current recommendations about when and how to use iron therapy for RLS/WED treatment are based on the conclusions of the meeting of a panel of experts in 2016 by the IRLSSG.[32]

The decision about when to initiate iron replacement therapy depends, for the moment, on the peripheral iron status. This could change in the future because new brain imaging techniques are in development.[39] Brain iron levels do not have a direct relation with peripheral iron levels; therefore frequently, individuals are found with brain iron deficiency, despite peripheral iron parameters within normal limits.[40]

Iron replacement therapy should be considered, to minimize the risk of iron overload whenever serum ferritin is less than or equal to 100 µg/mL or transferrin saturation is less than or equal to 45%.[32] Patients with serum ferritin levels greater than 100 µg/mL, however, might respond as well, because they still might have low brain iron.

Several IV and oral formulations are currently available on the market. Choosing between the oral or IV route depends on some factors that should be evaluated carefully and individually. The oral route has several limitations because iron absorption is autoregulated in response to body iron stores.

These following 6 questions can help with choosing between the oral versus IV routes:

1. Does any contraindication for the use of the oral route exist?
2. Does the patient suffer any disorder related to intestinal malabsorption (eg, celiac disease or inflammatory bowel disease)?
3. Has previous failure or intolerance with oral treatment been reported?
4. Is a more rapid response needed?
5. Is serum ferritin below 100 mg/mL?
6. Does chronic kidney disease coexist?

Should any of these questions be answered positively, then the IV administration is preferred over the oral route.

The main disadvantage of the oral route is that up to 70% of patients report gastrointestinal side effects, leading to a decrease in compliance.[41] The oral iron formulation, which has been most investigated in RLS/WED, is ferrous sulfate.[42–44] The recommended dose is 325 mg, once or twice a day.[32,42–44] The IV iron formulation with the best results in terms of safety and efficacy in RLS/WED is ferric carboxymaltose. The recommended dose is 1000 mg, administered in a single dose or 2 divided doses, of 500 mg each, 5 days to 7 days apart. Ferric carboxymaltose is considered 1 of the first-line treatments in patients with RLS/WED,[32] according to the results of 3 placebo-controlled trials.[45–47] Every patient receiving iron replacement therapy (both oral and IV) should have a strict follow-up because iron status changes over time, and iron deficiency can reoccur, which requires restarting iron therapy.

Finally, replenishment of brain iron stores using either oral or IV iron might lead to a reduction or even discontinuation of pharmacologic treatment, as has been suggested by recent studies.[39]

NEW DRUG DEVELOPMENTS

Based on recent findings of the role of glutamate in RLS/WED,[48] 2 substances have shown promising results in open studies: First, the selective AMPA glutamate receptor antagonist perampanel was evaluated in 20 RLS/WED patients over 8 weeks of treatment.[49] The IRLS scale score improved from a mean (±SD) 23.7 ± 4.2 to 11.5 ± 5.3 over an 8-week treatment period. Twelve of 20 patients were full responders (improvement 50% in IRLS scale total score), and 4 responded partially. The mean effective dose of perampanel at the end of treatment was 3.8 mg/d. Treatment with perampanel also caused an improvement in the mean (+SD) PLMI, from 27.8 ± 6.9 to 4.36 ± 2.0.

The use of dipyridamole[50] is based on recent studies showing that brain iron deficiency in an animal model is associated with hypoadenosinergic function, due to striatal down-regulation of adenosine A_1 receptors (A1Rs), leading to hypersensitive corticostriatal terminals. The authors hypothesize that an increase in the tonic A1R activation mediated by endogenous adenosine could represent a new alternative therapeutic strategy for RLS/WED. Because dipyridamole is an inhibitor of adenosine transport, it was thought that it could cause such an increase in extracellular adenosine and thereby exert a therapeutic effect on RLS/WED symptoms. Of 13 patients who completed the study, the IRLS scale score improved from a mean (±SD) of 23.4 ± 4.6 at baseline to 10.7 ± 4.5 at 8 weeks. Six of 13 patients were full responders and 4 were partial responders. The mean (±SD) effective dose of dipyridamole at 8 weeks was 281.8 (± 57.5) mg/d. Also, sleep variables improved, and the mean (±SD) PLMI decreased from 26.7 ± 7.2 to 4.3 ± 1.9.[51] These results support the hypothesis of adenosine playing a central role in the pathophysiology of RLS/WED, thus mediating the increase in the function of dopamine and glutamate in corticostriatal pathways. These results have recently been replicated in a double-blind, placebo-controlled, crossover study on 28 patients with RLS/WED.[52]

CLINICS CARE POINTS

- Choose α2δ ligands as the first line of treatment, avoiding the use of dopamine agonists whenever possible.
- It is important to identify early on any signs of dopaminergic augmentation, because treatment adjustment might be necessary.
- Factors aggravating RLS/WED symptoms should be identified and corrected whenever possible.

- Patients who might benefit from iron replacement therapy should be identified.
- Serum and brain iron levels should be monitored before and during treatment.

DISCLOSURE

D. Garcia-Borreguero has received research funding from Merck, Sharp and Dohme. The remaining authors have nothing to disclose.

REFERENCES

1. Akpinar S. Treatment of restless legs syndrome with levodopa plus benserazide. Arch Neurol 1982;39: 739.
2. Guilleminault C, Cetel M, Philip P. Dopaminergic treatment of restless legs and rebound phenomenon. Neurology 1993;43:445.
3. Garcia-Borreguero D, Kohnen R, Silber MH, et al. The long-term treatment of restless legs syndrome/ Willis-Ekbom disease: evidence-based guidelines and clinical consensus best practice guidance: a report from the International Restless Legs Syndrome Study Group. Sleep Med 2013;14:675–84.
4. Winkelman JW, Armstrong MJ, Allen RP, et al. Practice guideline summary: treatment of restless legs syndrome in adults: report of the guideline development, dissemination, and implementation subcommittee of the American Academy of Neurology. Neurology 2016;87(24):2585–93.
5. Högl B, Garcia-Borreguero D, Trenkwalder C, et al. Efficacy and augmentation during 6 months of double-blind pramipexole for restless legs syndrome. Sleep Med 2011;12:351–60.
6. Garcia-Borreguero D, Hogl B, Ferini-Strambi L, et al. Systematic evaluation of augmentation during treatment with ropinirole in restless legs syndrome (Willis-Ekbom disease): results from a prospective, multicenter study over 66 weeks. Mov Disord 2012; 27:277–83.
7. Garcia-Borreguero D, Cano-Pumarega I, Marulanda R. Management of treatment failure in restless legs syndrome (Willis-Ekbom disease). Sleep Med Rev 2018;41:50–60.
8. Silver N, Allen RP, Senerth J, et al. A 10-year, longitudinal assessment of dopamine agonists and methadone in the treatment of restless legs syndrome. Sleep Med 2011;12:440–4.
9. Lipford MC, Silber MH. Long-term use of pramipexole in the management of restless legs syndrome. Sleep Med 2012;13:1280–5.
10. Allen RP, Ondo WG, Ball E, et al. Restless legs syndrome (RLS) augmentation associated with

dopamine agonist and levodopa usage in a community sample. Sleep Med 2011;12:431–9.
11. Tzonova D, Larrosa O, Calvo E, et al. Breakthrough symptoms during the daytime in patients with restless legs syndrome (Willis-Ekbom disease). Sleep Med 2012;13:151–5.
12. Godau J, Spinnler N, Wevers AK, et al. Poor effect of guideline based treatment of restless legs syndrome in clinical practice. J Neurol Neurosurg Psychiatry 2010;81:1390–5.
13. Garcia-Borreguero D, Allen RP, Kohnen R, et al. Diagnostic standards for dopaminergic augmentation of restless legs syndrome: report from a World association of sleep medicine-international restless legs syndrome study group consensus conference at the Max Planck institute. Sleep Med 2007;8: 520–30.
14. Garcia-Borreguero D, Silber MH, Winkelman JW, et al. Guidelines for the first-line treatment of restless legs syndrome/Willis-Ekbom disease, prevention and treatment of dopaminergic augmentation: a combined task force of the IRLSSG, EURLSSG, and the RLS-foundation. Sleep Med 2016;21:1–11.
15. Walters AS, Hickey K, Maltzman J, et al. A questionnaire study of 138 patients with restless legs syndrome: the 'Night-Walkers' survey. Neurology 1996;46:92–5.
16. Winkelman JW, Johnston L. Augmentation and tolerance with long-term pramipexole treatment of restless legs syndrome (RLS). Sleep Med 2004;5: 9–14.
17. Mackie S, Winkelman JW. Long-term treatment of restless legs syndrome (RLS): an Approach to management of worsening symptoms, loss of efficacy, and augmentation. CNS Drugs 2015;29:351–7.
18. Allen RP, Chen C, Garcia-Borreguero D, et al. Comparison of pregabalin with pramipexole for restless legs syndrome. N Engl J Med 2014;370:621–31.
19. Ferini-Strambi L. Restless legs syndrome augmentation and pramipexole treatment. Sleep Med 2002; 3(Suppl):S23–5.
20. Garcia-Borreguero D, Kohnen R, Hogl B, et al. Validation of the Augmentation Severity Rating Scale (ASRS): a multicentric, prospective study with levodopa on restless legs syndrome. Sleep Med 2007; 8:455–63.
21. Ondo W, Romanyshyn J, Vuong KD, et al. Long-term treatment of restless legs syndrome with dopamine agonists. Arch Neurol 2004;61:1393–7.
22. Silber MH, Girish M, Izurieta R. Pramipexole in the management of restless legs syndrome: an extended study. Sleep 2003;26:819–21.
23. Silber MH, Shepard JW Jr, Wisbey JA. Pergolide in the management of restless legs syndrome: an extended study. Sleep 1997;20:878–82.
24. Frauscher B, Gschliesser V, Brandauer E, et al. The severity range of restless legs syndrome (RLS) and

augmentation in a prospective patient cohort: association with ferritin levels. Sleep Med 2009;10:611–5.

25. Trenkwalder C, Hogl B, Benes H, et al. Augmentation in restless legs syndrome is associated with low ferritin. Sleep Med 2008;9:572–4.

26. Allen RP, Earley CJ. Augmentation of the restless legs syndrome with carbidopa/levodopa. Sleep 1996;19:205–13.

27. Wijemanne S, Jankovic J. Restless legs syndrome: clinical presentation diagnosis and treatment. Sleep Med 2015;16:678–90.

28. Voon V, Napier TC, Frank MJ, et al. Impulse control disorders and levodopa-induced dyskinesias in Parkinson's disease: an update. Lancet Neurol 2017;16:238–50.

29. Heim B, Djamshidian A, Heidbreder A, et al. Augmentation and impulsive behaviors in restless legs syndrome: Coexistence or association? Neurology 2016;87:36–40.

30. Cornelius JR, Tippmann-Peikert M, Slocumb NL, et al. Impulse control disorders with the use of dopaminergic agents in restless legs syndrome: a case-control study. Sleep 2010;33:81–7.

31. Connor JR, Patton SM, Oexle K, et al. Iron and restless legs syndrome: treatment, genetics and pathophysiology. Sleep Med 2017;31:61–70.

32. Allen RP, Picchietti DL, Auerbach M, et al. Evidence-based and consensus clinical practice guidelines for the iron treatment of restless legs syndrome/Willis-Ekbom disease in adults and children: an IRLSSG task force report. Sleep Med 2018;41:27–44.

33. Winkelmann J, Allen RP, Hogl B, et al. Treatment of restless legs syndrome: evidence-based review and implications for clinical practice (Revised 2017)(section sign). Mov Disord 2018;33:1077–91.

34. Garcia-Borreguero D, Patrick J, DuBrava S, et al. Pregabalin versus pramipexole: effects on sleep disturbance in restless legs syndrome. Sleep 2014;37:635–43.

35. Hornyak M, Scholz H, Kohnen R, et al. What treatment works best for restless legs syndrome? Meta-analyses of dopaminergic and non-dopaminergic medications. Sleep Med Rev 2014;18:153–64.

36. Garcia-Borreguero D, Cano-Pumarega I, Garcia Malo C, et al. Reduced response to gabapentin enacarbil in restless legs syndrome following long-term dopaminergic treatment. Sleep Med 2019;55:74–80.

37. Silber MH, Becker PM, Buchfuhrer MJ, et al. The Appropriate Use of opioids in the treatment of Refractory restless legs syndrome. Mayo Clin Proc 2018;93:59–67.

38. Trenkwalder C, Benes H, Grote L, et al. Prolonged release oxycodone-naloxone for treatment of severe restless legs syndrome after failure of previous treatment: a double-blind, randomised, placebo-

controlled trial with an open-label extension. Lancet Neurol 2013;12:1141–50.

39. Garcia-Malo C. Quantitative transcranial sonography of the substantia nigra as a predictor of therapeutic response to intravenous iron therapy in restless legs syndrome. Sleep Med 2020;66:123–9.

40. Earley CJ, Connor J, Garcia-Borreguero D, et al. Altered brain iron homeostasis and dopaminergic function in restless legs syndrome (Willis-Ekbom disease). Sleep Med 2014;15:1288–301.

41. Tolkien Z, Stecher L, Mander AP, et al. Ferrous sulfate supplementation causes significant gastrointestinal side-effects in adults: a systematic review and meta-analysis. PLoS One 2015;10:e0117383.

42. Wang J, O'Reilly B, Venkataraman R, et al. Efficacy of oral iron in patients with restless legs syndrome and a low-normal ferritin: a randomized, double-blind, placebo-controlled study. Sleep Med 2009;10:973–5.

43. Lee CS, Lee SD, Kang SH, et al. Comparison of the efficacies of oral iron and pramipexole for the treatment of restless legs syndrome patients with low serum ferritin. Eur J Neurol 2014;21:260–6.

44. Davis BJ, Rajput A, Rajput ML, et al. A randomized, double-blind placebo-controlled trial of iron in restless legs syndrome. Eur Neurol 2000;43:70–5.

45. Allen RP, Adler CH, Du W, et al. Clinical efficacy and safety of IV ferric carboxymaltose (FCM) treatment of RLS: a multi-centred, placebo-controlled preliminary clinical trial. Sleep Med 2011;12:906–13.

46. Cho YW, Allen RP, Earley CJ. Clinical efficacy of ferric carboxymaltose treatment in patients with restless legs syndrome. Sleep Med 2016;25:16–23.

47. Trenkwalder C, Winkelmann J, Oertel W, et al. Ferric carboxymaltose in patients with restless legs syndrome and non-anemic iron deficiency. Mov Disord 2017;32(10):1478–82.

48. Ferre S, Garcia-Borreguero D, Allen RP, et al. New insights into the Neurobiology of restless legs syndrome. Neuroscientist 2019;25:113–25.

49. Garcia-Borreguero D, Cano I, Granizo JJ. Treatment of restless legs syndrome with the selective AMPA receptor antagonist perampanel. Sleep Med 2017;34:105–8.

50. Ferre S, Quiroz C, Guitart X, et al. Pivotal role of adenosine Neurotransmission in restless legs syndrome. Front Neurosci 2017;11:722.

51. Garcia-Borreguero D, Guitart X, Garcia Malo C, et al. Treatment of restless legs syndrome/Willis-Ekbom disease with the non-selective ENT1/ENT2 inhibitor dipyridamole: testing the adenosine hypothesis. Sleep Med 2018;45:94–7.

52. Garcia-Borreguero D, Garcia-Malo C, Granizo JJ, et al. Testing the adenosine hypothesis of restless legs syndrome: A randomized, cross-over, placebo-controlled study with dipyridamole. Mov Dis, 2021 (in press).

The Long-Term Psychiatric and Cardiovascular Morbidity and Mortality of Restless Legs Syndrome and Periodic Limb Movements of Sleep

Benjamin Wipper, BA[a], John W. Winkelman, MD, PhD[a,b,c],*

KEYWORDS

- Restless legs syndrome • Periodic limb movements of sleep • Psychiatric illness
- Cardiovascular disease • Mortality • Morbidity • Suicide • Depression

KEY POINTS

- Epidemiologic studies suggest that individuals with restless legs syndrome (RLS) face an increased risk of depression, anxiety, and other forms of psychiatric illness.
- Cross-sectional and longitudinal studies reveal that patients with RLS also may be at risk of developing cardiovascular disease, although studies yield contrasting results.
- Longitudinal studies provide evidence both for and against a relationship between RLS and increased mortality.
- Periodic limb movements of sleep also have been associated with psychiatric illness, cardiovascular disease, and mortality.

INTRODUCTION

Restless legs syndrome (RLS) is a sensory-motor neurologic disorder characterized by an irresistible urge to move the legs and associated leg discomfort. Symptoms are provoked by rest, typically relieved with movement or counter-stimulation, and worst in the evening or at night.[1] RLS can be either idiopathic (primary) or associated with an underlying medical condition, such as end-stage renal disease (ESRD) (secondary)[2] or iron deficiency,[3] although the syndrome phenotype is identical in primary RLS and secondary RLS. The leg sensations associated with RLS often are described by sufferers as unbearable and produce high levels of physical and emotional distress, lack of sleep, and daytime fatigue. RLS is a common disorder, with approximately 3% of the population experiencing clinically significant symptoms.[4] Most patients suffering from RLS experience at least initial clinical benefit with dopamine agonist medications (eg, ropinirole, pramipexole, and rotigotine) and $\alpha2\delta$ ligands (eg, pregabalin, gabapentin, and gabapentin encarbil); these medications improve the sensory and motor symptoms of RLS as well as sleep and quality of life.[5,6] Despite the high prevalence of RLS, the great distress that symptoms cause for afflicted individuals, and the

[a] Sleep Disorders Clinical Research Program, Massachusetts General Hospital, Harvard Medical School, One Bowdoin Square, 10th Floor, Boston, MA 02114, USA; [b] Department of Psychiatry, Massachusetts General Hospital, Harvard Medical School, 55 Fruit Street, Boston, MA 02114, USA; [c] Department of Neurology, Massachusetts General Hospital, Harvard Medical School, 55 Fruit Street, Boston, MA 02114, USA
* Corresponding author. One Bowdoin Square, 10th Floor, Boston, MA 02114.
E-mail address: jwwinkelman@mgh.harvard.edu

Sleep Med Clin 16 (2021) 279–288
https://doi.org/10.1016/j.jsmc.2021.02.005
1556-407X/21/© 2021 Published by Elsevier Inc.

typical clinical usefulness of medication therapy, the disorder is underdiagnosed.[4,7]

Periodic limb movements in sleep (PLMS) are repetitive, involuntary movements of the lower extremities that occur during sleep. Although individuals with PLMS typically are not aware of the movements (bed partners may report them), such movements can lead to brief arousals or frank awakenings during the night. This sleep disruption can lead to fatigue and somnolence during the day. Although PLMS often occur in the absence of other sleep disorders, they are especially common in those with RLS: whereas an estimated 4% to 60% of the general adult population have PLMS (depending on age),[8–10] these movements are observed in 80% to 90% of RLS patients.[11] Both dopamine agonists and $\alpha 2\delta$ ligands have been shown to also significantly reduce PLMS[12,13] in those with RLS.

In addition to the short-term detrimental effects that RLS has on sleep and quality of life, growing evidence suggests that the condition also is associated with long-term consequences. Various studies have proposed that PLMS also are linked to negative effects and that these movements may help explain the relationship between RLS and various health conditions. This article critically reviews an array of cross-sectional and longitudinal studies examining the long-term impacts of RLS and PLMS in 3 major domains: psychiatric illness, cardiovascular disease (CVD), and mortality.

PSYCHIATRIC ILLNESS

At least 25 studies have revealed a high prevalence of depressive symptoms and/or depressive disorders in patients with RLS.[14] In the Memory and Morbidity in Augsburg Elderly study,[15] 369 elderly individuals aged 65 to 83 were assessed for RLS by trained physicians. Compared with men without RLS, those with RLS had a higher prevalence of depression and lower mental health scores. Other cross-sectional studies have revealed a similar link between RLS and depressive symptoms both in women and in younger patients.[16,17] Recent studies have provided even more evidence for a link between RLS and depression. A community-based study of Korean adults (n = 7515) found that depressive symptoms were more prevalent in individuals with RLS.[18] Severe depression (Beck Depression Inventory score ≥24) was seen at especially high levels in those with RLS (odds ratio [OR] 56.54; P<.001). In a study of approximately 25,000 Danish blood donors,[19] men and women with RLS had a higher probability of both low mental health–related

quality of life (OR 1.71; P = .010) and depression (OR 1.99; P = .023). One contrasting study did find that a group of older individuals with RLS were not more depressed than patients of the same age and education without RLS.[20] These results may be explained partially, however, by the fact that the sample size was small (n = 26 in the RLS group) and that the sample of patients had relatively mild RLS. Research showing high rates of RLS in depressed individuals provides further evidence for a link between the 2 conditions: a population-based study of more than 1500 adults found that individuals with depression had an increased risk of experiencing RLS symptoms (OR 1.64; 95% CI: 1.07 -2.56").[21]

A pair of prospective studies have provided valuable insight into the temporal relationship between RLS and depression. During 6 years of follow-up of 56,399 women in a prospective study of female nurses (the Nurses' Health Study), participants with RLS had an increased risk of both incident clinical depression (relative risk [RR] 1.5; 1.1–2.1) and clinically relevant depression symptoms (CRDSs) (**Table 1**).[22] Similarly, analysis of a large-scale cohort study (Study of Health in Pomerania) confirmed this previous finding, showing that individuals with RLS at baseline were more likely to develop incident CRDSs after a median of 5.0 years of follow-up.[23] This study provided evidence for the reverse directionality as well: CRDSs at baseline were associated with increased risk of the new onset of RLS.

Considering the association between RLS and depression and the known link between depression and suicide, it might be expected that individuals with RLS are at an increased risk of suicidal behavior. Two recent longitudinal studies have provided evidence for increased suicidal ideation or behaviors in RLS patients. One cohort study utilizing longitudinal medical claim data from a large sample of US patients (n = 169373) found that those with physician-diagnosed RLS had an increased risk of suicide and self-harm during the 6-year follow-up period (adjusted hazard ratio [HR] 2.66, 1.70–4.15).[24] In a recent cross-sectional study,[25] more participants with RLS had lifetime suicidal ideation or behavior than controls (27.1% vs 7.0%, respectively; P<.00001). Furthermore, suicidality was linked to RLS severity: the probability of suicidal ideation or behavior increased if previous RLS symptoms were severe or very severe. These results suggest that increased suicidality seen in RLS patients may not simply be due to depression: even after adjusting for depression, participants with RLS had greater odds of lifetime suicidal ideation or behavior.

Table 1 Individuals with restless legs syndrome may be more likely to develop clinical depression				
	No Restless Legs Syndrome	Restless Legs Syndrome		P Value
		Relative Risk	95% CI	
No. of cases[a]	1235	33		
Person-years of follow-up	295,493	4662		
Crude incidence (per 100,000 person-years)	418	708		
Age-adjusted RR	1	1.66	1.18–2.35	0.004
Multivariate RR[b]	1	1.58	1.11–2.23	0.01
Multivariate RR[c]	1	1.51	1.07–2.14	0.02
Multivariate RR[d]	1	1.49	1.06–2.10	0.02

Adjusted RR of clinical depression according to baseline RLS status during 6 years of follow-up in a large-scale prospective study (Nurses' Health Study).

[a] Clinical depression was defined as reported regular use of antidepressant medication and physician-diagnosed depression.

[b] Adjusted for age (y), body mass index (weight [kg]/height [m]^2; continuous), ethnicity (white or other), smoking status (never, past, or current smoker), marital status (married/in a partnership, widowed, or separated/divorced/single), solitary living status (yes/no; binary), regular involvement in a social or community group (yes/no; binary), menopausal status (premenopausal or postmenopausal), menopausal hormone use (never, past, or current user), alcohol intake (0 g/d, 0.1–4.9 g/d, 5.0–9.9 g/d, 10.0–14.9 g/d, or $\geq$15 g/d), and physical activity (quintiles).

[c] Further adjusted for the presence of diabetes, arthritis, stroke, MI, angina, cancer, hypertension, high cholesterol level, or Parkinson disease (yes/no).

[d] Further adjusted for use of iron-specific supplements, sleep duration ($\leq$5, 6, 7, 8, or $\geq$9 h/24-h period), and snoring frequency (every night, most nights, a few nights per week, occasionally, or almost never).

From Li Y, Mirzaei F, O'Reilly EJ, et al. Prospective study of restless legs syndrome and risk of depression in women. American journal of epidemiology. 2012;176(4):279-288; with permission.

There also is a well-established relationship between RLS and anxiety. In a study analyzing data drawn from a community sample of Turkish adults, individuals with RLS had significantly higher symptoms of anxiety than control subjects.[26] There also was a significant positive correlation between symptoms of anxiety and RLS severity ($r = 0.21$; $P = .03$). Other cross-sectional studies have similarly revealed high rates of anxiety symptoms in patients with RLS.[27,28] In addition to anxiety symptoms, RLS patients may experience high rates of anxiety disorders. One community-based study found that individuals with RLS had an increased risk of panic disorder (PD),[29] and a recent cross-sectional study of approximately 1500 elderly participants found that probable RLS was associated with generalized anxiety disorder (GAD) (OR 2.17; 1.01–4.68).[30] Although the researchers in this latter study found a relationship between RLS and comorbid GAD depression, they did not find a link between RLS and depression alone; this suggests that anxiety may play a distinct role in driving the relationship between RLS and depressive disorders.

The temporal relationship between RLS and anxiety is not well understood. One cross-sectional study looking at 130 RLS patients, in which RLS was associated with increased risk of having 12-month PD (OR 4.7) and GAD (OR 3.5), provided some insight in this regard.[17] In a majority of the patients, in this sample who suffered from comorbid RLS and anxiety, RLS appeared first (this was the case in 60% of patients with PD and 64% with GAD). Although these results suggest that RLS commonly may precede anxiety disorders, large-scale longitudinal studies are needed in order to confirm this hypothesis.

There likely are numerous factors that underly the relationship between RLS and these various psychiatric ailments, and sleep disturbance may be one of them. RLS is known to disturb sleep, with sufferers experiencing both decreased sleep time and quality compared with controls.[31,32] Because many studies demonstrate the role of sleeplessness as a risk factor for the development of both mood disorders[33] and other psychiatric disorders,[34] it would not be surprising if sleep disturbance plays an important mediating role for RLS as well. A modeling study suggesting just this relationship used questions about RLS severity, sleep disturbance, and RLS-specific health-related quality of life. The strongest link was from RLS severity to sleep disturbance to emotional distress.[35]

Dopaminergic abnormalities also may underlie the relationship between RLS and psychiatric illness. As discussed previously, dopamine agonists effectively treat RLS symptoms. Additionally, a 2006 study revealed that RLS patients naïve to dopaminergic medications had PET results that were indicative of abnormal hypoactive dopaminergic transmission.[36] Although the current evidence is not conclusive, neuroimaging studies have suggested that both depressive and anxiety disorders also may be associated with abnormal dopamine functioning.[37,38] Additionally, dopamine agonist medications have been shown to be effective in some depressed patients.[39]

PLMS also may be an important factor in the relationship between RLS and psychiatric disorders. Numerous studies have linked PLMS to depression. One cross-sectional study found individuals with periodic limb movement disorder (PLMD) to have particularly high rates of previous depression treatment compared with other patients.[40] Another study found 26 individuals with PLMD (and no RLS) to have higher depression rating scores than controls.[41] More recent research has shown that PLMS may play a role in mediating the relationship between RLS and depression. In a cross-sectional study examining community-dwelling older men, there was a positive association between depressive symptoms and RLS severity in participants with a periodic limb movement index (PLMI) at or above the average.[42] This relationship between RLS severity and depressive symptoms was not observed in patients with lower PLMIs. Similar studies should assess whether PLMS mediate the link between RLS and both anxiety and suicidality.

RLS also may be associated with attention-deficit/hyperactivity disorder (ADHD). A large-scale cross-sectional study revealed that mothers of children with ADHD had a particularly high risk of having RLS (OR 1.27; 1.15–1.41).[43] In a recent cross-sectional study of more than 25,000 participants, RLS patients were more likely to suffer from ADHD symptoms than controls.[44] The risk of ADHD symptoms was particularly high among RLS patients who experienced involuntary leg movements during sleep, suggesting that PLMS may play a role in the relationship between the 2 disorders. Brain iron deficiency also may help explain the connection between RLS and ADHD. Low brain iron levels have been linked to both disorders.[45,46] One recent study specifically assessed the relationship between ADHD, RLS, and serum ferritin levels.[47] RLS was diagnosed in

a third of 200 adults with ADHD, and was linked to both early-onset ADHD and severe lifetime ADHD symptoms. Patients with both ADHD and RLS had low normal serum ferritin (<50 ng/mL) more frequently than other participants. PLMI was no different between those with ADHD with and without RLS. Although these results linking RLS and ADHD are intriguing, more research needs to be performed in this domain. The directionality of the relationship between the 2 disorders currently is unclear: well-designed prospective studies need to be conducted in order to determine whether individuals with RLS are at an increased risk of developing ADHD.

CARDIOVASCULAR DISEASE

Several cross-sectional studies have examined the relationship between RLS and CVD. The exact definition of CVD varies between studies but generally includes coronary artery disease (CAD), myocardial infarction (MI), stroke, and heart failure. Numerous studies also have suggested that individuals with RLS are at an increased risk of having hypertension,[48] which is a key risk factor for CVD.[49] In a study of 995 individuals residing in northern Finland, RLS (defined as experiencing RLS symptoms ≥ 1 time/week) was associated with coronary heart disease (CHD) (OR 2.92; 1.18–2.73).[50] Analysis of data from approximately 3000 participants in the Wisconsin Sleep Cohort showed that those with RLS symptoms had an increased prevalence of CVD (OR 2.58; 1.38–4.84).[27] In the Sleep Heart Health Study, another large-scale cross-sectional study (n >3000), multivariate logistic regression analysis revealed a heightened prevalence of CVD in RLS patients (OR 2.07; 1.43–3.00).[51] In the latter 2 studies, stratification by RLS frequency revealed that increased prevalence of CVD was present only in patients with regular RLS symptoms (daily in the Wisconsin Sleep Cohort and >15 d/mo in the Sleep Heart Health Study).

Other cross-sectional studies have produced conflicting results regarding the relationship between RLS and CVD. An analysis of 22,786 male physicians (the US Physicians' Health Study) found that RLS history (of undefined duration or frequency of symptoms) was not associated with the prevalence of major CVD events (multivariate adjusted OR 0.97; 0.79–1.20), although it was associated with the prevalence of stroke (OR 1.40; 1.05–1.86).[52] Contrary to the results of other studies, prevalent MI was associated with a decreased risk for RLS (OR 0.73; 0.55–0.97). In another large-scale study (n = 30,262) conducted by the same research team, RLS in female health professionals was not associated with overall major CVD events, MI, or stroke but was associated with coronary revascularization (OR 1.39; 1.10–1.77).[53]

Longitudinal studies have also provided mixed evidence regarding the relationship between RLS and CVD. A large propensity-matched prospective cohort study of US veterans (median follow-up = 8.1 years) showed that incident RLS was associated with higher risk of CHD (HR 3.97; 3.26–4.84) and stroke (HR 3.89; 3.07–4.94).[54] Analysis of data from 2823 men participating in the prospective Osteoporotic Fractures in Men Study (MrOS) (average follow-up = 8 years) revealed that RLS was not associated with composite CVD outcomes but was associated with incident MI.[55] Findings from a large retrospective study suggested that the distinction between primary and secondary RLS may be important in terms of the relationship between RLS and CVD. Analysis of the clinical records of 7621 patients with primary RLS found that these individuals did not have increased risk of incident CVD and CAD compared with controls, although they did have a 20% increased risk of incident hypertension.[56] Patients with secondary RLS (n = 4507), however, had an elevated risk of developing CVD, CAD, and hypertension. A 2012 study assessing 6-year follow-up data from the Nurses' Health Study found that duration of RLS may be a risk factor for CVD[57]: whereas women with physician-diagnosed RLS for less than 3 years at baseline did not have a higher risk of developing CHD compared with controls without RLS (HR 0.98; 0.44–2.19), those with RLS for ≥3 years did have an elevated risk (OR 1.72; 1.09–2.73). A similar pattern was observed for nonfatal MI.

Generally, the cross-sectional and longitudinal literature does provide evidence for an association between RLS and CVD, although the results certainly are nuanced. The variation seen between studies likely can be explained by several factors, such as differences in the study populations (eg, age and gender), methods of RLS diagnosis, specific cardiovascular conditions assessed, and, most importantly, RLS duration, frequency, and severity. **Fig. 1**, which was published in a recent review article,[58] shows possible routes through which RLS and CVD are linked. It is plausible that the sleep deprivation caused by RLS symptoms contributes to increased risk of CVD. Prospective studies suggest that short sleep duration (5 or fewer hours per night) may increase risk of developing both diabetes and hypertension,[59,60] 2 conditions that are known to be associated with increased prevalence of CVD. Additionally, analysis of data from the prospective

Nurses' Health Study directly established a link between short sleep duration and CVD: analysis of follow-up data at 10 years revealed that individuals who slept for 5 or fewer hours per night had an increased age-adjusted RR of developing CHD (RR 1.45; 1.10–1.92).[61]

PLMS also may play an important role in linking RLS and CVD. These movements have long been associated with the cardiovascular system: individual leg movements during sleep are associated with a significant (approximately 10%) rise in heart rate[62] as well as increases in systolic (approximately 20 mm Hg) and diastolic (approximately 10 mm Hg) blood pressure.[63] A pair of more recent studies have looked specifically at the relationship between PLMS and CVD. During a 4-year analysis of data from the MrOS, PLMI greater than or equal to 5 was associated with increased incidence of CVD (OR 1.83 for individuals with PLMI 5 to <30 and 1.89 for those with PLMI ≥30; P trend = 0.025), specifically in individuals without prevalent hypertension.[64] Similarly, an analysis of the MrOS data also found PLMI to predict incident MI. This result was unchanged after RLS status was added to the regression model.[55] Finally, a recent study[65] found that individual PLMs increased the risk of nonsustained ventricular tachycardia (OR 2.31; 1.02–5.25) during the sleep period, identifying PLMs as a potentially important trigger for arrhythmia and cardiovascular events. Although these studies suggest that PLMS independently may increase risk for CVD, more epidemiologic data on the topic are needed. Additionally, the exact mechanisms through which PLMS may increase CVD risk are unclear and need to be investigated further.

Lastly, iron deficiency also may help explain the relationship between RLS and CVD. As discussed previously, RLS is associated with low brain iron levels. Iron deficiency is also implicated in CVD: previous research has suggested that iron deficiency has harmful effects in individuals with CAD, heart failure, and other cardiovascular conditions.[66] Additionally, a mendelian randomization study found that individuals with lower iron status were at an increased risk of CAD.[67] Future research needs to further examine this potential relationship between RLS, CVD, and low iron status.

MORTALITY

A prospective cohort study of US men free of diabetes, arthritis, and renal failure showed that RLS was linked to increased mortality (HR 1.39; 1.19–1.62).[68] When these researchers looked specifically at individuals free of chronic diseases, a dose-response relationship between

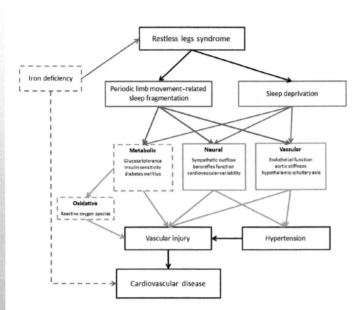

Fig. 1. Potential mechanisms linking RLS and CVD. Sleep deprivation, PLMS, and iron deficiency are 3 separate factors that may link RLS and CVD. (*From* Gottlieb DJ, Somers VK, Punjabi NM, Winkelman JW. Restless legs syndrome and cardiovascular disease: a research roadmap. Sleep medicine. 2017;31:10-17; with permission.)

RLS symptom frequency and mortality risk was observed (**Fig. 2**). The prospective study of US veterans conducted by Molnar and colleagues[54] also showed that RLS was associated with high mortality (HR 1.88; 1.70–2.08). In the Nurses' Health Study, with assessments of mortality after 10 years of follow-up, the relationship between physician-diagnosed RLS and overall mortality approached significance (HR 1.15; 0.98–1.34; $P = .09$),[69] and there was a significant positive association between RLS and cardiovascular mortality (HR 1.43; 1.02–2.00). Similarly, RLS symptoms also are associated with increased risk of death in patients with ESRD[70–73] (who have high rates of RLS), although there have also been studies that did not concur.[74,75]

Other studies assessing RLS and mortality risk have yielded contrasting results. A cohort study of more than 5000 participants in Sweden assessed mortality data over a 20-year period.[76] Although women with RLS and daytime sleepiness experienced higher mortality than those without, this same relationship was not seen in men. A 2012 analysis assessed all-cause mortality in 4

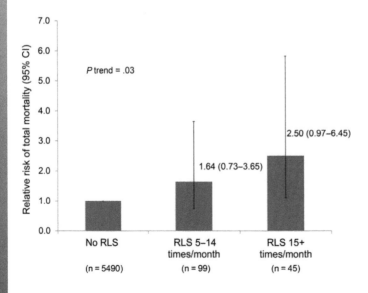

Fig. 2. There may be a dose-response relationship between RLS frequency and mortality in relatively healthy men. RR of total mortality by RLS frequency status after 8 years of follow-up in a large-scale prospective study. "Relatively healthy men" were free of cancer, diabetes, and other chronic health conditions. RR values were estimated from cox proportional hazards models and were adjusted for numerous potential confounding variables. (*From* Li Y, Wang W, Winkelman JW, Malhotra A, Ma J, Gao X. Prospective study of restless legs syndrome and mortality among men. Neurology. 2013;81(1):52-59; with permission.)

separate prospective cohort studies: the Dortmund Health Study, Study of Health in Pomerania, Women's Health Study, and Physicians' Health Study.[77] After adjusting for confounding factors, such as age, exercise, and other health conditions, these researchers found no relationship between RLS and mortality risk in any of the studies.

Increased mortality is the most concerning potential long-term effect of RLS and certainly needs to be studied in greater depth. As described previously for CVD, duration, frequency, and severity of RLS symptoms may modify mortality risk and such factors should be assessed in future long-term studies of RLS. Heightened mortality in RLS patients may be due to a plethora of factors. As suggested by the results of the Nurses' Health Study, increased incidence of CVD in RLS patients may lead to higher mortality rates. RLS is associated with reduced baroreflex gain,[78] which itself is a risk factor for cardiovascular mortality following MI.[79] Additionally, psychiatric illness (especially suicidal ideation) brought about by RLS symptoms may play an important role. Lastly, a pair of prospective studies suggest that PLMS may independently contribute to mortality. In a study of 29 patients with ESRD, the 20-month mortality rate was significantly higher for individuals with high PLMIs (>20) than for patients with lower PLMIs ($P = .007$).[80] Another study looked specifically at patients diagnosed with systolic heart failure[81] and revealed that individuals with a PLMI greater than or equal to 5 had a higher risk of death than individuals with a lower PLMI (HR 2.42; 1.16–5.02; $P = .018$). Knowing that high PLMI was a predictor of death in these populations with specific diseases, it seems plausible that it also is associated with death in the RLS population. Future prospective studies should assess whether this is the case.

SUMMARY

RLS is associated with poor sleep and decreased quality of life. Along with the high levels of short-term distress caused by the disorder, a body of evidence suggests that there also are long-term consequences: although there is contrasting evidence, observational studies suggest that RLS sufferers may face an increased risk of psychiatric illness, CVD, and death. Several studies further suggest that PLMS may play a role in mediating the relationship between RLS and long-term morbidity and mortality. These findings demonstrate the importance of increasing awareness of RLS and PLMS, which often can be treated effectively with pharmacologic therapy.

CLINICS CARE POINTS

- Patients with RLS may be at an increased risk of anxiety, depression, and suicide.
- RLS sufferers may also face a higher risk of developing myocardial infarction, coronary heart disease, and other cardiovascular diseases, although studies in this domain have yielded conflicting results.
- PLMS may play a role in linking RLS and cardiovascular disease.
- Clinicians should closely monitor patients with RLS and PLMS for symptoms of psychiatric illness and cardiovascular disease.

DISCLOSURE

Dr J.W. Winkelman reports acting as a consultant to Avadel, UpToDate, OrbiMed, and CVS and reports receiving research support from Luitpold, Merck and the RLS Foundation. Mr B. Wipper reports no disclosures. The authors did not receive any funding for the purposes of writing this review article.

REFERENCES

1. Allen RP, Picchietti DL, Garcia-Borreguero D, et al. Restless legs syndrome/Willis-Ekbom disease diagnostic criteria: updated International Restless Legs Syndrome Study Group (IRLSSG) consensus criteria–history, rationale, description, and significance. Sleep Med 2014;15(8):860–73.
2. Giannaki CD, Hadjigeorgiou GM, Karatzaferi C, et al. Epidemiology, impact, and treatment options of restless legs syndrome in end-stage renal disease patients: an evidence-based review. Kidney Int 2014;85(6):1275–82.
3. Allen RP, Auerbach S, Bahrain H, et al. The prevalence and impact of restless legs syndrome on patients with iron deficiency anemia. Am J Hematol 2013;88(4):261–4.
4. Allen RP, Walters AS, Montplaisir J, et al. Restless legs syndrome prevalence and impact: REST general population study. Arch Intern Med 2005; 165(11):1286–92.
5. Scholz H, Trenkwalder C, Kohnen R, et al. Dopamine agonists for restless legs syndrome. Cochrane Database Syst Rev 2011;(3):Cd006009.
6. Silber MH, Becker PM, Earley C, et al. Willis-Ekbom Disease Foundation revised consensus statement on the management of restless legs syndrome. Mayo Clin Proc 2013;88(9):977–86.

7. Allen RP, Stillman P, Myers AJ. Physician-diagnosed restless legs syndrome in a large sample of primary medical care patients in western Europe: prevalence and characteristics. Sleep Med 2010;11(1): 31–7.

8. Hornyak M, Feige B, Riemann D, et al. Periodic leg movements in sleep and periodic limb movement disorder: prevalence, clinical significance and treatment. Sleep Med Rev 2006;10(3):169–77.

9. Winkelman JW, Blackwell T, Stone K, et al. Genetic associations of periodic limb movements of sleep in the elderly for the MrOS sleep study. Sleep Med 2015;16(11):1360–5.

10. Haba-Rubio J, Marti-Soler H, Marques-Vidal P, et al. Prevalence and determinants of periodic limb movements in the general population. Ann Neurol 2016; 79(3):464–74.

11. Montplaisir J, Boucher S, Poirier G, et al. Clinical, polysomnographic, and genetic characteristics of restless legs syndrome: a study of 133 patients diagnosed with new standard criteria. Movement Disord 1997;12(1):61–5.

12. Garcia-Borreguero D, Larrosa O, de la Llave Y, et al. Treatment of restless legs syndrome with gabapentin: a double-blind, cross-over study. Neurology 2002;59(10):1573–9.

13. Inoue Y, Hirata K, Kuroda K, et al. Efficacy and safety of pramipexole in Japanese patients with primary restless legs syndrome: a polysomnographic randomized, double-blind, placebo-controlled study. Sleep Med 2010;11(1):11–6.

14. Hornyak M. Depressive disorders in restless legs syndrome: epidemiology, pathophysiology and management. CNS drugs 2010;24(2):89–98.

15. Rothdach AJ, Trenkwalder C, Haberstock J, et al. Prevalence and risk factors of RLS in an elderly population: the MEMO study. Memory and Morbidity in Augsburg Elderly. Neurology 2000; 54(5):1064–8.

16. Wesstrom J, Nilsson S, Sundstrom-Poromaa I, et al. Restless legs syndrome among women: prevalence, co-morbidity and possible relationship to menopause. Climacteric 2008;11(5):422–8.

17. Winkelmann J, Prager M, Lieb R, et al. Anxietas tibiarum". Depression and anxiety disorders in patients with restless legs syndrome. J Neurol 2005; 252(1):67–71.

18. Cho CH, Kim L, Lee HJ. Individuals with restless legs syndrome tend to have severe depressive symptoms: findings from a community-based cohort study. Psychiatry Investig 2017;14(6):887–93.

19. Didriksen M, Allen RP, Burchell BJ, et al. Restless legs syndrome is associated with major comorbidities in a population of Danish blood donors. Sleep Med 2018;45:124–31.

20. Driver-Dunckley E, Connor D, Hentz J, et al. No evidence for cognitive dysfunction or depression in

patients with mild restless legs syndrome. Mov Disord 2009;24(12):1840–2.

21. Foley D, Ancoli-Israel S, Britz P, et al. Sleep disturbances and chronic disease in older adults: results of the 2003 National Sleep Foundation Sleep in America Survey. J Psychosom Res 2004;56(5):497–502.

22. Li Y, Mirzaei F, O'Reilly EJ, et al. Prospective study of restless legs syndrome and risk of depression in women. Am J Epidemiol 2012;176(4):279–88.

23. Szentkiralyi A, Völzke H, Hoffmann W, et al. The relationship between depressive symptoms and restless legs syndrome in two prospective cohort studies. Psychosom Med 2013;75(4):359–65.

24. Zhuang S, Na M, Winkelman JW, et al. Association of restless legs syndrome with risk of suicide and self-harm. JAMA Netw Open 2019;2(8):e199966.

25. Para KS, Chow CA, Nalamada K, et al. Suicidal thought and behavior in individuals with restless legs syndrome. Sleep Med 2019;54:1–7.

26. Sevim S, Dogu O, Kaleagasi H, et al. Correlation of anxiety and depression symptoms in patients with restless legs syndrome: a population based survey. J Neurol Neurosurg Psychiatry 2004;75(2):226–30.

27. Winkelman JW, Finn L, Young T. Prevalence and correlates of restless legs syndrome symptoms in the Wisconsin Sleep Cohort. Sleep Med 2006;7(7): 545–52.

28. Sauerbier A, Sivakumar C, Klingelhoefer L, et al. Restless legs syndrome - the under-recognised non-motor burden: a questionnaire-based cohort study. Postgrad Med 2019;131(7):473–8.

29. Lee HB, Hening WA, Allen RP, et al. Restless legs syndrome is associated with DSM-IV major depressive disorder and panic disorder in the community. J Neuropsychiatry Clin Neurosci 2008;20(1):101–5.

30. Tully PJ, Kurth T, Elbaz A, et al. Convergence of psychiatric symptoms and restless legs syndrome: a cross-sectional study in an elderly French population. J Psychosom Res 2020;128:109884.

31. Hening W, Walters AS, Allen RP, et al. Impact, diagnosis and treatment of restless legs syndrome (RLS) in a primary care population: the REST (RLS epidemiology, symptoms, and treatment) primary care study. Sleep Med 2004;5(3):237–46.

32. Winkelman JW, Redline S, Baldwin CM, et al. Polysomnographic and health-related quality of life correlates of restless legs syndrome in the Sleep Heart Health Study. Sleep 2009;32(6):772–8.

33. Baglioni C, Battagliese G, Feige B, et al. Insomnia as a predictor of depression: a meta-analytic evaluation of longitudinal epidemiological studies. J Affect Disord 2011;135(1–3):10–9.

34. Hertenstein E, Feige B, Gmeiner T, et al. Insomnia as a predictor of mental disorders: a systematic review and meta-analysis. Sleep Med Rev 2019;43:96–105.

35. Kushida CA, Allen RP, Atkinson MJ. Modeling the causal relationships between symptoms associated

with restless legs syndrome and the patient-reported impact of RLS. Sleep Med 2004;5(5): 485–8.

36. Cervenka S, Pålhagen SE, Comley RA, et al. Support for dopaminergic hypoactivity in restless legs syndrome: a PET study on D2-receptor binding. Brain 2006;129(Pt 8):2017–28.

37. Schneier FR, Abi-Dargham A, Martinez D, et al. Dopamine transporters, D2 receptors, and dopamine release in generalized social anxiety disorder. Depress Anxiety 2009;26(5):411–8.

38. Sarchiapone M, Carli V, Camardese G, et al. Dopamine transporter binding in depressed patients with anhedonia. Psychiatry Res 2006;147(2–3): 243–8.

39. Fawcett J, Rush AJ, Vukelich J, et al. Clinical experience with high-dosage pramipexole in patients with treatment-resistant depressive episodes in unipolar and bipolar depression. Am J Psychiatry 2016; 173(2):107–11.

40. Mendelson WB. Are periodic leg movements associated with clinical sleep disturbance? Sleep 1996; 19(3):219–23.

41. Saletu M, Anderer P, Saletu B, et al. EEG mapping in patients with restless legs syndrome as compared with normal controls. Psychiatry Res 2002;115(1–2):49–61.

42. Koo BB, Blackwell T, Lee HB, et al. Restless legs syndrome and depression: effect mediation by disturbed sleep and periodic limb movements. Am J Geriatr Psychiatry 2016;24(11):1105–16.

43. Gao X, Lyall K, Palacios N, et al. RLS in middle aged women and attention deficit/hyperactivity disorder in their offspring. Sleep Med 2011;12(1):89–91.

44. Didriksen M, Thørner LW, Erikstrup C, et al. Self-reported restless legs syndrome and involuntary leg movements during sleep are associated with symptoms of attention deficit hyperactivity disorder. Sleep Med 2019;57:115–21.

45. Earley CJ, Connor JR, Beard JL, et al. Abnormalities in CSF concentrations of ferritin and transferrin in restless legs syndrome. Neurology 2000;54(8): 1698–700.

46. Bener A, Kamal M, Bener H, et al. Higher prevalence of iron deficiency as strong predictor of attention deficit hyperactivity disorder in children. Ann Med Health Sci Res 2014;4(Suppl 3):S291–7.

47. Lopez R, Micoulaud Franchi JA, Chenini S, et al. Restless legs syndrome and iron deficiency in adults with attention-deficit/hyperactivity disorder. Sleep 2019;42(5):zsz027.

48. Hwang IC, Na K-S, Lee YJ, et al. Higher prevalence of hypertension among individuals with restless legs syndrome: a meta-analysis. Psychiatry Investig 2018;15(7):701–9.

49. Kjeldsen SE. Hypertension and cardiovascular risk: general aspects. Pharmacol Res 2018;129:95–9.

50. Juuti AK, Läärä E, Rajala U, et al. Prevalence and associated factors of restless legs in a 57-year-old urban population in northern Finland. Acta Neurol Scand 2010;122(1):63–9.

51. Winkelman JW, Shahar E, Sharief I, et al. Association of restless legs syndrome and cardiovascular disease in the Sleep Heart Health Study. Neurology 2008;70(1):35–42.

52. Winter AC, Berger K, Glynn RJ, et al. Vascular risk factors, cardiovascular disease, and restless legs syndrome in men. Am J Med 2013;126(3):228–35. e2.

53. Winter AC, Schürks M, Glynn RJ, et al. Vascular risk factors, cardiovascular disease, and restless legs syndrome in women. Am J Med 2013;126(3): 220–7.e2.

54. Molnar MZ, Lu JL, Kalantar-Zadeh K, et al. Association of incident restless legs syndrome with outcomes in a large cohort of US veterans. J Sleep Res 2016;25(1):47–56.

55. Winkelman JW, Blackwell T, Stone K, et al. Associations of incident cardiovascular events with restless legs syndrome and periodic leg movements of sleep in older men, for the outcomes of sleep disorders in older men study (MrOS Sleep Study). Sleep 2017; 40(4):zsx023.

56. Van Den Eeden SK, Albers KB, Davidson JE, et al. Risk of cardiovascular disease associated with a restless legs syndrome diagnosis in a retrospective cohort study from Kaiser Permanente Northern California. Sleep 2015;38(7):1009–15.

57. Li Y, Walters AS, Chiuve SE, et al. Prospective study of restless legs syndrome and coronary heart disease among women. Circulation 2012;126(14): 1689–94.

58. Gottlieb DJ, Somers VK, Punjabi NM, et al. Restless legs syndrome and cardiovascular disease: a research roadmap. Sleep Med 2017;31:10–7.

59. Ayas NT, White DP, Al-Delaimy WK, et al. A prospective study of self-reported sleep duration and incident diabetes in women. Diabetes care 2003;26(2):380–4.

60. Gangwisch JE, Heymsfield SB, Boden-Albala B, et al. Short sleep duration as a risk factor for hypertension: analyses of the first National Health and Nutrition Examination Survey. Hypertension 2006; 47(5):833–9.

61. Ayas NT, White DP, Manson JE, et al. A prospective study of sleep duration and coronary heart disease in women. Arch Intern Med 2003;163(2):205–9.

62. Winkelman JW. The evoked heart rate response to periodic leg movements of sleep. Sleep 1999; 22(5):575–80.

63. Pennestri MH, Montplaisir J, Colombo R, et al. Nocturnal blood pressure changes in patients with restless legs syndrome. Neurology 2007;68(15): 1213–8.

64. Koo BB, Blackwell T, Ancoli-Israel S, et al. Association of incident cardiovascular disease with periodic limb movements during sleep in older men: outcomes of sleep disorders in older men (MrOS) study. Circulation 2011;124(11):1223–31.

65. May AM, May RD, Bena J, et al. Individual periodic limb movements with arousal are temporally associated with nonsustained ventricular tachycardia: a case-crossover analysis. Sleep 2019;42(11): zsz165.

66. von Haehling S, Jankowska EA, van Veldhuisen DJ, et al. Iron deficiency and cardiovascular disease. Nat Rev Cardiol 2015;12(11):659–69.

67. Gill D, Del Greco MF, Walker AP, et al. The effect of iron status on risk of coronary artery disease: a mendelian randomization study-brief report. Arterioscler Thromb Vasc Biol 2017;37(9):1788–92.

68. Li Y, Wang W, Winkelman JW, et al. Prospective study of restless legs syndrome and mortality among men. Neurology 2013;81(1):52–9.

69. Li Y, Li Y, Winkelman JW, et al. Prospective study of restless legs syndrome and total and cardiovascular mortality among women. Neurology 2018;90(2): e135–41.

70. Unruh ML, Levey AS, D'Ambrosio C, et al. Restless legs symptoms among incident dialysis patients: association with lower quality of life and shorter survival. Am J Kidney Dis 2004;43(5):900–9.

71. Winkelman JW, Chertow GM, Lazarus JM. Restless legs syndrome in end-stage renal disease. Am J Kidney Dis 1996;28(3):372–8.

72. La Manna G, Pizza F, Persici E, et al. Restless legs syndrome enhances cardiovascular risk and mortality in patients with end-stage kidney disease undergoing long-term haemodialysis treatment. Nephrol Dial Transplant 2011;26(6):1976–83.

73. Lin CH, Sy HN, Chang HW, et al. Restless legs syndrome is associated with cardio/cerebrovascular events and mortality in end-stage renal disease. Eur J Neurol 2015;22(1):142–9.

74. Stefanidis I, Vainas A, Giannaki CD, et al. Restless legs syndrome does not affect 3-year mortality in hemodialysis patients. Sleep Med 2015;16(9):1131–8.

75. Baiardi S, Mondini S, Baldi Antognini A, et al. Survival of dialysis patients with restless legs syndrome: a 15-year follow-up study. Am J Nephrol 2017;46(3): 224–30.

76. Mallon L, Broman JE, Hetta J. Restless legs symptoms with sleepiness in relation to mortality: 20-year follow-up study of a middle-aged Swedish population. Psychiatry Clin Neurosci 2008;62(4):457–63.

77. Szentkirályi A, Winter AC, Schürks M, et al. Restless legs syndrome and all-cause mortality in four prospective cohort studies. BMJ Open 2012;2(6): e001652.

78. Bertisch SM, Muresan C, Schoerning L, et al. Impact of restless legs syndrome on cardiovascular autonomic control. Sleep 2016;39(3):565–71.

79. De Ferrari GM, Sanzo A, Bertoletti A, et al. Baroreflex sensitivity predicts long-term cardiovascular mortality after myocardial infarction even in patients with preserved left ventricular function. J Am Coll Cardiol 2007;50(24):2285–90.

80. Benz RL, Pressman MR, Hovick ET, et al. Potential novel predictors of mortality in end-stage renal disease patients with sleep disorders. Am J Kidney Dis 2000;35(6):1052–60.

81. Yumino D, Wang H, Floras JS, et al. Relation of periodic leg movements during sleep and mortality in patients with systolic heart failure. Am J Cardiol 2011;107(3):447–51.

Periodic Leg Movements During Sleep

Stephany Fulda, PhD

KEYWORDS

- Periodic leg movements during sleep • Sleep • Polysomnography

KEY POINTS

- Different periodic leg movements during sleep (PLMS) scoring rules exist and will generate PLMS frequency counts with unsystematic and non-negligible differences.
- All PLMS scoring rules are excellent at identifying periodic leg movements, but are challenged by the need to reject nonperiodic leg movements.
- Leg movement activity varies along 2 dimensions: frequency and periodicity. Whether these dimensions are truly independent is currently unknown.
- Defining PLMS is an ongoing process with input both from clinical sleep medicine and from sleep research.

INTRODUCTION

Periodic leg movements during sleep (PLMS) are short, stereotypical movements that occur at strikingly regular intervals, typically between 20 and 40 seconds, in series of up to several hundreds of leg movements (LMs) in a single night[1,2] (see **Box 1** for nomenclature and common abbreviations). Most subjects affected by a restless legs syndrome (RLS) will show frequent PLMS during sleep.[3] Most subjects with frequent PLMS, however, will not suffer from RLS, as PLMS has been observed in a variable proportion of patients with various sleep disorders,[4,5] subjects with medical or neurologic disorders,[6–9] with many medications,[10,11] and also in a non-negligible proportion of the middle-aged or older general population.[12]

Nowadays, electromyography (EMG) of the bilateral tibialis anterior muscles is one of the standard biosignals in polysomnographic recordings.[13] From these EMG traces, leg movements (LMs) are manually or semi-automatically detected. These detected LMs are then classified into periodic leg movements and other leg movements according to specific rule sets, the PLMS scoring rules.[14] Currently, 2 major PLMS scoring rule sets coexist with the latest major updates to both sets in 2016.[15]

PLMS were first described in 1953 as nocturnal myoclonus,[16] and the first polysomnographic documentation was published in the 1960s in patients without[17] and with RLS.[18] In the 1980s, Coleman[19] published the first PLMS scoring rules and provided one of the first systematic descriptions in large and varied populations.[5] Despite PLMS being an active area of research ever since, the clinical significance of PLMS is still unclear. This may be partly due to perceived barriers, such as the existence of different rules sets, an under-appreciation of the importance and nature of the PLMS scoring rules, as well as several conceptual open questions that have been only incompletely addressed and are among the major future challenges.

The aim of this contribution is to illustrate key points regarding the PLMS scoring process, address the question of clinical significance of PLMS, and describe some of the key future challenges with the hope of contributing to a more differentiated understanding of the clinical

Sleep Medicine Unit, Neurocenter of Southern Switzerland, Via Tesserete 46, Lugano 6900, Switzerland
E-mail address: stephany.fulda@gmail.com

Sleep Med Clin 16 (2021) 289–303
https://doi.org/10.1016/j.jsmc.2021.02.004
1556-407X/21/© 2021 Elsevier Inc. All rights reserved.

Box 1
Nomenclature and common abbreviations

AASM	American Academy of Sleep Medicine
CLM	Candidate leg movements, leg movements with duration of 0.5–10 s (WASM 2016)
IMI	Intermovement interval, measured from the onset of the first to the onset of the second leg movement
iLM	Isolated leg movements
IRLSSG	International Restless Legs Syndrome Study Group
LM	Leg movements
LMA	Leg movement activity, all tibialis anterior muscle activity independent of duration
Non-CLM	Non-candidate LM; LM that are not counted for a PLM series but when observed end a PLM series. These are monolateral LM with duration longer than 10 s and bilateral LM with duration longer than 15 s or containing more than 4 monolateral LM or 1 or more monolateral LM with duration longer than 10 s
PLM	Periodic leg/limb movements
PLMS	Periodic leg/limb movements during sleep
rLM	Respiratory-event–related LM
WASM	World Association of Sleep Medicine
WASM 2006	PLMS scoring rules published in 2006 and created with the participation of the IRLSSG and adopted by the WASM
WASM 2016	PLMS scoring rules published in 2016 and created with participation of the IRLSSG and EURLSSG and adopted by the WASM and WSS
WSF	World Sleep Foundation
WSS	World Sleep Society formed in 2016 through the merging of the WASM and WSF

For PLM definition criteria see **Table 1**.

evaluation of PLMS and to facilitate scientific contributions to this intriguing field of research.[a]

PLMS Scoring Rules Are Important

PLMS scoring rules contain recommendations, specifications, definitions, and scoring criteria concerning 3 broad areas:

- *The registration of leg movement activity*: At the moment, bilateral EMG recordings of the tibialis anterior muscle during time in bed are the only internationally accepted way of recording sleep-related leg movement activity. Universally adopted specifications include minimum sampling rate (200 Hz), filter settings (10–100 Hz, notch filter to be avoided), recommended (5 kΩ) and acceptable (10 kΩ) impedances, as well as electrode placement (in the middle of the tibialis anterior muscles, 2–3 cm or one-third of the length of the muscle apart, whichever is shorter).
- *The detection of leg movements*: The identification of leg movements is based on criteria regarding duration and amplitude (**Table 1**). Leg movements are identified separately for each leg and fully visual scoring or visual supervision of automatic scoring of LMs is recommended[14] (see later in this article for a discussion of current barriers to fully automatic LM detection approaches).
- *PLM scoring*: PLM scoring is the classification of the detected LM into different, parallel but interrelated categories that include monolateral and bilateral LM, respiratory and nonrespiratory event-related LM (rLM and nrLM), candidate and non-candidate LM (CLM and non-CLM), and finally isolated and periodic LM (iLM and PLM), with PLM also being classified as associated or not with an electroencephalogram (EEG) arousal.

The first internationally adopted PLMS scoring rules were published by Coleman in 1982.[19] They were widely adopted and constituted the basis for the subsequent rules of the America Sleep Disorders Association created in 1993.[20] In 2006, the World Association of Sleep Medicine (WASM), together with the International Restless Legs Syndrome Study Group (IRLSSG), completely overhauled and modernized PLMS scoring rules, for example, taking into account that sleep recordings were by now fully digital.[21] One year later, in 2007, the American Academy of Sleep Medicine (AASM) published their first scoring manual that also included PLMS scoring rules[22] and whose PLMS scoring rules were similar but not identical to the

---

[a]This article focuses on periodic leg movements, not limb movements, in adults, and descriptions, arguments, and discussion points do not apply to children and adolescents.

Table 1
Key PLMS scoring criteria of the AASM manual (version 2.6. 2020) and the WASM/IRLSSG/EURLSSG 2016 rules

		AASM 2020	WASM/IRLSSG/EURLSSG 2016
LM detection criteria			
LM	Duration	0.5-10 s	$\geq$0.5 s
	Onset	$\geq$8 µV increase above resting EMG	$\geq$8 µV increase above resting EMG baseline
	Offset	decrease to $\leq$ 2µ above resting EMG for $\geq$0.5 s	decrease to <2 µV above resting EMG baseline for $\geq$0.5 s
	Amplitude	$\geq$0.5 s with amplitude $\geq$8 µV above resting EMG	$\geq$0.5 s with median amplitude $\geq$2 µV above resting EMG
PLMS scoring criteria			
Bilateral LM	LM involved	Only LM 0.5–10 s <5 s onset to onset	All LM $\geq$0.5 s <0.5 s offset to onset
CLM	Monolateral CLM	(= LM)	Duration: 0.5–10 s
	Bilateral CLM	(= LM)	Any bilateral LM with: $\leq$ 4 CLM, total duration $\leq$ 15 s, no LM >10 s
Non-CLM	Monolateral non-CLM		Duration >10 s
	Bilateral non-CLM		Duration >15 s or containing >4 LM or $\geq$1 LM >10 s
Respiratory event related LM	Any LM/CLM	0.5 s before start to 0.5 s after end of respiratory event	Recommended: −2 s to 10.25 s around the end of respiratory event Alternative: −0.5 s to 0.5 s around the end of respiratory event
PLM	Number in series	$\geq$4	$\geq$4
	IMI	5–90 s	10–90 s
	End of PLM series	IMI >90 s (IMI <5 s)	IMI >90 s, IMI <10 s, any non-CLM PLM series goes on, only PLM
	Sleep/Wake	LM during wake are ignored	during sleep are counted as PLMS

Abbreviations: AASM, American Academy of Sleep Medicine; CLM, candidate leg movement; EURLSSG, European Restless Legs Syndrome Study Group; IMI, intermovement interval; IRLSSG, International Restless Legs Syndrome Study Group; LM, leg movement; non-CLM, noncandidate leg movement; PLM, periodic leg movements; PLMS, periodic leg movements during sleep; WASM, World Association of Sleep Medicine.

WASM/IRLSSG 2006 rules. These, the WASM/IRLSSG 2006 rules, received a major update with several critical changes in 2016 and with additional participation of the European Restless Legs Syndrome Study Group (EURLSSG) creating the WASM/IRLSSG/EURLSSG 2016 rules[14] (for the sake of brevity, these rules are denoted as WASM 2006 and WASM 2016 in the following). The AASM manual, on the other hand, was updated annually or even biannually, with changes to the PLMS scoring rules introduced over several years and with the last major changes in 2016.[15] Both set of rules strive to be evidence-based and therefore future updates are to be expected.

Rather than a detailed description of the 2 sets of current scoring rules (see **Table 1**, the original publications[14,15] or reference[23] for a detailed description of the 2 rules sets and their differences), the following lists key clinical points and/or general considerations regarding the choice and application of the available PLMS scoring rules:

- *Completeness of scoring rules*: The minimum requirement for scoring rules is completeness, that is, the rules must specify what to do for any conceivable scenario. In this sense, the WASM/IRLSSG 2006 rules[21] were the first complete rules. Both the Coleman[19] and the ASDA rules[20] left key questions unspecified; it is therefore not technically possible to score according to these rules without adding self-made, undocumented specifications. The first AASM rules that were possibly complete for PLMS scoring were those in 2016[15] when it was finally specified whether and how PLMS series were affected by transitions from sleep to wake (but see later in this article for potential caveats). The key point here is that among all the available PLMS scoring rules only very few could actually be used as is (see also **Fig. 1**), for the majority one or more self-made specifications have to be added to allow their application in clinical or research settings. Clinicians and researchers alike are therefore well-advised to either chose one of the few complete scoring rules or fully explore and document the necessary added specifications.

- *Consideration of intervening LM:* The single most influential rule within any PLMS scoring rule set concerns the criteria that end an eventual PLM series. It is unequivocally accepted that a PLM series ends when there is no LM for 90 seconds or longer. There is, however, the more critical case in which one LM is observed shortly after another LM and the intermovement interval (IMI) of the 2 LMs is below the lower limit of the IMI acceptable for PLM (<5 seconds or <10 seconds, depending on rule set); these are called intervening LM[24] (or if occurring during sleep and with IMI <10 seconds also sometimes short interval leg movements during sleep [SILMS][25]). Whether or not such an intervening LM ends a PLM series had not been clearly specified (although possibly alluded

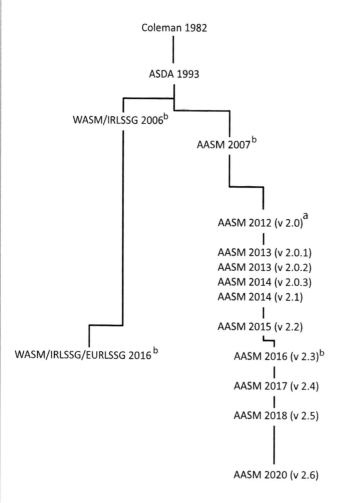

Fig. 1. History of PLMS scoring rules. Minor changes are marked by [a], major changes/updates to the rules are marked by [b]. AASM, American Academy of Sleep Medicine; ASDA, American Sleep Disorders Association; EURLSSG, European Restless Legs Syndrome Study Group; IRLSSG, International Restless Legs Syndrome Study Group; WASM, World Association of Sleep Medicine.

to) in the earlier scoring rules,[19,20] but the WASM 2006[21] rules clearly stated that these intervening LM are ignored and if there is another LM within the next 5 to 90 seconds, the PLM series goes on. The AASM 2007 manual[22] and all subsequent AASM manuals do not address this question directly but define a PLMS series by *consecutive leg movements* fulfilling the stated criteria, which could be interpreted as meaning that intervening LM end a PLMS series. However, when introducing the treatment of intermittent wake periods in 2016,[15] the AASM manual also stated that waking periods less than 90 seconds and all LMs within that period are ignored and a PLM series would go on, even in the case of one or more LMs during the waking period. This could call into question how exactly "consecutive leg movements" are defined and whether there are possible other LM that are exempt, such as intervening LM.

- *Intervening LM should be excluded*: Experience with the WASM 2006 rules has shown that ignoring intervening LM resulted in the PLMS scoring rules acting as a pattern extractor by ignoring all nonfitting LM (**Box 2**). The consequence of this was that the PLMS index was driven by the sheer number of LM and not necessarily by periodicity of these LMs. This has been corrected in the WASM 2016 rules and it is strongly recommended to choose a rule set that does not ignore intervening LMs.

- *Differences between PLMS scoring rule sets are not systematic and non-negligible*: It is important to realize that the differences between the different rule sets or between different versions of the same set may seem minor but can have major effects visible in only certain populations (see the next section: PLMS scoring rules are not about PLMS). For example, the rules to define bilateral LMs differ substantially between the WASM and the AASM scoring rules. Nevertheless, this has no discernible effect on the resulting LM and PLM counts, at least not in subjects with RLS and healthy control subjects.[26] On the other hand, the differences between WASM and AASM rules in defining rLM have major and clinically significant effects on PLMS parameter in moderate to severe obstructive sleep apnea.[27] The consequence is that depending on the specific choice of scoring rule set, results may not be comparable across scoring rules set.

Box 2
The effects of ignoring intervening leg movements

Intervening leg movements (LM) are LM that occur shortly after another LM with an inter-movement interval (IMI) shorter than the lower limit of the IMI acceptable for PLM (<5 s or <10 s, depending on rule set). The WASM 2006[21] rules were the first to explicitly state how to deal with those intervening LM namely that these were to be ignored and that PLM series would go on, provided there was another LM within 90 s. This rule was reversed in the updated WASM 2016[14] because subsequent experience showed that the unintended effect had been that the PLMS scoring rules acted like a pattern generator that ignored all nonfitting LMs. Here is a detailed illustration why this is the case:

Imagine a long series of 100 LMs, for simplicity's sake with 1 LM every 3 seconds; all IMIs are 3 seconds and none of the IMIs is within the PLM range. We are also assuming the lower limit for periodic IMIs is 5 seconds. The IMI from the first to the second LM is 3 seconds and therefore the second LM is ignored; the IMI from the first to the third LM is 6 seconds and therefore within our PLM range. The IMI from the third to the fourth LM will be ignored again and so on, ignoring every second LM (LM numbers 2,4, 6, 8, until 100) will leave 50 LMs (LM numbers 1, 3, 5, 7, until 99) with IMIs of 6 seconds between each, a valid PLM series. Similar examples can easily be constructed also for a minimum periodic IMI of 10 seconds.

Although none of the IMIs were within the PLM range, ignoring nonfitting LM resulted in a formally valid PLM series. This serves to illustrate the two important consequences of this rule: a significant number of PLMS will be identified even in completely arrhythmic leg movement activity given a large enough number of LM and increasing the number of LM can only increase the number of identified PLM. By ignoring intervening LM, scoring according to the WASM 2006 rules has confounded PLM with nonperiodic increased LM.

- *PLMS scoring rules have zero degree of freedom and should be automated*: PLMS scoring, the classification of detected LM, can be seen as post-processing. Rules that are complete are fully specified and although complicated, their application requires no expert judgment, is completely standardized, and can be automatically produced by any suitable, automated program. It is therefore strongly recommended to score all LM during time in bed, preferably with no maximum duration of LM. This will allow the post hoc application of any and all PLMS scoring rule sets including potentially future, updated rule sets, at least as long as the criteria for LM detection do not substantially change.

- *A word of caution*: many clinicians and researchers do not choose a PLMS scoring rule set but have to rely on the output that their commercial polysomnography systems provide. The rules implemented or chosen in these systems may or may not fully correspond to a specific internationally adopted rule system and the user is well advised to consider the following points:
  - *Software updates*: as is clear from the development of scoring rules over time, if your polysomnography program has not been updated in or after 2016, it does not implement the current PLMS scoring rules, independent of whether you have chosen to use the WASM or AASM rule set.
  - *Variable key parameter*: many programs have options to set key parameters for LM detection and PLMS classification. Often these are restricted to just a few parameters, such as duration of movements or intermovement intervals, leaving inaccessible the more intricate or complicated parameters such as the definition of bilateral movements or conditions that end PLM series. It may be prudent to regularly control accessible parameters, especially in a multiuser environment, and to find out about the more hidden parameters through manuals, direct inquiries, or trial and error with simple, constructed test cases.
  - *Non-PLM parameters with unintended effects*: polysomnography systems are complex programs that have to coordinate multiple areas (EEG, electrooculogram, respiration, movement, and more), each with its own fixed and variable key parameters. Users should be aware that there might be parameter settings from other areas with direct or indirect consequences for PLM scoring.[b]

The development of PLMS scoring rules is a dynamic process that is evidence based and reflects critical progress in this field. The choice and implementation of a specific scoring rule set for clinical and research purposes deserves careful attention and should be an informed choice.

PLMS Scoring Rules Are Not About PLMS

PLMS scoring rules have been created in a top-down manner: first, PLMS were observed and then rules were created to identify the observed phenomenon. And in this respect, all rules are very successful: no matter whether from 1982[19] or 2020,[13] the overwhelming majority of "classic" PLMS will be correctly identified with all of them. These "classic" PLMS are those most often found in subjects with RLS, long series of LM with strikingly regular intermovement intervals, typically between 20 and 40 seconds (**Fig. 2**, left part).

It turns out that identification of PLMs is the easy part, the difficult part is the rejection of non-periodic leg movement activity. **Fig. 2** illustrates the scope of the problem: the two 5-minute excerpts show nocturnal leg movements, in the form of PLM on the left and non-periodic but increased LM on the right. The regular PLM on the left will be correctly scored by any and all, past and present scoring rules with little difference between the rules. Scoring the non-periodic increased LM on the right for the presence of PLM, however, will show significant differences between the different rules and for some might even generate PLM counts that are higher than for the periodic PLM on the left.

This is what is meant by the provocative title of this section: the continuous update of PLMS scoring rules is no longer motivated by improved identification of PLM, that was achieved already by Coleman in 1982,[19] it is the need to reject non-periodic LM. This was one of the main motivations for the 2016 update of the WASM rules,[14] which introduced several evidence-based changes to address this issue: the treatment of intervening LMs,[24] the introduction of a range of conditions that end a PLM series, and the change of the IMI from 5 to 90 seconds to 10 to 90 seconds.[28–30] First studies have demonstrated that these rules or parts of it do indeed reduce PLM counts in populations or conditions, such as wakefulness, where non-periodic increased LM activity is frequently encountered.[29,31,32] Future studies

---

[b]One very trivial example is the option to exclude events when the subject is standing. Although this seems a sensible setting, it is also easy to imagine the effects of malfunctioning or other scenarios in which this will lead to an unwanted reduction of LM/PLM counts. At the very least, the LM/PLM count now also depends on the correct functioning of the position sensor. This might be more of a concern for research projects that process a large number of recordings and where such occasional malfunctions of unrelated sensors might go unnoticed.

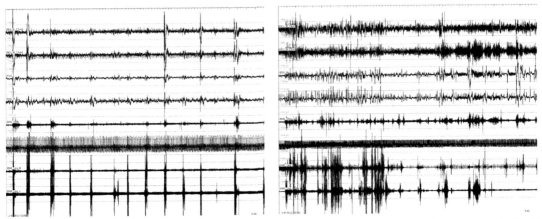

Fig. 2. Five-minute examples of nocturnal LM activity with regular PLMs in the left example and non-periodic LM in the right example. The distinction between the 2 types of frequent LMs is the main challenge for PLMS scoring rules. The excerpts show electroencephalogram (EEG, 2 channels), electrooculogram (EOG, 2 channels), chin electromyogram (EMG, 1 channel), electrocardiogram (ECG, 1 channel), and right and left anterior tibialis EMG.

are needed to show whether this increase in specificity for PLM is already sufficient.

Sleep-related leg movement activity varies along (at least) 2 fundamental dimensions (**Fig. 3**): frequency and periodicity. In populations or conditions with frequent but periodic LM, such as PLM during sleep in subjects with RLS, all scoring rules will correctly identify the PLMS with little appreciative difference between them; this is because most LMs during sleep are indeed periodic in subjects with RLS.[28] However, there is also a group with frequent LMs that are little periodic. At least for the WASM 2006 rules, the PLM index alone was not able to distinguish sufficiently between the 2 cases: frequent LMs that are periodic versus those that are not periodic.[28,29] This has indirect repercussions also for the group with frequent PLMS because the theoretic existence of this group alone, with frequent, non-periodic LM, is enough to be wary of all high PLM indices unless periodicity is documented in another way.

So how can periodicity be demonstrated? The most informative but possibly underappreciated measure, advocated already by Coleman in the 1980s[5,19,33] and highly valued by experts ever since,[2,14] is the IMI distribution, the distribution of all intermovement intervals (**Box 3** for construction and interpretation of IMI distributions). The advantage of the IMI distribution is that periodic and non-periodic movements are easily recognized visually. The disadvantage is the need to evaluate them visually on a case-by-case basis. One prominent attempt to distill the salient information of the IMI distribution into a single measure, is the periodicity index created in 2006[28] and updated within the WASM 2016 rules.[14] The combination of the PLM index with either the IMI distribution and/or the periodicity index provides a more differentiated description of PLM and both measures continue to be among the recommended descriptive measures of PLM.[14]

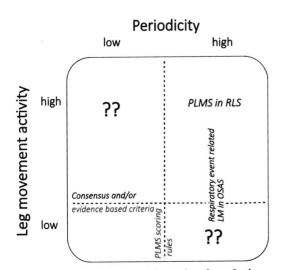

Fig. 3. Sleep-related LM activity varies along 2, theoretically independent dimensions: the frequency of the movements and their periodicity. Although frequent and very periodic LM in subjects with RLS are well described, subjects or conditions with frequent but non-periodic LM or vice versa, infrequent but highly periodic LM, have not received equal attention (see main text: open question).

Box 3
The value of the intermovement interval (IMI) distribution

Available PLMS scoring rules identify periodicity as IMI between 10 seconds (or 5 seconds) and 90 seconds, a very broad range. Having many consecutive LMs with IMIs between 10 and 90 seconds is a necessary but not necessarily sufficient condition for what is generally understood to be periodic behavior. In fact, the "classic" PLMS, often seen in subjects with RLS, have IMIs that are predominantly between 20 and 40 seconds and that also do not show a lot of variability. These 2 features, the variability of the IMI over the PLM range and the existence and strength of the peak IMI, are readily appreciated when visually evaluating the distribution of all suitable IMIs (for examples between LM during sleep) (**Fig. 4**).

The IMI distribution on the left shows a distribution typical for PLMS in subjects with RLS: a peak around 20 seconds and another peak in the 2-second to 10-second range. The IMI distribution on the right also shows frequent LMs; however, no clear peak in the PLM range is visible. The IMI distribution may even offer further information not yet systematically used but potentially valuable in a clinical setting when evaluating PLMS. For example, it has been shown that in subjects with RLS, the very first peak of the distribution in the 2-second to 10-second range is not responsive to dopaminergic treatment, whereas the second, "periodic" peak is.[30]

Technical specifications for constructing the intermovement interval distribution

The IMI is measured from the onset of one LM to the onset of the next LM but the IMI is attributed to the latter LM. In a series of 3 LM, the IMI of the first LM is undetermined, the IMI of the second LM is the interval between the onset of the first LM and the second LM, and the IMI of the third LM is the interval between onsets of the second and the third LM.

When constructing an IMI distribution for selected LM, such as those during sleep, the IMI of all LM during sleep will be considered, with the associated IMI as specified previously, that is, the IMI from the last LM during wake to the first LM during sleep will be included, but the interval from the last LM during sleep to the first LM during wake will not. According to the same principle, when encountering a non-CLM (see **Box 1**), the IMI of the LM following the non-CLM is not defined.

For all selected IMIs, a frequency distribution is constructed that counts the number of times an IMI is observed within a specific interval range. Conventionally, these intervals are 2-second bins in the range from 0 to ≥90 s, with special specifications for the first and last bin. The first bin, which would be from 0 to 2 seconds, can only assume values from 1 to 2 seconds, because the minimum IMI is 1 second (0.5-second minimum duration of LM + 0.5-second minimum interval between the offset of one LM and the onset of the next LM). The following bins, 2 to 4 seconds, 4 to 6 seconds, and so on until 88 to 90 seconds, are in the form (2 – 4s], meaning they include 2.001 (but not 2.000) up to and including 4.0 seconds, with the second to last category including intervals from 88.001 to 90.000 seconds. The last category includes IMI with greater than 90-second duration; this category is normally not shown in the IMI distribution plot.

The IMI distribution plot graphs the frequency for all frequency bins (see **Fig. 4**). Typically, bars are choosing to represent frequencies when the IMI distribution if graphed for a single subject and points/symbols when the distribution describes groups of subjects.

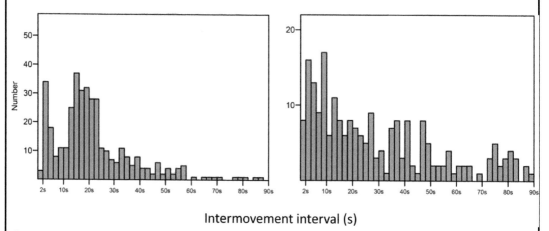

Fig. 4. Two typical IMI distributions of periodic (left) and non-periodic LM. Please note difference in scale.

Clinical Significance of Periodic Leg Movements During Sleep

So far, the accumulated evidence does not support the assumption that frequent PLMS are causing clinically significant consequences in the vast majority of subjects with frequent PLMS. Even if not a causal risk factor, PLMS might still be useful markers for other conditions because of systematic associations to these conditions. Ideally, such an association would mean that the presence of PLMS would have high predictive value for the presence of the condition, whereas the absence of PLMS would also be predictive for the absence of the condition.

A prominent example, of course, is RLS. Most subjects with RLS will have PLMS,[3,34,35] and PLMS is therefore sensitive for the presence of RLS, but most subjects with PLMS will not have RLS and the presence of PLMS has little (positive) predictive value for the presence of RLS in unselected populations. However, the registration of PLMS still has clinical value because the negative predictive value is considerably higher, that is, the absence of PLMS is a good predictor for the absence of RLS.[36]

A large-scale, systematic role of PLMS in objective or subjective sleep disturbances is questionable. In particular, the notion that PLMS cause cortical arousals and are therefore a major cause of sleep disturbances has been critically reevaluated, at least in subjects with RLS.[37] Among the arguments against a causal link between PLMS and arousals are the observations that only approximately a third of PLMS are associated with arousals and only approximately a third of arousals are concurrent with PLMS,[38] leg movements precede the onset of arousals in only 40% to 50%.[39,40] In addition, in subjects with RLS, PLMS and arousal can be pharmacologically dissociated with the dopamine agonist pramipexole reducing PLMS but leaving arousal frequency unchanged, whereas the benzodiazepine clonazepam reduced arousals but had no effect on PLMS frequency.[41]

There is, however, accumulating evidence that suggests that frequent PLMS could be a candidate cardiovascular risk factor. The main argument is the consistent observation that PLMS are accompanied by transient increases in blood pressure[42–45] and heart rate.[46–52] Given the frequency of PLMS, these frequent sympathetic system activations could indeed increase the risk for cardiovascular diseases.[53,54] It must, however, be mentioned that not all PLMS are followed by blood pressure increases and most transient blood pressure increases are neither associated with PLMS nor with arousals.[55] Nevertheless, in patients with RLS and frequent PLMS, treatment with rotigotine significantly reduced not only the number of PLMS-associated blood pressure increases but also the total number of increases during sleep.[56]

There is also an increasing number of studies linking frequent PLMS to cardiovascular disease[57–59] or to mortality in patients with end-stage renal disease[60,61] or heart failure.[62–64] It deserves mentioning, however, that the preceding populations also included a large percentage of subjects with sleep-related breathing disorders (SRBD), which raises the question of whether the leg movements that were identified as PLMS could be partly or completely respiratory event-related LM (rLM). As detailed in the section later in this article on rLM, rLM will be misclassified as PLM when non–evidence-based definition criteria are used to identify them[27] and the presence of rLM could signal a more severe form of sleep-related breathing disorder.[31,65] In addition, the most consistent association of PLMS is with age. The prevalence of frequent PLMS increases significantly after the age of 40 years[63] and the presence of PLMS in unselected groups often identifies subjects that tend to be older than subjects without PLMS, with age differences even being as large as 5 to 10 years (eg, Ref.[12]). Finally, also the presence of RLS had not been excluded in the preceding studies addressing mortality,[60–64,66] a differential diagnosis that has also been reported to be associated with increased mortality.[59]

Future research will hopefully show whether the presence of PLMS can reliably identify subgroups of subjects with more specific or more severe morbidity or could serve as a warning sign, identifying subjects at risk for future morbidity. For PLMS to be classified as a causal risk factor, however, it would need to be demonstrated that the specific treatment of PLMS has indeed a systematic effect on clinically significant outcomes. This also applies to clinical practice: PLMS is a frequent finding in polysomnographic recordings and a possible clinical significance must be carefully evaluated on a case-by-case basis. In individual cases, in which PLMS are strongly suspected to be the cause of sleep or other disturbances (eg, Ref.[67]) and a periodic limb movement disorder (PLMD)[68] is considered, treating PLMS and critically evaluating and documenting a positive and sustained treatment response of sleep and/or other disturbances is fundamental, not only for demonstrating the reasonable cause-effect relationship needed for the diagnosis of PLMD[23,68] but also to justify the potential risks associated with long-term dopaminergic treatment.[69,70]

Open Questions and Future Challenges

Sleep medicine and sleep research is now fully digital, coding literacy is increasing, and visionary and exemplary efforts such as the National Sleep Research Resource[71] that are making available thousands of well-documented polysomnographies, already have and continue to have major effects on clinical sleep research.

The next decade will offer unprecedented opportunities for sleep research, and among the questions to be addressed are a more complete appreciation of the full range of sleep-related LMs including but not limited to respiratory event–related LMs and the creation of internationally accepted benchmarks for LM scoring.

Characterization of the full range of sleep-related leg movement activity

As depicted in **Fig. 3**, sleep-related leg movement activity varies along 2, possibly independent dimensions: frequency and periodicity. Although highly frequent and periodic LMs such as those encountered in RLS, are well described, the opposite group of highly frequent but non-periodic LM, are so far not systematically described. However, the first question asked must be whether there are indeed subjects that exhibit highly frequent LMs during sleep that are not periodic? Or are most LMs periodic, once they surpass a certain threshold of frequency? It is clear that such LM, highly frequent but nonperiodic, are easily observed during wakefulness, but they might not be compatible with sleep. Delineating the limits of frequent, non-periodic LM compatible with sleep could also have repercussions for the interpretation of PLMS: most studies up to now have compared subjects with PLMS, that is, frequent LM that were periodic, with subjects without PLMS but also without frequent LM. The critical comparison of periodic with nonperiodic but equally frequent LMs will allow a more complete exploration of the unique properties of PLMS.

There is also another group of subjects that has received little attention: subjects with only a few but highly periodic LM. In case of less frequent LM, is it relevant that these are organized in a periodic fashion? How large is this group and could these be subjects in whom the known night-to-night variability[72–75] has sampled from the lower end of the distribution? Are these subjects more or less likely to exhibit more frequent PLMS when multiple nights are recorded?

Already now, besides PLM there are different LM described, such as alternative leg muscle activity (ALMA),[76] hypnagogic foot tremor (HFT),[77,78] short interval leg movements,[25] or general high-frequency leg movements (HFLMs).[79,80] However, just like with PLMS, definition criteria were mostly created post hoc, based on the properties of the observed phenomena. We are lacking large scale studies that systematically consider and characterize all leg movement activity during sleep and generate purely evidence-based classifications. And the challenging null hypothesis would be that it is the totality of sleep-related LMs rather than a specific form such as PLMS that has clinical significance.

Respiratory event–related leg movements

Among the full range of sleep-related LM, rLM occupy a very special place because they are often periodic, but not counted as such. The rLM are LM that occur near respiratory events and their definition, characterization, and significance is already an area of active research[27,31,65] and lively discussion,[81,82] whose key points can be summarized as follows:

- *Definition of rLM*: The definition of rLM differs substantially between the WASM 2006 and all AASM rules, although none of the rules had been evidence based (see **Table 1**). Research has shown that the empirical distribution of LMA is systematically increased at the end but not the beginning of respiratory events.[27,65] The distribution is rather wide and extends from 2 seconds before the end of the event to approximately 10.25 seconds after the end of the respiratory events. Importantly, the LMA distribution is unimodal with a peak shortly after the end of the respiratory event and without visual indication that it is composed of more than one distribution.

- *rLM misclassification has a direct effect on PLM counts*: LMA is strongly suppressed during a respiratory event.[27] Because the minimum duration of respiratory events are 10 seconds, rLMs at the end of the respiratory events will formally satisfy periodicity criteria because their IMI is necessarily 10 seconds or longer and will also visually appear periodic in the frequent case that the respiratory events occur in a series. Misclassification or disregard of rLM status will therefore result in a proportional increase of LMs classified as PLMs.

- *The absolute but not the relative frequency of rLM is determined by respiratory event frequency*: Because there can be only so many LM at the end of a respiratory event, typically only a single one,[27,65] the number of respiratory events limits the absolute number of rLM. Within this upper absolute limit, however, the rLM probability, that is, the percentage of respiratory events that are accompanied by an rLM, varies widely. In fact, apnea/hyponea frequency, ie, the apnea-hypopnea index (AHI), is not correlated with rLM probability.[27,31,65]

- *Two types of rLM*: Recent research suggests that there are likely 2 types rLM: in subjects with frequent non–respiratory-related PLMS (nrPLMS), the rLM are likely PLM paced or displaced by the respiratory event. This is based on the repeated observation[31,65] that rLM in these subjects behave PLMS-like: their probability decreases over the course the night, they are relatively suppressed during rapid-eye movement (REM) sleep compared with non-REM (NREM) sleep, and are less influenced by respiratory factors. On the other hand, in subjects without nrPLMS, rLM are most likely periodic appearing but respiratory-driven events, as their probability is significantly influenced by the type of respiratory event (being higher in obstructive events compared with all other events), increased with increasing duration of the respiratory event, and less or not influenced by sleep-related variables such as the NREM-REM sleep distinction or the time of the night.[31,65] In both groups equally, rLM probability is significantly increased when there is an arousal at the end of the respiratory event.[31,65]

The existence of 2 types of rLM and their differential association with sleep and respiratory-related factors suggests that in subjects without nrPLMS, rLM probability could be an AHI-independent marker of obstructive sleep apnea syndrome (OSAS) severity, with a higher rLM probability signaling a more severe form. Another hypothesis is the prediction that OSAS subjects with frequent nrPLMS will be highly likely to show PLMS also when OSAS is adequately treated, whereas in those without nrPLMS, in whom periodic-appearing rLMs are mostly respiratory driven, no PLMS will be observed in the treated state. This may not appear to be a novel hypothesis, however, as detailed previously, rLMs are particularly prone to be confounded with and erroneously classified as PLM, so that a careful choice of definition criteria is fundamental and it is likely that previous studies on this topic have at least partly confounded respiratory and periodic LM.[83–89] So far, the distinction between periodic and periodic-appearing rLMs has been based on the observation of frequent nrPLMS. Further research is needed to explore whether there are alternative measures of distinction, possibly on the level of the individual LMs, that allows classification of rLM into periodic or respiratory driven LM.

Leg movement scoring and automatic detection

The marking of individual LM, leg movement activity equal to or longer than 0.5 seconds without maximum duration, separately for each leg and during sleep and wakefulness, is currently the most important bottleneck for PLMS research. It is very likely, that LM detection will be fully automated in the future; already now there is no lack of approaches to automatic LM/PLM detection,[90–94] and more are expected to follow. However, for any automatic detector to become internationally accepted and/or adopted, a sufficiently high agreement with the gold standard in the field needs to be demonstrated and it is our lack of knowledge regarding the characteristics and limits of this gold standard that is currently holding the field back. Although it is generally accepted that expert visual detection and/or supervision of LM detection is the gold standard, we know very little about interrater agreement,[91,95–97] especially with regard to interlaboratory comparisons. Without such data, we have no clear idea whether or not to trust scorings from a single or a limited number of centers.

We tend to think that manual LM detection is tedious but not difficult, but this may be true for only a subset of LM, possibly for PLMS. The detection of LM during wakefulness or during periods with technical artifacts can certainly be a challenge and it is currently unknown whether human scorers can reliably identify LMs in such difficult circumstances and what are the limits of visual scoring.

It is important to stress that we need LM and not PLM detection algorithms that accurately detect single LM and not PLM, that is, LM that a human scorer thinks are PLM. As detailed previously, PLM classification is post-processing and subject to change. If all LM in a single night are identified, any classification rule can be flexibly applied post hoc. In addition, and in contrast to PLM classification, LM detection has changed little over time, apart from duration criteria, and therefore LM but not PLM detectors are expected to be sustainable applications.

A complicating factor is that there is no international consensus or clear guidance on how agreement between different visual and/or automatic LM detections should be calculated. Should accuracy be quantified on an event level and if yes, by what criteria? Is any overlap between detections enough to label this an accurate detection, or should we set precision limits? After all, we evaluate associations of LM to arousals based on 0.5 seconds or less between them, so should that be our lower limit of precision? And is precision in the onset as important as precision in the offset? Do we weight them differently when calculating agreement? Or should we quantify time with over-lapping detections? Even in the case that a specific measure of agreement is chosen, there is no clear consensus on what is a desirable or even minimally acceptable level of agreement.

Because we need LM and not PLM detectors, and we will also need to ask for research-level precision for human detection of LM, such data sets will need to be newly created. International efforts are currently under way to create a large gold standard data set, in which international expert scorers will identify LM during sleep and wakefulness in leg EMG traces. Such data are expected to not only provide crucial data on interrater reliability and to inform future updates to little or ill-defined constructs, such as baseline EMG levels, but will also be available for the development and validation of LM detection algorithms.

SUMMARY

In summary, defining PLMS is an ongoing, dynamic process with input both from clinical sleep medicine and from sleep research. There is no support for the assumption that frequent PLMS are causing clinically significant consequences in the vast majority of subjects with frequent PLMS, however, PLMS are at least nonspecific markers for advanced age and general morbidity.

CLINICS CARE POINTS

- Clinicians and sleep researchers should be aware of the existence of different rule sets for the scoring of PLMS as well as the non-negligible consequences of choosing a specific rule set.
- The clinical significance of frequent PLMS is still unclear and must be carefully evaluated on a case-by-case basis.
- Future studies should characterize the full range of sleep-related leg movement activity to allow a deeper understanding of the unique role of PLMS.

DISCLOSURE

Dr S. Fulda is supported by Swiss National Science Foundation (SNSF) grants No. 320030-160009 and 320030-179194.

REFERENCES

1. Ferri R, Koo BB, Picchietti DL, et al. Periodic leg movements during sleep: phenotype, neurophysiology, and clinical significance. Sleep Med 2017;31:29–38.
2. Ferri R. The time structure of leg movement activity during sleep: the theory behind the practice. Sleep Med 2012;13(4):433–41.
3. Montplaisir J, Boucher S, Poirier G, et al. Clinical, polysomnographic, and genetic characteristics of restless legs syndrome: a study of 133 patients diagnosed with new standard criteria. Mov Disord 1997;12:61–5.
4. Plazzi G, Ferri R, Franceschini C, et al. Periodic leg movements during sleep in narcoleptic patients with or without restless legs syndrome. J Sleep Res 2012;21(2):155–62.
5. Coleman RM, Pollak CP, Weitzman ED. Periodic movements in sleep (nocturnal myoclonus): relation to sleep disorders. Ann Neurol 1980;8(4):416–21.
6. Wetter TC, Collado-Seidel V, Pollmächer T, et al. Sleep and periodic leg movement patterns in drug-free patients with Parkinson's disease and multiple system atrophy. Sleep 2000;23:361–7.
7. Happe S, Pirker W, Klösch G, et al. Periodic leg movements in patients with Parkinson's disease are associated with reduced striatal dopamine transporter binding. J Neurol 2003;250(1):83–6.
8. Hanly PJ, Zuberi-Khokhar N. Periodic limb movements during sleep in patients with congestive heart failure. Chest 1996;109(6):1497–502.
9. Javaheri S. Sleep disorders in systolic heart failure: a prospective study of 100 male patients. The final report. Int J Cardiol 2006;106(1):21–8.
10. Hoque R, Chesson AL. Pharmacologically induced/exacerbated restless legs syndrome, periodic limb movements of sleep, and REM behavior disorder/REM sleep without atonia: literature review, qualitative scoring, and comparative analysis. J Clin Sleep Med 2010;6(1):79–83.
11. Yang C, White DP, Winkelman JW. Antidepressants and periodic leg movements of sleep. Biol Psychiatry 2005;58(6):510–4.
12. Haba-Rubio J, Marti-Soler H, Marques-Vidal P, et al. Prevalence and determinants of periodic limb movements in the general population. Ann Neurol 2016;79(3):464–74.
13. Berry R, Quan SF, Abreu A. The AASM manual for the scoring of sleep and associated events: rules, terminology and technical specifications. Version 2.6. Darien, (IL): American Academy of Sleep Medicine; 2020.
14. Ferri R, Fulda S, Allen RP, et al. World Association of Sleep Medicine (WASM) 2016 standards for recording and scoring leg movements in polysomnograms developed by a joint task force from the International and the European Restless Legs Syndrome Study Groups (IRLSSG and EURLSSG). Sleep Med 2016;26:86–95.
15. Berry R, Brooks R, Gamaldo C, et al. The AASM manual for the scoring of sleep and associated events: rules, terminology and technical specifications, version 2.3.

Darien, (IL): American Academy of Sleep Medicine; 2016.

16. Symonds CP. Nocturnal myoclonus. J Neurol Neurosurg Psychiatry 1953;16(3):166–71.

17. Lugaresi E, Coccagna G, Gambi D, et al. [Apropos of some nocturnal myoclonic manifestations. (Symonds' nocturnal myoclonus)]. Rev Neurol (Paris) 1966;115(3):547–55.

18. Lugaresi E, Coccagna G, Tassinari CA, et al. [Polygraphic data on motor phenomena in the restless legs syndrome]. Riv Neurol 1965;35(6):550–61.

19. Coleman R. Periodic movements in sleep (nocturnal myoclonus) and restless legs syndrome. In: Guilleminault C, editor. Sleeping and waking disorders: indications and techniques. Menlo Park: Addison-Wesley; 1982. p. 265–95.

20. American Sleep Disorders Association. Recording and scoring leg movements. The Atlas task force. Sleep 1993;16(8):748–59.

21. Zucconi M, Ferri R, Allen R, et al. The official World Association of Sleep Medicine (WASM) standards for recording and scoring periodic leg movements in sleep (PLMS) and wakefulness (PLMW) developed in collaboration with a task force from the International Restless Legs Syndrome Study Group (IRLSSG). Sleep Med 2006;7(2):175–83.

22. Iber C, Ancoli-Israel S, Chesson A, et al. The AASM manual for the scoring of sleep and associated events: rules, terminology and technical specifications. 1st edition. Darien, (IL): American Academy of Sleep Medicine; 2007.

23. Fulda S. Periodic limb movement disorder: a clinical update. Curr Sleep Med Rep 2018;4(1):39–49.

24. Hiranniramol K, Fulda S, Skeba P, et al. Intervening leg movements disrupt PLMS sequences. Sleep 2017;40(1):zsw023.

25. Ferri R, Rundo F, Silvani A, et al. Short-interval leg movements during sleep entail greater cardiac activation than periodic leg movements during sleep in restless legs syndrome patients. J Sleep Res 2017; 26(5):602–5.

26. Ferri R, Manconi M, Rundo F, et al. Bilateral leg movements during sleep: detailing their structure and features in normal controls and in patients with restless legs syndrome. Sleep Med 2017;32:10–5.

27. Manconi M, Zavalko I, Fanfulla F, et al. An evidence-based recommendation for a new definition of respiratory-related leg movements. Sleep 2015; 38(2):295–304.

28. Ferri R, Zucconi M, Manconi M, et al. New approaches to the study of periodic leg movements during sleep in restless legs syndrome. Sleep 2006;29(6):759–69.

29. Ferri R, Rundo F, Zucconi M, et al. Putting the periodicity back into the periodic leg movement index: an alternative data-driven algorithm for the computation of this index during sleep and wakefulness. Sleep Med 2015;16(10):1229–35.

30. Manconi M, Ferri R, Feroah TR, et al. Defining the boundaries of the response of sleep leg movements to a single dose of dopamine agonist. Sleep 2008; 31(9):1229–37.

31. Schipper MH, Alvarez-Estevez D, Jellema K, et al. Sleep-related leg movements in obstructive sleep apnea: definitions, determinants, and clinical consequences. Sleep Med 2020;75:131–40.

32. Elena H, Leslie B, Skeba P, et al. Effects of new PLM scoring rules on PLM rate in relation to sleep and resting wake for RLS and healthy controls. Sleep Breath 2021;25:381–6.

33. Coleman RM, Pollack CP, Weitzman ED. Periodic nocturnal myoclonus in a wide variety of sleep-wake disorders. Trans Am Neurol Assoc 1978;103: 230–3.

34. Ferri R, Rundo F, Zucconi M, et al. Diagnostic accuracy of the standard and alternative periodic leg movement during sleep indices for restless legs syndrome. Sleep Med 2016;22:97–9.

35. Ferri R, Manconi M, Lanuzza B, et al. Age-related changes in periodic leg movements during sleep in patients with restless legs syndrome. Sleep Med 2008;9(7):790–8.

36. Allen RP, Picchietti D, Hening WA, et al. Restless legs syndrome: diagnostic criteria, special considerations, and epidemiology. A report from the restless legs syndrome diagnosis and epidemiology workshop at the National Institutes of Health. Sleep Med 2003;4(2):101–19.

37. Allen RP, Picchietti DL, Garcia-Borreguero D, et al. Restless legs syndrome/Willis– Ekbom disease diagnostic criteria: updated International Restless Legs Syndrome Study Group (IRLSSG) consensus criteria – history, rationale, description, and significance. Sleep Med 2014;15:860–73.

38. Fulda S. The role of periodic limb movements during sleep in restless legs syndrome: a selective update. Sleep Med Clin 2015;10(3):241–8, xii.

39. Karadeniz D, Ondze B, Besset A, et al. EEG arousals and awakenings in relation with periodic leg movements during sleep. J Sleep Res 2000; 9(3):273–7.

40. Ferri R, Rundo F, Zucconi M, et al. An evidence-based analysis of the association between periodic leg movements during sleep and arousals in restless legs syndrome. Sleep 2015;38(6):919–24.

41. Manconi M, Ferri R, Zucconi M, et al. Dissociation of periodic leg movements from arousals in restless legs syndrome. Ann Neurol 2012;71(6):834–44.

42. Ali NJ, Davies RJ, Fleetham JA, et al. Periodic movements of the legs during sleep associated with rises in systemic blood pressure. Sleep 1991;14(2): 163–5.

43. Pennestri M-H, Montplaisir J, Fradette L, et al. Blood pressure changes associated with periodic leg movements during sleep in healthy subjects. Sleep Med 2013;14(6):555–61.

44. Siddiqui F, Strus J, Ming X, et al. Rise of blood pressure with periodic limb movements in sleep and wakefulness. Clin Neurophysiol 2007;118(9):1923–30.

45. Pennestri MH, Montplaisir J, Colombo R, et al. Nocturnal blood pressure changes in patients with restless legs syndrome. Neurology 2007;68(15):1213–8.

46. Winkelman JW. The evoked heart rate response to periodic leg movements of sleep. Sleep 1999;22(5):575–80.

47. Ferri R, Zucconi M, Rundo F, et al. Heart rate and spectral EEG changes accompanying periodic and non-periodic leg movements during sleep. Clin Neurophysiol 2007;118(2):438–48.

48. Allena M, Campus C, Morrone E, et al. Periodic limb movements both in non-REM and REM sleep: relationships between cerebral and autonomic activities. Clin Neurophysiol 2009;120(7):1282–90.

49. Gosselin N, Lanfranchi P, Michaud M, et al. Age and gender effects on heart rate activation associated with periodic leg movements in patients with restless legs syndrome. Clin Neurophysiol 2003;114(11):2188–95.

50. Lavoie S, de Bilbao F, Haba-Rubio J, et al. Influence of sleep stage and wakefulness on spectral EEG activity and heart rate variations around periodic leg movements. Clin Neurophysiol 2004;115(10):2236–46.

51. Manconi M, Ferri R, Zucconi M, et al. Effects of acute dopamine-agonist treatment in restless legs syndrome on heart rate variability during sleep. Sleep Med 2011;12(1):47–55.

52. Sforza E, Nicolas A, Lavigne G, et al. EEG and cardiac activation during periodic leg movements in sleep: support for a hierarchy of arousal responses. Neurology 1999;52(4):786–91.

53. Alessandria M, Provini F. Periodic limb movements during sleep: a new sleep-related cardiovascular risk factor? Front Neurol 2013;4:116.

54. Walters AS, Rye DB. Review of the relationship of restless legs syndrome and periodic limb movements in sleep to hypertension, heart disease, and stroke. Sleep 2009;32(5):589–97.

55. Cassel W, Kesper K, Bauer A, et al. Significant association between systolic and diastolic blood pressure elevations and periodic limb movements in patients with idiopathic restless legs syndrome. Sleep Med 2016.

56. Bauer A, Cassel W, Benes H, et al. Rotigotine's effect on PLM-associated blood pressure elevations in restless legs syndrome. Neurology 2016;86(19):1785–93.

57. Mirza M, Shen W-K, Sofi A, et al. Frequent periodic leg movement during sleep is associated with left ventricular hypertrophy and adverse cardiovascular outcomes. J Am Soc Echocardiogr 2013;26(7):783–90.

58. Mirza M, Shen W-K, Sofi A, et al. Frequent periodic leg movement during sleep is an unrecognized risk factor for progression of atrial fibrillation. PLoS One 2013;8(10):e78359.

59. Kendzerska T, Kamra M, Murray BJ, et al. Incident cardiovascular events and death in individuals with restless legs syndrome or periodic limb movements in sleep: a systematic review. Sleep 2017;40(3):zsx013.

60. Benz RL, Pressman MR, Hovick ET, et al. Potential novel predictors of mortality in end-stage renal disease patients with sleep disorders. Am J Kidney Dis 2000;35(6):1052–60.

61. Jung HH, Lee J, Baek HJ, et al. Nocturnal hypoxemia and periodic limb movement predict mortality in patients on maintenance hemodialysis. Clin J Am Soc Nephrol 2010;5(9):1607–13.

62. Yumino D, Wang H, Floras JS, et al. Relation of periodic leg movements during sleep and mortality in patients with systolic heart failure. Am J Cardiol 2011;107(3):447–51.

63. Yoshihisa A, Suzuki S, Kanno Y, et al. Prognostic significance of periodic leg movements during sleep in heart failure patients. Int J Cardiol 2016;212:11–3.

64. Yatsu S, Kasai T, Suda S, et al. Association between periodic leg movements during sleep and clinical outcomes in hospitalized patients with systolic heart failure following acute decompensation. J Am Coll Cardiol 2015;65(10, Supplement):A822.

65. Fulda S, Heinzer R, Haba-Rubio J. Characteristics and determinants of respiratory event–associated leg movements. Sleep 2018;41(2):zsx206.

66. Kendzerska T, Gershon AS, Hawker G, et al. Obstructive sleep apnea and risk of cardiovascular events and all-cause mortality: a decade-long historical cohort study. Plos Med 2014;11(2):e1001599.

67. Gaig C, Iranzo A, Pujol M, et al. Periodic limb movements during sleep mimicking REM sleep behavior disorder: a new form of periodic limb movement disorder. Sleep 2017;40(3):zsw063.

68. American Academy of Sleep Medicine. International classification of sleep disorders. 3rd edition. Darien, (IL): American Academy of Sleep Medicine; 2014.

69. Santamaria J, Iranzo A, Tolosa E. Development of restless legs syndrome after dopaminergic treatment in a patient with periodic leg movements in sleep. Sleep Med 2003;4(2):153–5.

70. Allen RP, Earley CJ. Augmentation of the restless legs syndrome with carbidopa/levodopa. Sleep 1996;19(3):205–13.

71. Zhang G-Q, Cui L, Mueller R, et al. The national sleep research resource: towards a sleep data commons. J Am Med Inform Assoc 2018;25(10):1351–8.

72. Ferri R, Fulda S, Manconi M, et al. Night-to-night variability of periodic leg movements during sleep

in restless legs syndrome and periodic limb movement disorder: comparison between the periodicity index and the PLMS index. Sleep Med 2013;14(3): 293–6.

73. Haba-Rubio J, Staner L, Krieger J, et al. What is the clinical significance of periodic limb movements during sleep? Neurophysiol Clin Clin Neurophysiol 2004;34(6):293–300.

74. Bliwise DL, Carskadon MA, Dement WC. Nightly variation of periodic leg movements in sleep in middle aged and elderly individuals. Arch Gerontol Geriatr 1988;7(4):273–9.

75. Edinger JD, McCall WV, Marsh GR, et al. Periodic limb movement variability in older DIMS patients across consecutive nights of home monitoring. Sleep 1992;15(2):156–61.

76. Chervin RD, Consens FB, Kutluay E. Alternating leg muscle activation during sleep and arousals: a new sleep-related motor phenomenon? Mov Disord 2003;18(5):551–9.

77. Broughton R. Pathological fragmentary myoclonus, intensified hypnic jerks and hypnagogic foot tremor: three unusual sleep-related movement disorders. Sleep 1988;86:240–3.

78. Wichniak A, Tracik F, Geisler P, et al. Rhythmic feet movements while falling asleep. Mov Disord 2001; 16(6):1164–70.

79. Yang C, Winkelman JW. Clinical and polysomnographic characteristics of high frequency leg movements. J Clin Sleep Med 2010;6(5):431–8.

80. Frauscher B, Gabelia D, Mitterling T, et al. Motor events during healthy sleep: a quantitative polysomnographic study. Sleep 2014;37(4):763–73, 773A-773B.

81. Walters AS. The new WASM rules for respiratory-related leg movements lack clinical or polysomnographic validation. Sleep Med 2017;34:253.

82. Ferri R. Leg movements during sleep and respiratory events are not causally linked. Sleep Med 2017;34:254–5.

83. Aritake-Okada S, Namba K, Hidano N, et al. Change in frequency of periodic limb movements during sleep with usage of continuous positive airway pressure in obstructive sleep apnea syndrome. J Neurol Sci 2012;317(1–2):13–6.

84. Baran AS, Richert AC, Douglass AB, et al. Change in periodic limb movement index during treatment of obstructive sleep apnea with continuous positive airway pressure. Sleep 2003;26(6):717–20.

85. Benz RL, Pressman MR, Wu X. Periodic limb movements in sleep revealed by treatment of sleep apnea

with continuous positive airway pressure in the advanced chronic kidney disease population. Clin Nephrol 2011;76(6):470–4.

86. Carelli G, Krieger J, Calvi-Gries F, et al. Periodic limb movements and obstructive sleep apneas before and after continuous positive airway pressure treatment. J Sleep Res 1999;8(3):211–6.

87. Fry JM, DiPhillipo MA, Pressman MR. Periodic leg movements in sleep following treatment of obstructive sleep apnea with nasal continuous positive airway pressure. Chest 1989;96(1):89–91.

88. Drigo R, Fontana M, Coin A, et al. APAP titration in patients with mild to moderate OSAS and periodic limb movement syndrome. Monaldi Arch Chest Dis 2006;65(4):196–203.

89. Hedli LC, Christos P, Krieger AC. Unmasking of periodic limb movements with the resolution of obstructive sleep apnea during continuous positive airway pressure application. J Clin Neurophysiol 2012; 29(4):339–44.

90. Alvarez-Estevez D. A new automatic method for the detection of limb movements and the analysis of their periodicity. Biomed Signal Process Control 2016;26:117–25.

91. Carvelli L, Olesen AN, Brink-Kjær A, et al. Design of a deep learning model for automatic scoring of periodic and non-periodic leg movements during sleep validated against multiple human experts. Sleep Med 2020;69:109–19.

92. Huang AS, Skeba P, Yang MS, et al. MATPLM1, A MATLAB script for scoring of periodic limb movements: preliminary validation with visual scoring. Sleep Med 2015;16(12):1541–9.

93. Stefani A, Heidbreder A, Hackner H, et al. Validation of a leg movements count and periodic leg movements analysis in a custom polysomnography system. BMC Neurol 2017;17(1):42.

94. Moore H, Leary E, Lee S-Y, et al. Design and validation of a periodic leg movement detector. PLoS One 2014;9(12):e114565.

95. Bliwise DL, Keenan S, Burnburg D, et al. Inter-rater reliability for scoring periodic leg movements in sleep. Sleep 1991;14(3):249–51.

96. Kazenwadel J, Pollmächer T, Trenkwalder C, et al. New actigraphic assessment method for periodic leg movements (PLM). Sleep 1995;18(8):689–97.

97. Rauhala E, Erkinjuntti M, Polo O. Detection of periodic leg movements with a static- charge-sensitive bed. J Sleep Res 1996;5(4):246–50.

Pediatric Restless Legs Syndrome

Rosalia Silvestri, MD[a],*, Lourdes M. DelRosso, MD[b]

KEYWORDS

- RLS • Children • Pediatric sleep

KEY POINTS

- Pediatric restless legs syndrome (RLS) is still an underdiagnosed and undertreated disorder.
- RLS pediatric symptoms need to be carefully screened for a differential diagnosis with mimics.
- RLS in children impacts academic abilities and behavior and is comorbid with mood and neurodevelopmental disorders, including attention-deficit hyperactivity disorder and autism spectrum disorders.
- Brain-iron deficiency and dopamine dysregulation are essential factors in the pathophysiology of RLS.

 Video content accompanies this article at http://www.sleep.theclinics.com.

HISTORY/BACKGROUND AND DEFINITION

Originally described only in middle-aged adults or seniors, restless legs syndrome (RLS) was first reported in children and adolescents in 1994.[1] Despite recent increased awareness and implementation of specific diagnostic criteria adapted to age,[2] the syndrome remains largely underdiagnosed with a consequent delay of appropriate treatment and access to specialized tertiary care. RLS pediatric diagnostic criteria have been revised and simplified by the International Restless Legs Syndrome – Study Group (IRLS-SG) just before the latest International Classification of Sleep Disorders (ICSD-3)[3] (**Box 1**).

Supportive diagnostic features, especially important in early-onset cases,[4] include a positive family history for RLS, periodic limb movements (PLMs), or periodic limb movement disorder (PLMD) among first-degree relatives and the objective diagnosis of a PLMs index >5/h.

The same investigators report the convenient classification of probable and possible RLS: the former, in children who meet all diagnostic criteria except the circadian factor; the latter, in children who manifest behaviors and discomfort compatible with all RLS criteria without adequate verbalization of urgency.

PREVALENCE AND PREDISPOSING FACTORS

The prevalence of pediatric RLS is approximately 2% to 4%,[5,6] and is slightly more prevalent and more severe in adolescents.

Unlike the adult population in which an evident female prevalence has been established, no gender differences have been reported until late adolescence, with the exception of a Chinese study[7] reporting a female prevalence of 2.7% versus 1.7% in boys in a cohort of 8-year-old to 17-year-old subjects. Because of the specifics of diagnostic criteria, 17% of children were diagnosed in a general pediatric clinic versus 5.9% in a sleep clinic, independently of the referral motive.

Pediatric RLS is highly familial, as demonstrated by the common occurrence in monozygotic twins and first-degree siblings.[8]

[a] Department of Clinical and Experimental Medicine, Sleep Medicine Center, University of Messina, AOU G Martino, Pad. H, Via Consolare Valeria 1, Messina, Messina 98125, Italy; [b] Seattle Children's Hospital, OC.7. 720 - Pulmonary, 4800 Sand Point Way Northeast, Seattle, WA 98105, USA
* Corresponding author.
E-mail address: rsilvestri@unime.it

Sleep Med Clin 16 (2021) 305–314
https://doi.org/10.1016/j.jsmc.2021.02.006
1556-407X/21/© 2021 Elsevier Inc. All rights reserved.

Box 1
Definition, diagnostic criteria, and special consideration for restless leg syndrome (RLS)

RLS is a sensory-motor disorder referring to an urge to move the legs caused by unpleasant sensations, paresthesias, or dysesthesias.

A. Symptoms must

   a. Begin or worsen during resting or inactivity periods, such as sitting or lying down.

   b. Be partially relieved by active movements as long as the activity continues.

   c. Occur predominantly at night or in the evening, rather than all day long.|

B. May not exclusively be accounted for by another medical or behavioral disorder.

C. Cause distress, functional impairment, and sleep disturbance.

Special considerations to aid childhood RLS diagnosis include the following:

- The patient's description of symptoms in his or her own words.

- The awareness of typical children's language to describe symptoms.

- The applicability of diagnostic criteria depending on language and cognitive development rather than age.

- The possibility that some adult-specifiers, such as circadian distribution, may not apply.

- A relatively greater impairment of behavioral and educational domains with respect to mood, sleep, and global functioning.

Both linkage and genotype analyses, as well as extensive cross-sectional studies, show a positive family history in 87% to 90.9% of probands. Among the different genes associated with adult RLS (*MEIS1*, *BTBD9*, *NAP2K5/SKOR1*), only *MEIS1* and *SKOR1*, supporting the sensory component of RLS, were found in association with the pediatric form. Whereas, an association to BTBD9, which seems to be linked to low ferritin and RLS motor aspects, has not been found in pediatric RLS.[8]

Risk factors for pediatric RLS development include low iron stores[9] and vitamin D deficiency, both seen in celiac disease correlating with a younger onset and more severe symptoms.[10] Furthermore, chronic kidney disease and the presence of PLMs with an index (number of PLMs/h of sleep) >5 seem to be positively correlated with pediatric RLS onset.

Precipitating factors include prolonged immobility, such as hospitalization and several medications, in particular, sedative antihistamines, central dopaminergic receptor antagonists, and most antidepressants, especially selective serotonin reuptake inhibitors (SSRIs).

CLINICAL CHARACTERISTICS AND RELEVANCE

As previously stated, the urge to move in children may be accompanied by sensations that are difficult to describe, particularly for young children. Uncomfortable, often painful feelings, frequently expanding to all 4 limbs, may be referred to as feeling "uncomfortable," "restless," "funny," or needing "to kick." Sometimes, asking a child to draw his symptoms may ensure more fruitful results.[11]

Symptoms may start earlier during the day in children and adolescents because of the long hours of motor inactivity at school.

RLS in children impacts 4 main domains, which are specifically probed by the pediatric RLS severity scale (P-RLS-SS).[12] These include sleep, due to prolonged sleep latency and intermittent insomnia for which motor restlessness and PLMs are mostly responsible (See Video 1). In fact, the latter induce multiple arousals with consequent detrimental effects on slow-wave sleep (N3).

A second domain affected by pediatric RLS is mood, with a consistently increased incidence of both anxiety (11.5%) and, even more so, depression (29%).[13]

A third domain refers to cognition and the negative impact of RLS on academic performance and the ability to concentrate, leading to frequent interruptions of both schoolwork and homework. Behavioral aspects comprise the fourth domain affected by pediatric RLS. In particular, the restlessness of children with RLS can lead to a mistaken diagnosis of attention-deficit hyperactivity disorder (ADHD). Indeed, some features of RLS in children with impulsive behavior and lack of inhibition are part of the ADHD spectrum. Increased rates of ADHD (25%) are reported among children with RLS.[13] Likewise, RLS symptoms are frequently reported in children and adolescents with ADHD, with different prevalence ranging from 43% to 33% when the IRLS-SG criteria are used.[14]

ADHD, rather than attention-deficit disorder, seems to be more frequently linked to RLS.

Although a joint genetic dysfunction may be hypothesized, a genetic linkage has been explored but not confirmed thus far.[15]

The most recent study corroborating the prevalence of pediatric RLS and its mimic conditions in

ADHD[16] reports an RLS prevalence of 11% versus 23% for RLS mimic conditions. Subjects with ADHD and RLS share a significant relationship with a positive family history for RLS. On multivariate linear regression, comorbid subjects did worse in terms of school and life-skills.

There is also an increased prevalence of RLS in autism spectrum disorders (ASD) where bedtime resistance could sometimes be interpreted as possible RLS, an underrecognized cause of insomnia in children with autism.[17] Other comorbid disorders include renal failure and iron depletion anemia, both aggravating children's symptoms, RLS prognosis, and life quality.

Among sleep comorbidities, pediatric RLS is often comorbid with other sleep-related movement disorders, such as bruxism and PLMD, and with obstructive sleep apnea syndrome, within[18] or independently from a diagnosis of neurodevelopmental disorders[19]; OSAS, in particular, may exacerbate inattention and cognitive/academic disadvantage of children with RLS.

Early-onset RLS is usually, but not univocally, recognized as a slower progressing form than late-onset RLS (ICSD 3).[3]

Cardiovascular and metabolic impact is undoubtedly less extensive than mood and academic/behavioral consequences.

PATHOPHYSIOLOGY

At present, the iron deficiency–metabolic theory represents the most acclaimed explanation for the nature and distribution of RLS symptoms.[20]

Animal models,[21] imaging,[22,23] and postmortem studies[24] all substantiate this theory.

Brain-iron deficiency (BID), due to impaired iron transport across the blood-brain barrier, primarily affects the substantia nigra[22] and, to a lesser extent, the caudate, putamen, and thalamus, with the activation of the hypoxic pathway. The latter, in turn, increases dopaminergic activity with subsequent post-synaptic downregulation. BID also increases glutamate and reduces adenosine, resulting in hyperarousal and sleep fragmentation unresponsive to dopaminergic treatment.

The circadian turnover of dopamine and iron metabolism also explains the circadian night distribution of symptoms and induces overcompensation via an adaptive post-synaptic mechanism.[25]

Iron deficiency is currently recognized as an integral component of many neurodevelopmental and sleep disorders. In fact, it has been shown to strongly correlate with so-called hyperactive behaviors,[26] including restless sleep disorder (RSD),[27] ADHD,[14] and ASD.[28]

DIAGNOSTIC EVALUATION AND DIFFERENTIAL DIAGNOSIS
Diagnostic and Severity Scales

An extensive and thorough review of diagnostic instruments to assess pediatric RLS has been published this year.[29] As previously stated, an accurate history taken in the presence of parents or caregivers should confirm the presence of essential criteria, stimulate the child's description of symptoms in his or her own words, and look for supportive criteria (a positive family history, objective impairment of sleep) whenever adult criteria cannot be met.

Compared with the ICSD-3,[3] the IRLS-SG criteria,[30] updated according to the suggestion of the IRLS-SG Pediatric task force,[2] states that frequency (chronic-persistent or intermittent) and duration (persistent or intermittent over 1 year) criteria may be waived in children, and that functional impairment may be present but is not required.

Several diagnostic questionnaires have been designed to aid the diagnosis of adult RLS, of which only a few have been used in children (**Box 2**). These include the single question for RLS,[31] the Pediatric Emory RLS diagnostic questionnaire,[32] and the RLS questionnaire (RLSQ).[33]

The single question for RLS diagnosis: "When you try to relax in the evening or sleep at night,

---

Box 2
Pediatric RLS diagnostic tools

Diagnostic Interview

- Single question for RLS
- Pediatric Emory RLS diagnostic questionnaire
- The Restless Legs Syndrome questionnaire (RLSQ)

Severity Scales

- International Restless Legs Scale (IRLS)
- Clinical Global Impressions Rating Scales (CGI)
- RLS-6 scale of restless legs syndrome/ Willis-Ekbom disease
- Pediatric Restless Legs Syndrome Severity Scale (P-RLS-SS)
- Rating the 4 RLS diagnostic criteria

Contributing Instrumental Tools

- Video polysomnography (vPSG)
- Actimetry
- Suggested Immobilization Test (SIT)
- Suggested Clinical Immobilization Test (SCIT)

do you ever have unpleasant, restless feelings in your legs that can be relieved by walking or movement?" was developed by Ferri and coworkers[31] and has been validated[34] in children and adolescents against an in-person interview by 2 clinicians. This single question has a positive predictive value of 86.9% and a negative predictive value of 100%.

A specific instrument for diagnosing RLS in children is the Pediatric Emory RLS diagnostic questionnaire, which adapts questions from the Cambridge-Hopkins diagnostic questionnaire, the RLS-Expanded Questionnaire, and the Phenotypic Presentation of Restless Legs Syndrome Questionnaire, modifying them according to pediatric use. Two different age groups are considered, 8 to 12 and 13 to 18, with 47 and 46 questions to be addressed, respectively. For the first group, questions are directed at the child in the presence of parents/caregivers. The first 5 items are screening questions that, besides investigating classic criteria, also inquire about the presence of growing pains and a history of rubbing-massage to relieve symptoms. A series of age-specific queries follow if any screening question is answered affirmatively. Specific attention is granted to rule out mimics and assess the quality of sleep and medication use. There is also the possibility of indicating the most affected body parts by shading them on a printed image of the human body. Instructions for the correct classification into definite and probable RLS are provided. The Pediatric Emory RLS questionnaire has been used to evaluate children with chronic kidney disease,[32] but has yet to be fully validated.

The RLSQ[33] is an 11-item parent-report questionnaire whose validation details are not available with the original report. However, it is judged reliable, exhibiting an internal consistency of 65% and repeat-measure reliability (rho = 0.58).

As far as severity scales are concerned, several measures have been used but have yet to be validated in children and adolescents. The International Restless Legs Scale (IRLS) is a 10-item scale to be administered by an examiner with the scope of obtaining the patient's severity rating.[35] Among a panoply of severity scales, it represents the most used instrument in clinical, academic, and pharmaceutical trials. The IRLS allows a distinction based on the sum of scores (0–4) of single questions into mild, moderate, severe, and very severe. It was initially validated in adults by comparing the Clinical Global Impression (CGI) and Patient Global Impression.[35] Several studies have used it in adolescents,[10,36,37] but only a few in children.[38]

A self-administered version of the IRLS-SG severity rating scale (sIRLS) has been recently validated in adults,[39] but not yet in adolescents, despite its foreseeably accessible and advantageous use in this age group.

Despite its lack of specificity for RLS, the CGI is among the most administered tools in adult RLS patients, but it has also been used in adolescents with RLS, along with the RLS-6 scale of RLS/Willis-Ekbom disease.[37] The latter is a 6-item rating scale that asks participants to rate the severity of RLS symptoms over the course of the past week from 0 to 10. The questions selectively probe RLS severity during different daytime and nighttime activities and quality of sleep. The correlation coefficients with the IRLS total score ranged from 0.35 to 0.67.[40]

Among other adult scales assessing severity, no use has been reported of the John Hopkins Restless Legs Severity Scale[41] and the Augmentation Severity Rating Scale[42] in pediatric populations.

A specific severity scale for pediatric use, as implied by its name, is the P-RLS-SS.[12] Composed of 41 Likert-type items, it is a self-administered tool for children 9 years and older. The P-RLS-SS is based on interviews of 6-year-old to 17-year-old subjects obtained at multiple tertiary centers and entails debriefing both children and parents. As previously mentioned, it measures RLS symptoms and impact on 4 domains: sleep, wake activities (behavioral aspects), emotion (mood), and tiredness (cognitive ramifications). It also includes a separate complementary questionnaire for parents to provide observations of their child's sleep and mood. The P-RLS-SS still needs to be validated and possibly shorted from its original version through field testing to assess the appropriateness and comprehension of the separate items.

A promising but not yet validated instrument used for both diagnostic and severity assessment is rating the 4 RLS diagnostic criteria in children.[43] This is a modified version of the P-RLS-SS that proceeds to rate symptom severity from 4 to 16, only after the child qualifies for definite RLS.

Quality-of-life scales specific for RLS, such as the Kohen RLS Quality-of-Life Instrument,[44] the RLS Quality-of-Life Questionnaire – Abetz,[45] and the RLS Quality-of-Life Instrument,[46] have not been used in children. The same is true for the quality of sleep scales used in RLS adult patients, such as the Post-Sleep Questionnaire for RLS[47] and the RLS-Next Day Impact Questionnaire.[48]

In fact, to date, no validated instrument exists to assess the quality of life in children with RLS. However, the Peds Quality-of-Life Inventory for children aged 2 to 18 has 4 subscales (physical, emotional, social, and school functioning) that have been used either alone[36,49] or in combination with the Sleep Behavior Questionnaire[50] to assess the quality of life in children and adolescents with RLS.

Clinical and Polysomnographic Evaluation

Laboratory testing for anemia, iron profile, ferritin, and vitamin D levels should be part of the clinical evaluation.

Physical and neurologic examination of children with RLS should prove within normal limits, whereas behavioral observation, along with quantification of movements, could be assessed by the Suggested Immobilization Test (SIT)[51] in older, cognitively competent children or the Suggested Clinical Immobilization Test (SCIT) in neurodevelopmentally challenged children or those younger than 8 years.[52]

SIT evaluates PLMs during wakefulness and sensory symptoms during resting-wake 1 hour before bedtime. The child is instructed to sit in bed with his or her legs outstretched, while symptoms are ascertained on a visual analog scale to confirm the diagnosis. PLMs are simultaneously recorded and confirmed via an actimeter[53] or standard polysomnography (PSG).

Instead, the SCIT encourages children to sit freely on the floor with their parents while the doctor annotates or video-records their movements and posture related to possible underlying tension.

A supportive objective criterion to strengthen the diagnosis of pediatric RLS may be obtained by (formally unrequired) PSG assessment of a PLMs index greater than 5/h, along with proof of altered sleep onset and/or maintenance, with increased wake after sleep onset and number of awakenings per night. PLMs are extremely rare in children, albeit in specific conditions, one of which is RLS. Limb movements also have limited periodicity in younger subjects compared with older patients. The presence of a PLM index greater than 5/h may help as a supportive criterion for the diagnosis of possible RLS (see History/background and definition section).

Only one-third of PLM-related arousals is cortical, whereas most are classified as autonomic arousals. A parameter to be possibly evaluated through PSG to assess a periodicity index (PI = number of sequences of 3 leg movement [LM] intervals [10–90 s]/total number of inter-LM intervals) is the intermovement interval (IMI). In children, IMIs are short and variable, often less than 10 seconds in duration, showing night-to-night variability. Total LMs and PLMs are higher in younger children and decrease with age. The PI is low, especially in ADHD-comorbid RLS, where non–rapid eye movement sleep alteration does not respond to dopaminergic therapy.

Differential Diagnosis and Pediatric Restless Legs Syndrome Mimics

The primary differential diagnosis of RLS is PLMD, which refers to the presence of objectively demonstrated PLMs via PSG recording with a frequency of greater than 5/h in children, causing significant sleep disturbance and/or daytime consequences. Unlike RLS, children do not report any subjective sensory symptoms or urge to walk and are often unaware of their altered sleep.

The most common pediatric RLS mimics include growing pains, leg cramps, positional discomfort, arthritis, and dermatitis.

Less common mimics that are also considered in the differential diagnosis of PLMD include sleep starts, fragmentary myoclonus, and myoclonic epilepsy. Given the specific scope of this article, only growing pains and leg cramps are addressed.

Growing pains refer to intermittent nonarticular pain occurring mostly at night with a more extensive prevalence (3%–49%) than RLS, peaking at age 5 (range 4–14 years). Pain is bilateral, involving the legs both proximally and distally. Laboratory, objective, and neurologic evaluations are unrevealing. Symptoms include all features of RLS, with the exception of urgency or relief from walking the floor. Pain, more than discomfort, is referred by the patient.[54] Vitamin D supplementation, rather than iron, proves helpful. Genetic-observational studies suggest a possible overlap between growing pains and RLS.[55]

Leg cramps refer to brief, painful tightness of the calf. They often occur at night, mostly idiopathic, but they may also be secondary to diabetes, neurologic disorders, or iatrogenic causes. Leg cramps usually occur with low frequency in children, almost exclusively unilaterally. Forceful or passive stretching out of bed, rather than walking the floor, alleviates symptoms.[56]

It is imperative to consider that mimics may also co-occur in children with RLS.

Associated conditions/comorbidities of RLS, besides iron depletion anemia and chronic kidney disease, include "secondary" RLS in the context of diabetes/peripheral neuropathy, myopathies, and dysthyroidism. Among less commonly reported comorbidities, sickle cell anemia and fibromyalgia are also to be mentioned.

TREATMENT

A recent article published last year by DelRosso and Bruni[57] reviewed all possible treatment options for pediatric RLS, including nonpharmacologic and pharmacologic management (**Box 3**). With respect to the former, the investigators stress the importance of instructing children and parents about sleep hygiene after assessing inadequate or poor sleep habits. This approach is particularly beneficial to adolescents, even if it is seldom resolutive alone. Dietary modifications include avoidance of caffeine-containing substances from the early afternoon onward. Pediatricians and general practitioners should also be aware of the iatrogenic risks for the precipitating or worsening of RLS due to sedative antihistamines, tricyclic antidepressants, SSRIs, neuroleptics, nicotine, and alcohol. Stretching before bedtime, without strenuous exercise, may relieve symptoms by 63%,[58] possibly by improving circulation and increasing endorphin release.[59]

Furthermore, cool or heating pads, rubbing, and massaging may provide some relief via a possible increase of dopamine urinary excretion.

Pharmacologic treatment options primarily include iron supplementation, dopaminergic drugs, antiepileptic medications, benzodiazepines, and clonidine.

As previously mentioned, BID, best expressed by low ferritin levels, is often associated with pediatric RLS unless infection or inflammation is present. Children with low ferritin levels (<35–50 ng/mL) receiving iron supplementation in the form of oral ferrous sulfate (3 mg/kg per day) improve their RLS symptoms after 3.8 months of therapy,[60] showing an inverse correlation with their ferritin levels.[61] Dye and colleagues[62] reported long-lasting (2 years) benefits of long-term iron supplementation for symptoms and PSG-wise in children with RLS and PLMs.

Side effects include difficulty swallowing pills in children, constipation, or reflux. In celiac disease or whenever oral absorption is challenged or ferritin is very low, intravenous supplementation is advised. A beneficial effect is reported with 1.21–6.8 mg/kg (maximum 120 mg) iron sucrose in patients 2 to 16 years old.[63]

Guidelines endorsing the use of iron supplementation in children with RLS were published in 2018.[64] Although there is not enough evidence to formally accredit iron as a treatment option for RLS in children, it is nevertheless considered first-line for pediatric RLS.

Iron insufficiency is a broadly generic, often underrecognized condition, commanding clinical attention and treatment. Determinants of ferritin response to oral supplementation in children with sleep-related movement disorders including RLS, PLMD, restless sleep disorder, obstructive sleep apnea, and neurodevelopmental disorders, depend strictly on therapy adherence hindered by possible side effects, such as constipation and treatment duration in respondents only.[65]

However, some investigators have recently questioned the benefit of iron supplementation because the substantial improvement of low ferritin levels was not paralleled by an equal lessening of nocturnal symptoms in supplemented children.[43] However, suboptimal ferritin levels do not necessarily correlate with improved symptoms after iron supplementation.[66]

Only a few studies, mostly case reports and small open-label studies, support dopaminergic treatment in children with RLS with and without ADHD.[67,68]

A small randomized study[69] showed benefits for RLS and PLMs but not ADHD symptoms

---

Box 3
Pediatric RLS treatment

Nonpharmacologic Management	Pharmacologic Treatments
• Dietary modifications	• Iron supplementation
• Physical activity	• Dopaminergic drugs
• Sensory stimulation	• Anticonvulsants
• Avoidance of medications	○ Alpha 2 Delta (α2δ) ligands
• Sleep hygiene	○ Levetiracetam
	• Benzodiazepines
	• Clonidine

with L-Dopa. Rotigotine has been successfully used in adolescents,[37] also in combination with iron.[62] There are significant limitations to using dopaminergic drugs in adults with RLS, owing to side effects, withdrawal symptoms, and possible augmentation. Minimal data are available in pediatrics, with no report of augmentation.

Anticonvulsants used to control RLS in children include levetiracetam,[38] but mostly gabapentin (GBP), although it is not approved by the Food and Drug Administration (FDA) for use in children. The extant literature on successful GBP use in RLS children is scarce, with only 1 indication of partial resolution of symptoms[61] and a case report on a 14-month-old toddler describing complete disappearance of symptoms with increased dosing of GBP from 50 to 200 mg.[70]

Clonazepam (0.1–1 mg) has proven effective in improving sleep and reducing arousals in children with RLS, without a substantial effect on associated motor and sensory abnormalities.[71]

Clonidine, an alpha-2-adrenergic agonist, used for insomnia in children with neurodevelopmental disorders and hyperactivity, has proven readily effective and well-tolerated in children with RLS, alone or in association with iron supplementation,[62] despite no FDA approval.

Exogenous melatonin (MLT) has been shown to decrease PLMs in children with a delayed circadian phase.[72] However, no evidence supports MLT use in children with RLS, as is also true for magnesium, vitamin D, and opioids.

Dye and colleagues[73] suggest that choosing and personalizing therapy for children with RLS is crucially important. Hence, prospective randomized studies should be encouraged in this population.

First-line therapy should consist of 3 to 6 months of iron supplementation with slow tapering. Both alpha-2-delta-1 ligands and dopaminergic medications should be considered as second-line treatment. In particular, L-dopa and dopaminergics should be restricted to older children and adolescents suffering from refractory, severe RLS. All other cases should benefit from GBP (5–15 mg/kg 1.5 hours before bedtime) or pregabalin (2–6 mg/kg before bedtime).

FUTURE DIRECTIONS

Pediatric RLS, as a highly familial disorder, should be more explored in terms of genetic research in different geographic areas, also to assess the relevance of epigenetic factors such as climate and diet that have been proposed to account for the pathophysiology of adult RLS.

Specific diagnostic tools for assessing severity and quality of life should be developed and validated for this age group. Alternative, nonconventional testing, probing nonverbal communication, such as drawings and behavioral observation, should be further cultivated and explored in very young and neurodevelopmentally challenged subjects.

A strong effort to educate general practitioners, parents, and teachers should underscore the importance of a healthy diet and sleep hygiene. This educational effort should also promote adequate knowledge of the underestimated risk of iatrogenic RLS in children.

SUMMARY

RLS is an underrecognized pediatric disorder characterized by sensory-motor symptoms occurring mostly at night and affecting children's sleep, mood, behavior, and academic performance. Because of its possible mimics, it is critical to refer potential patients to pediatricians with sleep medicine expertise. Treating brain-iron deficiency in children with low ferritin is a harmless and beneficial approach despite no FDA-approved treatments exist for the management of RLS in children.

CLINICS CARE POINTS

- A thorough medical and familial history and behavioral observation are key to the diagnosis of RLS in children.
- Pediatric RLS should be suspected in all cases of initial/maintenance pediatric insomnia.
- Particular attention should be directed toward mimicking behaviors, such as growing pains and leg cramps.
- Testing ferritin levels and iron profile is highly recommended.
- Best practices: nonpharmacologic treatment and iron supplementation if ferritin is <50 ng/mL.

DISCLOSURE

The authors have nothing to disclose.

SUPPLEMENTARY DATA

Supplementary data related to this article can be found online at https://doi.org/10.1016/j.jsmc.2021.02.006.

REFERENCES

1. Walters AS, Picchietti DL, Ehrenberg BL, et al. Restless legs syndrome in childhood and adolescence. Pediatr Neurol 1994;11(3):241–5.
2. Picchietti DL, Bruni O, de Weerd A, et al. Pediatric restless legs syndrome diagnostic criteria: an update by the international restless legs syndrome study group. Sleep Med 2013;14(12):1253–9.
3. Darien I. The International Classification of Sleep Disorders (ICSD-3). 2014.
4. Simakajornboon N, Dye TJ, Walters AS. Restless legs syndrome/Willis-Ekbom disease and growing pains in children and adolescents. Sleep Med Clin 2015;10(3):311–22.
5. Picchietti D, Allen RP, Walters AS, et al. Restless legs syndrome: prevalence and impact in children and adolescents - the peds REST study. Pediatrics 2007;120(2):253–66.
6. Turkdogan D, Bekiroglu N, Zaimoglu S. A prevalence study of restless legs syndrome in Turkish children and adolescents. Sleep Med 2011;12(4):315–21.
7. Xue R, Liu G, Ma S, et al. An epidemiologic study of restless legs syndrome among Chinese children and adolescents. Neurol Sci 2015;36(6):971–6.
8. Muhle H, Neumann A, Lohmann-Hedrich K, et al. Childhood-onset restless legs syndrome: clinical and genetic features of 22 families. Mov Disord 2008;23(8):1113–21.
9. Halac G, Sezer GM, Saglam NO, et al. The relationship between Willis-Ekbom disease and serum ferritin levels among children in northwestern Turkey. Neurosciences 2015;20(4):336–40.
10. Işıkay S, Işıkay N, Per H, et al. Restless leg syndrome in children with celiac disease. Turk J Pediatr 2018;60(1):70–5.
11. Picchietti DL, Arbuckle RA, Abetz L, et al. Pediatric restless legs syndrome: analysis of symptom descriptions and drawings. J Child Neurol 2011;26(11):1365–76.
12. Arbuckle R, Abetz L, Durmer JS, et al. Development of the pediatric restless legs syndrome severity scale (P-RLS-SS)©: a patient-reported outcome measure of pediatric RLS symptoms and impact. Sleep Med 2010;11(9):897–906.
13. Pullen SJ, Wall CA, Angstman ER, et al. Psychiatric comorbidity in children and adolescents with restless legs syndrome: a retrospective study. J Clin Sleep Med 2011;7(6):587–96.
14. Oner P, Dirik EB, Taner Y, et al. Association between low serum ferritin and restless legs syndrome in patients with attention deficit hyperactivity disorder. Tohoku J Exp Med 2007;213(3):269–76.
15. Schimmelmann BG, Friedel S, Nguyen TT, et al. Exploring the genetic link between RLS and ADHD. J Psychiatr Res 2009;43(10):941–5.
16. Srifuengfung M, Bussaratid S, Ratta-apha W, et al. Restless legs syndrome in children and adolescents with attention-deficit/hyperactivity disorder: prevalence, mimic conditions, risk factors, and association with functional impairment. Sleep Med 2020;73:117–24.
17. Kanney ML, Durmer JS, Trotti LM, et al. Rethinking bedtime resistance in children with autism: is restless legs syndrome to blame? J Clin Sleep Med 2020. https://doi.org/10.5664/jcsm.8756.
18. Silvestri R, Gagliano A, Aricò I, et al. Sleep disorders in children with attention-deficit/hyperactivity disorder (ADHD) recorded overnight by video-polysomnography. Sleep Med 2009;10(10):1132–8.
19. Romero-Peralta S, Cano-Pumarega I, Garcia-Malo C, et al. Treating restless legs syndrome in the context of sleep disordered breathing comorbidity. Eur Respir Rev 2019;28(153). https://doi.org/10.1183/16000617.0061-2019.
20. Earley CJ, Connor J, Garcia-Borreguero D, et al. Altered brain iron homeostasis and dopaminergic function in restless legs syndrome (Willis-Ekbom disease). Sleep Med 2014;15(11):1288–301.
21. Qu S, Le W, Zhang X, et al. Locomotion is increased in A11-lesioned mice with iron deprivation: a possible animal model for restless legs syndrome. J Neuropathol Exp Neurol 2007;66(5):383–8.
22. Godau J, Schweitzer KJ, Liepelt I, et al. Substantia nigra hypoechogenicity: definition and findings in restless legs syndrome. Mov Disord 2007;22(2):187–92.
23. Earley CJ, Barker P B, Horská A, et al. MRI-determined regional brain iron concentrations in early- and late-onset restless legs syndrome. Sleep Med 2006;7(5):458–61.
24. Connor JR, Ponnuru P, Wang XS, et al. Profile of altered brain iron acquisition in restless legs syndrome. Brain 2011;134(4):959–68.
25. Allen RP. Restless leg syndrome/Willis-Ekbom disease pathophysiology. Sleep Med Clin 2015;10(3):207–14.
26. Ipsiroglu OS, Wind K, Hung YH, Amy), et al. Prenatal alcohol exposure and sleep-wake behaviors: exploratory and naturalistic observations in the clinical setting and in an animal model. Sleep Med 2019;54:101–12.
27. Delrosso LM, Bruni O, Ferri R. Restless sleep disorder in children: a pilot study on a tentative new diagnostic category. Sleep 2018;41(8). https://doi.org/10.1093/sleep/zsy102.
28. Leung W, Singh I, McWilliams S, et al. Iron deficiency and sleep – a scoping review. Sleep Med Rev 2020;51. https://doi.org/10.1016/j.smrv.2020.101274.
29. Stubbs PH, Walters AS. Tools for the assessment of pediatric restless legs syndrome. Front Psychiatry 2020;11. https://doi.org/10.3389/fpsyt.2020.00356.

30. Allen RP, Picchietti DL, Garcia-Borreguero D, et al. Restless legs syndrome/Willis-Ekbom disease diagnostic criteria: updated International Restless Legs Syndrome Study Group (IRLSSG) consensus criteria - history, rationale, description, and significance. Sleep Med 2014;15(8):860–73.

31. Ferri R, Lanuzza B, Cosentino FII, et al. A single question for the rapid screening of restless legs syndrome in the neurological clinical practice. Eur J Neurol 2007;14(9):1016–21.

32. Riar SK, Leu RM, Turner-Green TC, et al. Restless legs syndrome in children with chronic kidney disease. Pediatr Nephrol 2013;28(5):773–95.

33. Evans A, Blunden S. Development of a parental report questionnaire for restless legs syndrome (RLS) in children: the RLSQ. J Foot Ankle Res 2011;4(S1). https://doi.org/10.1186/1757-1146-4-s1-o15.

34. Zhang J, Lam SP, Li SX, et al. Restless legs symptoms in adolescents: epidemiology, heritability, and pubertal effects. J Psychosom Res 2014;76(2):158–64.

35. Walters AS, LeBrocq C, Dhar A, et al. Validation of the international restless legs syndrome study group rating scale for restless legs syndrome. Sleep Med 2003;4(2):121–32.

36. Silva GE, Goodwin JL, Vana KD, et al. Restless legs syndrome, sleep, and quality of life among adolescents and young adults. J Clin Sleep Med 2014;10(7):779–86.

37. Elshoff JP, Hudson J, Picchietti DL, et al. Pharmacokinetics of rotigotine transdermal system in adolescents with idiopathic restless legs syndrome (Willis–Ekbom disease). Sleep Med 2017;32:48–55.

38. Gagliano A, Aricò I, Calarese T, et al. Restless leg syndrome in ADHD children: levetiracetam as a reasonable therapeutic option. Brain Dev 2011;33(6):480–6.

39. Sharon D, Allen RP, Martinez-Martin P, et al. Validation of the self-administered version of the International Restless Legs Syndrome study group severity rating scale – the sIRLS. Sleep Med 2019;54:94–100.

40. Kohnen R, Martinez-Martin P, Benes H, et al. Rating of daytime and nighttime symptoms in RLS: validation of the RLS-6 scale of restless legs syndrome/Willis-Ekbom disease. Sleep Med 2016;20:116–22.

41. Allen RP, Earley CJ. Validation of the Johns Hopkins restless legs severity scale. Sleep Med 2001;2(3):239–42.

42. García-Borreguero D, Kohnen R, Högl B, et al. Validation of the Augmentation Severity Rating Scale (ASRS): a multicentric, prospective study with levodopa on restless legs syndrome. Sleep Med 2007;8(5):455–63.

43. Rosen GM, Morrissette S, Larson A, et al. Does improvement of low serum ferritin improve symptoms of restless legs syndrome in a cohort of pediatric patients? J Clin Sleep Med 2019;15(8):1149–54.

44. Kohnen R, Martinez-Martin P, Benes H, et al. Validation of the Kohnen restless legs syndrome–quality of life instrument. Sleep Med 2016;24:10–7.

45. Abetz L, Vallow SM, Kirsch J, et al. Validation of the restless legs syndrome quality of life questionnaire. Value Heal 2005;8(2):157–67.

46. Atkinson MJ, Allen RP, DuChane J, et al. Validation of the restless legs syndrome quality of life instrument (RLS-QLI): findings of a consortium of national experts and the RLS Foundation. Qual Life Res 2004;13(3):679–93.

47. Canafax DM, Bhanegaonkar A, Bharmal M, et al. Validation of the post sleep questionnaire for assessing subjects with restless legs syndrome: results from two double-blind, multicenter, placebo-controlled clinical trials. BMC Neurol 2011;11. https://doi.org/10.1186/1471-2377-11-48.

48. Lasch KE, Abraham L, Patrick J, et al. Development of a next day functioning measure to assess the impact of sleep disturbance due to restless legs syndrome: the restless legs syndrome-next day impact questionnaire. Sleep Med 2011;12(8):754–61.

49. Furudate N, Komada Y, Kobayashi M, et al. Daytime dysfunction in children with restless legs syndrome. J Neurol Sci 2014;336(1–2):232–6.

50. Sander HH, Eckeli AL, Costa Passos AD, et al. Prevalence and quality of life and sleep in children and adolescents with restless legs syndrome/Willis-Ekbom disease. Sleep Med 2017;30:204–9.

51. Garcia-Borreguero D, Kohnen R, Boothby L, et al. Validation of the multiple suggested immobilization test: a test for the assessment of severity of restless legs syndrome (Willis-Ekbom disease). Sleep 2013;36(7):1101–9.

52. Ipsiroglu OS, Beyzaei N, Berger M, et al. "Emplotted narratives" and structured "behavioral observations" supporting the diagnosis of Willis-Ekbom disease/restless legs syndrome in children with neurodevelopmental conditions. CNS Neurosci Ther 2016;22(11):894–905.

53. Plante DT. Leg actigraphy to quantify periodic limb movements of sleep: a systematic review and meta-analysis. Sleep Med Rev 2014;18(5):425–34.

54. Walters AS, Gabelia D, Frauscher B. Restless legs syndrome (Willis-Ekbom disease) and growing pains: are they the same thing? A side-by-side comparison of the diagnostic criteria for both and recommendations for future research. Sleep Med 2013;14(12):1247–52.

55. Champion D, Pathirana S, Flynn C, et al. Growing pains: twin family study evidence for genetic susceptibility and a genetic relationship with restless legs syndrome. Eur J Pain (United Kingdom) 2012;16(9):1224–31.

56. Leung AKC, Wong BE, Chan PYH, et al. Nocturnal leg cramps in children: incidence and clinical characteristics. J Natl Med Assoc 1999;91(6):329–32.

57. DelRosso L, Bruni O. Treatment of pediatric restless legs syndrome. Adv Pharmacol 2019;84:237–53. https://doi.org/10.1016/bs.apha.2018.11.001.

58. Dinkins EM, Stevens-Lapsley J. Management of symptoms of restless legs syndrome with use of a traction straight leg raise: a preliminary case series. Man Ther 2013;18(4):299–302.

59. Bega D, Malkani R. Alternative treatment of restless legs syndrome: an overview of the evidence for mind-body interventions, lifestyle interventions, and neutraceuticals. Sleep Med 2016;17:99–105.

60. Mohri I, Kato-Nishimura K, Kagitani-Shimono K, et al. Evaluation of oral iron treatment in pediatric restless legs syndrome (RLS). Sleep Med 2012; 13(4):429–32.

61. Amos LB, Grekowicz ML, Kuhn EM, et al. Treatment of pediatric restless legs syndrome. Clin Pediatr (Phila) 2014;53(4):331–6.

62. Dye TJ, Jain SV, Simakajornboon N. Outcomes of long-term iron supplementation in pediatric restless legs syndrome/periodic limb movement disorder (RLS/PLMD). Sleep Med 2017;32:213–9.

63. Grim K, Lee B, Sung AY, et al. Treatment of childhood-onset restless legs syndrome and periodic limb movement disorder using intravenous iron sucrose. Sleep Med 2013;14(11):1100–4.

64. Allen RP, Picchietti DL, Auerbach M, et al. Evidence-based and consensus clinical practice guidelines for the iron treatment of restless legs syndrome/Willis-Ekbom disease in adults and children: an IRLSSG task force report. Sleep Med 2018;41: 27–44.

65. DelRosso LM, Yi T, Chan JHM, et al. Determinants of ferritin response to oral iron supplementation in children with sleep movement disorders. Sleep 2020; 43(3).

66. Ingram DG, Al-Shawwa B. Serum ferritin in the pediatric sleep clinic: what's normal anyway? J Clin Sleep Med 2019;15(11):1699–700.

67. Konofal E, Arnulf I, Lecendreux M, et al. Ropinirole in a child with attention-deficit hyperactivity disorder and restless legs syndrome. Pediatr Neurol 2005; 32(5):350–1.

68. Walters AS, Mandelbaum DE, Lewin DS, et al. Dopaminergic therapy in children with restless legs/periodic limb movements in sleep and ADHD. Pediatr Neurol 2000;22(3):182–6.

69. England SJ, Picchietti DL, Couvadelli BV, et al. L-Dopa improves restless legs syndrome and periodic limb movements in sleep but not attention-deficit-hyperactivity disorder in a double-blind trial in children. Sleep Med 2011;12(5):471–7.

70. Bruni O, Angriman M, Luchetti A, et al. Leg kicking and rubbing as a highly suggestive sign of pediatric restless legs syndrome. Sleep Med 2015;16(12): 1576–7.

71. Manconi M, Ferri R, Zucconi M, et al. Dissociation of periodic leg movements from arousals in restless legs syndrome. Ann Neurol 2012;71(6):834–44.

72. Kunz D, Bes F. Exogenous melatonin in periodic limb movement disorder: an open clinical trial and a hypothesis. Sleep 2001;24(2):183–7.

73. Dye TJ, Gurbani N, Simakajornboon N. How does one choose the correct pharmacotherapy for a pediatric patient with restless legs syndrome and periodic limb movement disorder? Expert guidance. Expert Opin Pharmacother 2019;20(13):1535–8.

Sleep-Related Rhythmic Movement Disorder

Lourdes M. DelRosso, MD[a],*, Irene Cano-Pumarega, MD, PhD[b,c],
Samantha S. Anguizola E, MD[d,1]

KEYWORDS

- Sleep related rhythmic movement disorder • Headbanging • Body rocking • Head rolling

KEY POINTS

- Sleep-related rhythmic movement disorder must have a complaint of sleep interference, impaired daytime function, or self-inflicted bodily injury.
- It is typically considered a benign pediatric sleep disorder that usually resolves spontaneously as the child ages.
- The diagnosis is clinical and based on history, physical examination, and fulfillment of the diagnostic criteria.
- In most cases, treatment consists of reassurance, ensuring safety, adequate sleep, and injury prevention.

INTRODUCTION

Sleep-related rhythmic movement disorders (SRRMD) comprise a group of movement disorders that are characterized by repetitive, stereotyped, and rhythmic motor behaviors that occur predominantly early in childhood with an average age of onset of 9 months of age, although can also be seen in adults. SRRMD are characterized under Movement Disorder in the *International Classification of Sleep Disorders* (Third Edition) (*ICSD-3*).[1] **Fig. 1** demonstrates the taxonomy of sleep-related movement disorders described in the *ICSD-3*, showing the subtype "sleep related rhythmic movement disorders." Unlike rhythmic movements during sleep, which are usually benign and self-resolving, SRRMD has significant effect on daytime or nighttime impairment. To fit the diagnostic criteria for SRRMD, the patient must present with the following clinical symptoms:

1. Rhythmic, stereotyped, and repetitive movements involving large muscle groups (especially neck and trunk muscles)

2. Movements that occur predominantly during drowsiness or sleep
3. A complaint of sleep interference, impaired daytime function, or self-inflicted bodily injury
4. Movements that are not better explained by seizures or another medical disorder[1]

The *ICSD-3* diagnostic criteria for SRRMD is summarized in **Fig. 2**. The American Academy of Sleep Medicine Scoring Manual has further characterized the movements as having a frequency of 0.5 to 2 Hz, and with a minimum number of 4 clustered movements. **Fig. 3** illustrates the typical artifact seen on electroencephalography (EEG) and electromyography in patients exhibiting SRRMD during a sleep study.

SRRMD was initially described in 2 case reports in children ages 3 and 6 in 1905 and called "jactation capitis nocturna," a name still used for headbanging.[2] SRRMD are often subdivided into categories depending on the type of movements involved. The most common categories of SRRMD are headbanging and body rocking. Headbanging is characterized by repetitive lifting of the head

[a] Seattle Children's Hospital, 4800 Sand Point Way NE, Seattle, WA 98105, USA; [b] Sleep Research Institute, Calle del Padre Daniel 44 - 28036 Madrid, Spain; [c] Sleep Unit, Respiratory Department, Hospital Ramón y Cajal (IRYCIS), CIBERES, Ctra.Colmenar Viejo km 9,100, 28034 Madrid, Spain; [d] European Sleep Instituto, Panama, Panama
[1] Present address: 51 Street, Bella Vista, Habitats Plaza, Panama City, Panama.
* Corresponding author.
E-mail address: lourdesdelrosso@me.com

Sleep Med Clin 16 (2021) 315–321
https://doi.org/10.1016/j.jsmc.2021.02.007
1556-407X/21/© 2021 Elsevier Inc. All rights reserved.

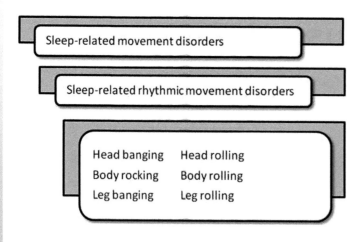

Fig. 1. Subtypes of SRRMD.

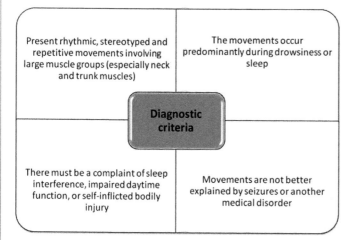

Fig. 2. Diagnostic criteria of SRRMD.

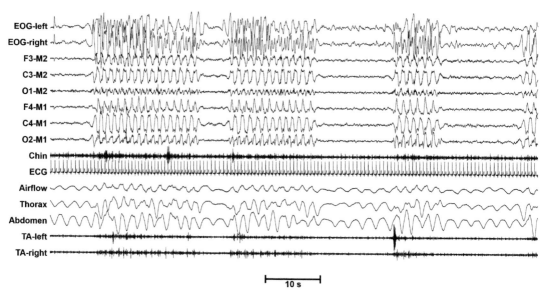

Fig. 3. Polysomnographic findings during SRRMD. Note the artifact on the EEG leads (F3-M2, F4-M1, C3-M2, C4-M1, O1-M2, O2-M1).

with banging the head into the pillow or mattress. Body rocking consists of a rhythmic forward and backward movement of the trunk that can occur in the sitting or quadruped position. Other less common SRRMD types include head rolling, leg banging, body rolling, or leg rolling. On rare occasions, several forms of rhythmic movements are seen in a single patient.[3] The subtypes of SRRMD are described in **Fig. 1**.

In this article, the authors discuss SRRMD, their prevalence, pathophysiology, characteristics, and treatment options, emphasizing the differences between children and adult presentations.

DEMOGRAPHICS

SRRMD is typically considered a benign pediatric sleep disorder that usually resolves spontaneously as the child ages. The prevalence at 9 months of age is up to 66%, decreasing to 5% at age 5, with most cases resolving by age 10; nevertheless, it can persist into adulthood.[4,5] SRRMD can occur in a wide variety of patient populations ranging from normal asymptomatic patients, patients with comorbid sleep disorders, and patients with developmental delay or mental retardation. In adults, SRRMD is more likely to be reported with comorbid sleep disorders, such as narcolepsy, rapid eye movement (REM) sleep behavior disorder, restless legs syndrome, or obstructive sleep apnea (OSA).

The prevalence of SRRMD is the same for boys and girls at a younger age, but in adults, a male predominance has been suggested.[4]

PATHOPHYSIOLOGY

The pathophysiology of SRRMD is unknown, but there are several postulated mechanisms.

Self-Soothing

Because SRRMD occurs with a high prevalence in young normally developing children, it is likely that rhythmic movements during sleep represent a normal physiologic phenomenon. It has been suggested that rhythmic movements constitute a positive vestibular stimulation for a self-soothing effect or a stimulus for motor development in the early stages of life.[6] This hypothesis is supported by the fact the rhythmic movements during sleep are common in the early years of life and self-resolve without any adverse consequences.

Sleep Instability

Polysomnography (PSG) findings have demonstrated a close relationship between SRRMD and arousals, leading to studies exploring sleep instability in patients with SRRMD. Cyclic alternating pattern (CAP) is the periodic EEG activity occurring during non–rapid eye movement (NREM) sleep. CAP is a marker of sleep instability and has standardized rules and criteria for its visual scoring.[7] A CAP cycle is composed of phase A and phase B. Phase A is subdivided into A1, A2, and A3 phases. Phase A represents neural synchronization and has been associated with various movements during sleep (periodic limb movements, bruxism, and sleepwalking).[8,9] Manni and Terzaghi[10] showed that rhythmic movements during sleep occurred shortly after phase A regardless of sleep stage. Similarly, a case report of a 9-year-old with SRRMD showed a relationship between phases A2 and A3 of the cycling alternating pattern and rhythmic movements during NREM sleep.[11]

Central Pattern Generators

The basal ganglia may play a role in rhythmic movements during sleep.[12] The basal ganglia forms part of a system called "central pattern generators" (CPG). CPG have been hypothesized to play a role in motor phenomena during sleep, including leg movements and parasomnias. The CPG is a neural network involved in the control of early motor function thought to be under the inhibitory control of the cortex. It has been postulated that immaturity of the inhibitory cortical system in early infancy might be associated with rhythmic movements during sleep in the first year of life.[13] In this model, the loss of inhibitory cortex function could also be secondary to specific pathologic conditions, which would explain the persistence, relapse, various manifestations, or later onset of SRRMD.

Genetics

Familial case series have been reported in the literature. The exact genetics is unknown.[14]

DIAGNOSIS

The diagnosis of SRRMD is mainly clinical and based on history, physical examination, and fulfillment of the diagnostic criteria (see **Fig. 2**).

During sleep, patients who exhibit rhythmic movements are unresponsive to commands, but if awakened, they are alert, are oriented, and deny dream recall. Patients can present with 1 type of rhythmic movement, a couple of coexisting different types, or resolution of 1 type with persistence of another type of movement as the patient grows older. The clinical presentation of SRRMD is usually mild and sporadic. It consists of single episodes of rhythmic movements occurring at bedtime before sleep onset. Rarely, persistent movements through the night or more severe forms exist.

Cases of atypical SRRMD, with head slapping or head punching, have been reported in both adults and children.[15,16] Because of these atypical presentations and the stereotypic nature of the movements, a differential diagnosis of epilepsy is often considered, and in some cases, patients with SRRMD warrant a referral to rule out seizures.[5] Epilepsy can be stereotypic, simple, or complex, can occur during sleep, during wakefulness, or during both. Epilepsy can therefore mimic a sleep disorder. Nocturnal paroxysmal dystonia, for example, initially thought to be a sleep-related movement disorder, is now considered to be a form of frontal lobe epilepsy.[17] In SRRMD, unlike epilepsy, there is no autonomic changes, and the movements stop upon awakening or can be stopped on request when occurring during wakefulness. Rhythmic movements are also not associated with tongue biting, urinary incontinence, tonic-clonic activity, automatisms, or other activity resembling seizure.[18] The differential diagnosis IS summarized in **Box 1** and also includes parasomnias, other movement disorders, such as periodic limb movement disorder, REM-sleep behavior disorder, and sleep myoclonus.[2] Many times the diagnosis can be made with a clinical evaluation alone, but when atypical features are present, video-PSG will aid in the diagnosis.

The features of rhythmic movement seen by home video recording and a full-night PSG examination may be useful, particularly in differentiating SRRMD from other sleep-related diseases (bruxism, periodic leg movements during sleep) or in identifying comorbid sleep disorders (OSA). Full night PSG has shown that SRRMD can occur during wakefulness and in every stage of sleep.[19] Rhythmic movements can occur during the sleep-wake transition or any sleep stage with various prevalences per sleep stage. It has been reported in 46% of NREM sleep, 30% of both NREM and REM sleep, and in 24% of only REM

sleep,[2] with most events occurring in N2.[18] The reporting of SRRMD occurring exclusively during REM sleep can raise the question of a possible relationship between SRRMD and REM behavior disorder.[20] However, there is no current documentation of REM without atonia observed in patients with REM-related SRRMD, and studies in patients with SRRMD exclusively during REM sleep have demonstrated normal atonia during REM.[21]

Fig. 3 shows several characteristic findings of SRRMD on PSG. Each individual run or episode of RMD is characterized by a unique artifact created by the repetitive movements, consisting of high-amplitude waveforms on the electrooculogram and EEG channels. As seen in **Fig. 3**, the waveforms are synchronous with the repetitive movements of SRRMD. The video monitoring can also aid in the identification of these movements. The electromyogram channels also show a transient increase in muscle tone, and the audio can reveal associated vocalizations when present. The authors recommend that technicians comment on the presence of SRRMD in PSG. The total time spent in episodes of rhythmic movements during PSG ranged from 1 to 59 minutes. Periods of rhythmic movements are interspersed between periods of normal NREM or REM sleep stages. The sleep architecture is usually normal, with normal sleep stage distributions of REM and all stages of NREM sleep. Each type of rhythmic movement is typical for each child. The movements did not occur in any particular sleep cycle or time of the night. On the day after the studies, all patients were amnestic for the previous night's episodes.[18]

In cases in which a larger work up has been done, including MRI, computed tomography (CT), and EEG, in most cases the work up has been normal.[19]

CLINICAL FEATURES AND COMORBIDITIES

In children, SRRMD has been reported to be a benign self-limiting condition seen in most cases in normally developing children. However, there are some associations with comorbidities. Dyken and colleagues[18] reported the association between SRRMD and attention-deficit/hyperactivity disorder (ADHD) in 3 out of 7 children ages 1 to 12 years. SRRMD was confirmed with video-PSG. Other researchers found that ADHD, predominantly of the inattentive type, cooccurred with SRRMD, but the combined inattentive and hyperactive type was still seen in 2 of the 6 children with ADHD.[19]

Rhythmic movements during sleep can be seen in children with autism spectrum disorder, in

---

Box 1
Differential diagnosis of sleep-related rhythmic movement disorders
Epilepsy
Parasomnia
Other sleep-related movement disorders
Sleep myoclonus

children with mental retardation, and in children with psychiatric disorders. Rhythmic movements as explained above, by themselves, do not constitute a disorder unless associated with sleep disruption, daytime sleepiness, or injuries. Furthermore, in some children with neurodevelopmental disorders, rhythmic movements are also seen during the day.

Early reports noted that SRRMD was not unique to childhood. When reported in adolescents,[22] a full work up, including laboratory, brain computed tomography, MRI, and resting EEG, was normal.

On rare occasions, SRRMD persist into adulthood or can start de novo. Stepanova and colleagues[19] studied 10 patients from age 7 to 24 and followed them up to 6 years. All patients had symptoms since infancy. The investigators confirmed that movements occurred in all sleep stages and varied by sleep stage. During wakefulness or NREM stage 1, movements were longer, whereas during NREM stage 2, NREM stage 3, and REM sleep, the movements were shorter. The investigators also found that in those 19 to 24 years old, there was comorbid depression and obsessive-compulsive disorder. A case report in a 24-year-old man showed that symptoms of headbanging worsened with stress and with chocolate, occurred nightly, and were associated with significant daytime sleepiness despite getting adequate sleep at night. PSG was obtained, and headbanging was recorded during 14% of the epochs with 54% of N1 spent headbanging but also with episodes occurring during N2 and N3.[23]

In adults, cases of SRRMD occurring exclusively during REM sleep have been reported,[4,24] which is intriguing, in particular, because of the atonia that is part of REM sleep. Furthermore, SRRMD has also been reported with concomitant REM behavior disorder. A hypothesis for the coexistence of both disorders can be the involvement of CPG in both SRRMD and REM behavior disorder.[25]

A case series of 5 adults with sleep-disordered breathing and RMD showed that all but 1 patient reported SRRMD since childhood. Initially, rhythmic movements occurred mainly at sleep-onset transition, but as the patients grew into adulthood, the SRRMD started occurring in deeper sleep and persisted across the entire night. In this cohort of adults with sleep-disordered breathing, 81.4% of the rhythmic movements were triggered by a respiratory event. In only 1 case, SRRMD improved after continuous positive airway pressure (CPAP) therapy.[26]

Although some investigators have suggested an association between RMD and psychopathologies when RMD persists beyond childhood, this association remains controversial, and the pathophysiology of this possible association remains unknown; furthermore, Mayer and colleagues showed that most adult patients with SRRMD did not have abnormal psychopathology.[4]

TREATMENT OPTIONS

Currently, there are no evidence-based treatment guidelines or recommendations for the treatment of SRRMD in children or adults. In most cases, SRRMD does not result in significant concern or significant daytime symptoms and do not warrant treatment, but in rare instances, headbanging in particular has resulted in soft tissue, eye, and skull injuries, hemoglobinuria with acute renal failure, internal carotid artery dissection, and subdural hemorrhage.[27] A single case report studied brain MRI in a 27-year-old woman with a history of headbanging and found enlarged sulci in the occipital lobes, enlarged diploic space in the posterior parietal and occipital bones, and loss of gray matter without loss of the adjacent white matter, a finding associated with superficial atrophy secondary to chronic headbanging.[28] Treatment options found in the literature are summarized in **Table 1**.

Prescription Medication

Benzodiazepines have been used in children with various degrees of success. Oxazepam 10 to 20 mg at bedtime was used to treat body rocking and headbanging in an 8-year-old girl with symptoms since age 7 months.[29] In other reports, clonazepam has shown partial improvement in frequency or severity of movements,[4,22] and in others, there has been no improvement in symptoms.[16] Imipramine and phenytoin were unsuccessful in a 27 month old.[30] A single case report showed worsened symptoms with dopaminergics with resolution of movements with antipsychotics (antidopaminergics).[16]

Nonprescription

Etzioni and colleagues[31] successfully treated 6 children with SRRMD using mild sleep deprivation (1 hour less than the habitual total sleep time) and chloral hydrate with improvement in sleep latency and SRRMD. The investigators postulated that their success supported the hypothesis that SRRMD is a voluntary self-soothing behavior rather than an involuntary one, because shortening sleep latency with chloral hydrate and mild sleep deprivation eliminated SRRMD in almost all children with the exception of one.

Melatonin was reported in an 8-year-old girl with ADHD and SRRMD, showing improvement in

Table 1
Treatment options of sleep-related rhythmic movement disorders found in the literature

Prescription Medication	Nonprescription	Behavioral Strategies
Short-acting benzodiazepines (Oxazepam)[29] and intermediate-acting (Clonazepam)[4,22]; improves frequency and severity of movements[4,22,29]	Melatonin,[32] improves the frequency of SRRMD	Behavior modification
Antipsychotics[16]	If OSA is present: improves with CPAP treatment[34]	Injury prevention
	Hypnosis[33]	Psychotherapy
		Sleep restriction[31]

frequency of RMD.[32] The investigators postulated that melatonin may modulate dopaminergic pathways involved in movement disorders among other properties. Circadian entrainment can help stabilize sleep, and antioxidant properties may play an important role in locomotor activity during sleep.

Hypnosis was reported as successful in a case report of a 26-year-old woman with body rocking since infancy.[33]

If comorbid OSA is present, CPAP may decrease the severity of SRRMD.[34]

SUMMARY

Rhythmic movements are common during sleep in young children and in most cases resolve spontaneously by 10 years of age. In a small number of cases, the sleep-related rhythmic movements can persist into adulthood.

Most cases are benign and do not fit criteria for SRRMD. If sleep disruption, injury, or daytime sleepiness are present, then the patient is diagnosed with SRRMD. Further evaluation with laboratory work up, imaging, PSG, or EEG is not needed when the diagnosis is clear and the history and clinical presentation are typical. Atypical, frequent, injurious, or other activity suspicious for seizures warrants further evaluation. In other cases, a comorbid sleep disorder may be suspected, such as sleep-disordered breathing, and PSG is indicated.

There are currently no guidelines in the treatment of SRRMD, but various medications and methods have been used with some degree of success. Ensuring safety, adequate sleep, and injury prevention should be a general recommendation.

CLINICS CARE POINTS

- Sleep-related rhythmic movement disorder occurs predominantly early in childhood with an average age of onset of 9 months of age.
- Symptoms resolve spontaneously in most children.
- In most children, treatment options include conservative measures to ensure safety and parental reassurance.
- If a concomitant sleep disorder is suspected or if features of another disorder are present (epilepsy), further evaluation is recommended, including a sleep study or referral to neurology.
- When the onset of sleep-related rhythmic movement disorder is in adulthood, consider evaluation of other sleep disorders.
- There are no current treatment guidelines, but medications including benzodiazepines are an option for presentations with significant symptoms or sleep disruption.

DISCLOSURE

The authors have nothing to disclose.

REFERENCES

1. International classification of sleep disorders. 3rd edition. Darien (IL): American Academy of Sleep Medicine; 2014.
2. Hoban TF. Rhythmic movement disorder in children. CNS Spectr 2003;8(2):135–8.

3. Su C, Miao J, Liu Y, et al. Multiple forms of rhythmic movements in an adolescent boy with rhythmic movement disorder. Clin Neurol Neurosurg 2009; 111(10):896–9.

4. Mayer G, Wilde-Frenz J, Kurella B. Sleep related rhythmic movement disorder revisited. J Sleep Res 2007;16(1):110–6.

5. Happe S, Ludemann P, Ringelstein EB. Persistence of rhythmic movement disorder beyond childhood: a videotape demonstration. Mov Disord 2000; 15(6):1296–8.

6. Sallustro F, Atwell CW. Body rocking, head banging, and head rolling in normal children. J Pediatr 1978; 93(4):704–8.

7. Terzano MG, Parrino L, Sherieri A, et al. Atlas, rules, and recording techniques for the scoring of cyclic alternating pattern (CAP) in human sleep. Sleep Med 2001;2(6):537–53.

8. Terzano MG, Parrino L. Origin and significance of the cyclic alternating pattern (CAP). REVIEW ARTICLE. Sleep Med Rev 2000;4(1):101–23.

9. Parrino L, Smerieri A, Spaggiari MC, et al. Cyclic alternating pattern (CAP) and epilepsy during sleep: how a physiological rhythm modulates a pathological event. Clin Neurophysiol 2000;111(Suppl 2): S39–46.

10. Manni R, Terzaghi M. Rhythmic movements during sleep: a physiological and pathological profile. Neurol Sci 2005;26(Suppl 3):s181–5.

11. Manni R, Terzaghi M, Sartori I, et al. Rhythmic movement disorder and cyclic alternating pattern during sleep: a video-polysomnographic study in a 9-year-old boy. Mov Disord 2004;19(10):1186–90.

12. Freund HJ, Hefter H. The role of basal ganglia in rhythmic movement. Adv Neurol 1993;60:88–92.

13. Grillner S, Wallen P. Central pattern generators for locomotion, with special reference to vertebrates. Annu Rev Neurosci 1985;8:233–61.

14. Attarian H, Ward N, Schuman C. Case report: a multigenerational family with persistent sleep related rhythmic movement disorder (RMD) and insomnia. J Clin Sleep Med 2009;5(6):571–2.

15. Yeh SB, Schenck CH. Atypical headbanging presentation of idiopathic sleep related rhythmic movement disorder: three cases with video-polysomnographic documentation. J Clin Sleep Med 2012;8(4):403–11.

16. Lee SK. A case with dopamine-antagonist responsive repetitive head punching as rhythmic movement disorder during sleep. J Epilepsy Res 2013; 3(2):74–5.

17. Walters AS. Clinical identification of the simple sleep-related movement disorders. Chest 2007; 131(4):1260–6.

18. Dyken ME, Lin-Dyken DC, Yamada T. Diagnosing rhythmic movement disorder with video-polysomnography. Pediatr Neurol 1997;16(1):37–41.

19. Stepanova I, Nevsimalova S, Hanusova J. Rhythmic movement disorder in sleep persisting into childhood and adulthood. Sleep 2005;28(7):851–7.

20. Kempenaers C, Bouillon E, Mendlewicz J. A rhythmic movement disorder in REM sleep: a case report. Sleep 1994;17(3):274–9.

21. Kohyama J, Matsukura F, Kimura K, et al. Rhythmic movement disorder: polysomnographic study and summary of reported cases. Brain Dev 2002;24(1): 33–8.

22. Hashizume Y, Yoshijima H, Uchimura N, et al. Case of head banging that continued to adolescence. Psychiatry Clin Neurosci 2002;56(3):255–6.

23. Chisholm T, Morehouse RL. Adult headbanging: sleep studies and treatment. Sleep 1996;19(4): 343–6.

24. Anderson KN, Smith IE, Shneerson JM. Rhythmic movement disorder (head banging) in an adult during rapid eye movement sleep. Mov Disord 2006; 21(6):866–7.

25. Manni R, Terzaghi M. Rhythmic movements in idiopathic REM sleep behavior disorder. Mov Disord 2007;22(12):1797–800.

26. Chiaro G, Maestri M, Riccardi S, et al. Sleep-related rhythmic movement disorder and obstructive sleep apnea in five adult patients. J Clin Sleep Med 2017;13(10):1213–7.

27. Mackenzie JM. "Headbanging" and fatal subdural haemorrhage. Lancet 1991;338(8780):1457–8.

28. Carlock KS, Williams JP, Graves GC. MRI findings in headbangers. Clin Imaging 1997;21(6):411–3.

29. Walsh JK, Kramer M, Skinner JE. A case report of jactatio capitis nocturna. Am J Psychiatry 1981; 138(4):524–6.

30. Freidin MR, Jankowski JJ, Singer WD. Nocturnal head banging as a sleep disorder: a case report. Am J Psychiatry 1979;136(11):1469–70.

31. Etzioni T, Katz N, Hering E, et al. Controlled sleep restriction for rhythmic movement disorder. J Pediatr 2005;147(3):393–5.

32. Metin O, Eynalli-Gok E, Kuygun-Karci C, et al. The effectiveness of melatonin in head banging: a case report. Sleep Sci 2019;12(1):53–6.

33. Rosenberg C. Elimination of a rhythmic movement disorder with hypnosis–a case report. Sleep 1995; 18(7):608–9.

34. Chirakalwasan N, Hassan F, Kaplish N, et al. Near resolution of sleep related rhythmic movement disorder after CPAP for OSA. Sleep Med 2009;10(4): 497–500.

Sleep Disorders in Parkinson Disease

Ambra Stefani, MD, Birgit Högl, MD*

KEYWORDS

- Parkinson disease • PD • RBD • Insomnia • Movement disorders

KEY POINTS

- All categories of sleep disorders are found in patients with Parkinson disease (PD).
- Insomnia is the most frequent sleep disorder in PD patients and its frequency increases over time.
- Increased daytime sleepiness or involuntary falling asleep frequently have been described in PD patients.
- Disturbance of sleep-wake rhythmicity is common in PD.
- Rapid eye movement sleep behavior disorder (RBD) is particularly relevant to PD, and an accurate and safe diagnosis of RBD excluding mimics is mandatory.

INTRODUCTION

Sleep disorders were included in the very first description of Parkinson disease (PD) by James Parkinson[1] and have been mentioned by many pioneer investigators since the late 1960s.[2–14]

Multiple factors contribute to the manifestation of sleep and wakefulness disturbances in patients with PD.[10,15,16] These range from the motor manifestations of the disease itself (eg, nocturnal akinesia, intermittent tremor manifestations, and painful OFF phenomena) to the intrinsic pathophysiology of the disease (eg, disturbance of motor and sleep-wake regulating neural circuits and neurotransmitters). Other contributing factors also can affect sleep and circadian rhythmicity as can the presence of frequent comorbidities; these include the adverse effects of treatment, genetic susceptibilities, and behavioral consequences of PD and its treatment.

The sleep disorders seen in patients with PD include several types of insomnia, multiple and varying degrees of sleep-related breathing disorders, disorders of daytime hypersomnolence, circadian rhythm disorders, parasomnias of rapid eye movement (REM) sleep and non-REM sleep, and motor disorders of sleep. Although the effect of PD on sleep and wakefulness has been studied extensively, a reverse effect of sleep on PD motor symptoms also exists but has been less investigated.

INSOMNIA

Insomnia is the most frequent sleep disorder in patients with PD and can manifest as disordered sleep onset, sleep maintenance, or early morning awakening. A diagnosis of insomnia is clinical, based on subjective symptoms. In patients with PD and insomnia alterations in sleep, however, macrostructure and microstructure also are present. In the 1980s, polysomnographic studies already had described specific patterns of light and fragmented sleep in patients with PD.[2] Reduced sleep efficiency and less slow wave sleep also often are areported.[17]

Insomnia is a progressive phenomenon in patients with PD; its frequency increases over time and also increases with longer duration of treatment, presence of depression, age, and certain sleep-related comorbidities.[18–20] Although several studies have indicated that insomnia may precede the onset of PD symptoms,[21–24] others report that the duration of nocturnal sleep is not affected in prediagnostic cases.[19,20] There is controversy about whether there is abnormal sleep structure

Department of Neurology, Medical University of Innsbruck, Anichstr. 35, Innsbruck 6020, Austria
* Corresponding author.
E-mail address: birgit.ho@i-med.ac.at

Sleep Med Clin 16 (2021) 323–334
https://doi.org/10.1016/j.jsmc.2021.03.001
1556-407X/21/© 2021 Elsevier Inc. All rights reserved.

in early PD.[20,25] Priano and coworkers[26] demonstrated that non-REM sleep instability is present in PD and can be quantified using a cyclic alternating pattern. Wetter and colleagues[27] performed electroencephalogram (EEG) frequency analysis during REM sleep and found increased alpha wave activity in de novo PD patients during the first third of the night.

During the course of the disease, the influence of specific PD medications on sleep structure has been documented extensively,[10] for example, the induction of arousals by dopamine agonists.[28,29]

Sleep quality not only is relevant to patients' quality of life but also likely has a prognostic value. A recent study found a significant association between sleep efficiency and global cognitive performance in patients with PD.[30] Another study reported that a higher accumulated power of slow waves during sleep was associated with slower motor progression in PD.[31] It has been shown that slow wave activity in non-REM sleep still shows the physiologic decrease between early sleep and late sleep in patients with PD, except in patients with dyskinesia, in whom it was interpreted as inadequate synaptic downscaling.[32]

Assessment of Insomnia in Parkinson Disease

In a structured sleep history, sleep habits (going to bed, getting up, and daytime naps), the subjective time it takes to fall asleep, the estimated number of nocturnal awakenings and their estimated durations (specifically, prolonged awakenings), and timing (eg, presence of any early morning awakenings) must be assessed. This structured sleep history enables an estimation of the circadian timing of the sleep episode; the subjective duration of total nocturnal sleep both gives an estimate of real sleep duration alerts to a potential misperception of sleep state.

In addition to a thorough sleep history, several scales are recommended for assessing sleep impairment in patients with PD: the Pittsburgh Sleep Quality Index, the Scales for Outcomes in Parkinson's Disease-Sleep, and the Parkinson's Disease Sleep Scale.[10,33–35]

Treatment of Insomnia

If specific medications to help sleep are used in PD, multiple caveats and interactions need to be kept in mind.[10] Hypnotics might be indicated in some cases but potential worsening of a sleep-related breathing disorder and daytime sleepiness should be taken into account. Although evidence for drug treatment of insomnia in PD is insufficient, eszopiclone and melatonin (3–5 mg) have been suggested by some investigators.[36] Although it might seem counterintuitive to apply cognitive-behavior therapy in patients with PD, where insomnia has a large organic component, recent studies have shown that cognitive-behavior therapy, if professionally administered,[37–40] also is specifically useful in patients with PD.

DAYTIME SLEEPINESS AND INVOLUNTARY NAPPING

Increased daytime sleepiness or involuntary falling asleep frequently has been described in PD patients,[13,41,42] often in association with disease duration or medications, although this always has been controversial. Some well-designed studies failed to show any association with nighttime sleep duration, clinical variables, or medications,[19,43–46] and other studies pointed to the disease itself or suspected comorbid sleep-related breathing disorders as causes of daytime sleepiness in PD.[42] Although apomorphine-induced yawning was an early observed phenomenon[47] and levodopa-induced sleepiness has been reported[48] and was suggested to be prominent particularly in multiple system atrophy compared with PD,[49] dopamine agonist–induced daytime sleepiness first was reported with nonergoline dopamine agonists 2 decades ago.[50]

Concerning daytime sleepiness, it is important to understand that patients often are unaware and that it is necessary to disentangle subjective and caregiver-observed daytime sleepiness.[44,51] Potential underlying causes for daytime sleepiness should be evaluated, such as sleep deprivation and circadian disorders, including those induced by therapy and potentially related to impulse control disorders (ICDs),[43] undiagnosed relevant sleep-related breathing disorders, and side effects of dopaminergic therapy (reviewed by Stefani and Högl, 2020[10]). It has been shown that excessive daytime sleepiness relates to extensive topographic Lewy pathology expansion in patients with PD.[52]

A study from the Parkinson's Progression Markers Initiative cohort showed that de novo untreated PD patients compared with controls did not have a different prevalence of excessive daytime sleepiness but that sleepiness was related to mood and autonomic function.[53] Moreover, daytime sleepiness increased over time in longitudinal assessment over several years.[54]

Assessment of Excessive Daytime Sleepiness

For the assessment of daytime sleepiness, the Epworth Sleepiness Scale is the instrument used most frequently and covers the recent period, often specified as 1 week or 2 weeks.[33] Suggestions to add additional questions accounting for so-called sleep attacks on dopaminergic medications have been made[33,55]; however, there is low awareness of sleepiness,[56] discrepancies between self-assessment and caregiver assessment of daytime sleepiness, and a significant difference between self-awareness of sleepiness and objective sleepiness.[57] Therefore, objective assessment of daytime sleepiness is helpful, specifically the assessment of sleep propensity with a multiple sleep latency test or of the capacity to remain awake with the maintenance of wakefulness test, although these tests sometimes are cumbersome for PD patients.

In some cases, daytime sleepiness is particularly severe, which has led to the description of a "narcolepsy-like phenotype"; in few patients at the onset of sleep, REM (resembling sleep-onset REM sleep episodes) can be observed.[56]

Treatment of Daytime Sleepiness

If there is no otherwise treatable cause of daytime sleepiness in patients with PD (eg, severe comorbid obstructive sleep apnea [OSA]), symptomatic vigilance enhancing treatment, for instance, with modafinil, has been used with limited success.[58–60]

SLEEP-RELATED BREATHING DISORDERS

Although the presence of snoring[42,61,62] and OSA has been described in multiple studies in PD (reviewed by Stefani and Högl[10]), the clinical relevance of OSA in PD sometimes has been questioned[63–65] or reported to be less severe or abortive in a significant part of the patients,[66] possibly related to decreased body mass index in many PD patients.[63,67]

Specific PD-related factors might contribute to OSA in these patients. Vincken and Cosio[68] suggested that hypokinesia and rigidity also involve the upper airway muscles and thus contribute to upper airway obstruction during sleep in PD. Furthermore, sleeping exclusively in the supine position can aggravate sleep-related breathing disorders in PD.[64]

In general, it must be acknowledged that in patients with parkinsonian syndromes beyond PD, namely multiple system atrophy, the spectrum of sleep-related breathing disorders is even wider and includes central apnea, impaired rhythmicity of breathing,[69] and stridor.[70]

Assessment of Sleep-Related Breathing Disorders in Parkinson Disease

Suspected sleep-related breathing disorder should be evaluated with polysomnography. If it is not available, cardiorespiratory polygraphy with transcutaneous oxygen saturation and respiratory channels can give a first impression of the presence or severity of sleep-related breathing disorders.

Treatment of Sleep Apnea

Regarding treatment, the gold standard for sleep apnea continues to be nasal continuous positive airway pressure (CPAP); it also is used in PD patients if there is clinically significant sleep apnea.[33,55] Other modalities, for instance, intraoral mandibular advancement devices, are difficult to use in advanced patients because of the presence of dyskinesia and abnormal salivation.

In general, daytime sleepiness and/or cognitive impairment in patients with PD often are multifactorial, and CPAP treatment alone is not able to solve these concerns.[71]

CIRCADIAN DISORDERS

Disturbance of sleep-wake rhythmicity is common in PD and may manifest as the flattened amplitude of rest-activity rhythm, circadian phase advance or delay, and other sleep-wake rhythmicity alterations.[72] Contributing factors include the lack of bright light exposure in institutionalized patients with impaired mobility[73] but also treatment effects, particularly in patients with ICDs, as an effect of dopamine agonists.[43,74] Videnovic and coworkers[75] reported a relation between circadian melatonin secretion rhythm and excessive daytime sleepiness in PD with reduced melatonin amplitude. Independently of ICDs, earlier studies showed that dopaminergic drugs per se seem to have an advancing effect on sleep.[76–78] Genetic factors also contribute to susceptibility to the circadian disturbance.[78,79]

Assessment of Circadian Disorders in Parkinson Disease

For the assessment of circadian disturbances, actigraphy over 2 weeks is a useful instrument[80] and can be combined with dim light melatonin onset determination and genetics.[81] In patients with apparent circadian abnormalities, ICDs should be ruled out and polysomnography performed in case it is unclear if the reported nocturnal behaviors occur during wakefulness or sleep.

Treatment of Circadian Disorders

Light treatment has been shown to improve sleep, increase alertness, and even improve mood and motor activity.[82–84] A study in mice with alpha-synuclein A53T missense mutation, however, showed impaired light entrainment of the circadian system,[85] suggesting that in some genetic PD forms light therapy might not be helpful.

A placebo-controlled study evaluating the effect of melatonin in 26 patients with PD showed an increase in 1 clock gene (BMAL1) but not in another 1 (PER1) and neither daytime sleepiness nor abnormal nighttime sleepiness changed after intervention.[86]

In summary, it seems that chronotherapeutics, in particular light therapy, is an underappreciated approach to improving sleep and wakefulness in PD.[78]

RAPID EYE MOVEMENT SLEEP BEHAVIOR DISORDER AND OTHER PARASOMNIAS

The steepest increase in knowledge of sleep and PD has been seen in REM sleep behavior disorder (RBD). RBD is characterized by repeated episodes of different vocalization and various motor behaviors, including single jerks,[87,88] during REM sleep[89] and can involve serious injuries for the patient or the bed partner, including falling out of bed.[90] This issue includes a specific article on isolated RBD, Iranzo A, Ramos LA, Sabela N. The isolated form of REM sleep behavior disorder: The upcoming challenges. Although RBD can precede PD symptoms—and is called in this case (clinically) isolated RBD,[91–93] it also may manifest simultaneously with the motor manifestations of PD,[94] or appear only later, after a diagnosis of PD has long been made.[95] Although the Braak and colleagues'[96] theory often is used to explain the early occurrence of RBD prior to PD manifestation,[96] a possible explanation of why RBD can precede or succeed PD motor symptoms has been provided by Lai and Siegel.[97] They found that the onset of the neurodegenerative process can be either in the midbrain or in the rostroventral junction; thus, this determines which symptoms manifest earlier.[91,92,94,97–103] Recently, another hypothesis has been proposed, with a brain-first (top-down) and a body-first (bottom-up) type of PD. According to this hypothesis, isolated RBD is a prodromal phenotype for the body-first type.[104]

Prevalence of RBD in PD ranges from 16% to 47%.[91,94,95] and an even larger proportion of patients have REM sleep without atonia on polysomnography, without meeting the criteria for RBD.[94,95] Although nightmares are common in RBD, a detailed analysis of dream content in PD reported no differences in action-filledness, vividness, or threat content of dreams of PD patients with and without RBD. Dreams, however, were more often negatively than positively toned in PD patients with RBD.[105]

As discussed previously, if RBD manifests prior to/in the absence of PD, it is called isolated (previously idiopathic).[91] In general, 80% to 90% of patients with initially clinically isolated RBD later manifest an alpha-synuclein–related disease, most often PD or dementia with Lewy bodies,[92,93,102] and certain biomarkers are useful in indicating that the risk of phenoconversion is higher or even imminent.[91,101] In particular, dopamine transporter single-photon emission computer tomography[106,107] and olfactory dysfunction[99] are well-investigated predictors of imminent conversion, but multiple other promising biomarkers have been reviewed extensively elsewhere.[91] The assessment of biomarkers will be of outstanding help in assessing the risk of conversion in patients with isolated RBD.[101] In those patients with very long-standing isolated RBD, however, signs of neurodegeneration always are present if the examination is detailed enough.[108]

Assessment of Rapid Eye Movement Sleep Behavior Disorder

Although the current version of the *International Classification of Sleep Disorders–Third Edition* (*ICSD-3*) makes the performance of polysomnography to assess REM sleep without atonia obligatory, the *Diagnostic and Statistical Manual of Mental Disorders* (Fifth Edition), allows for a diagnosis of RBD in the context of PD without polysomnography if it is not available.[45] This diagnosis should be made while keeping in mind significant caveats, however, namely, the confounding of RBD with severe periodic limb movements (PLMs) or severe sleep apnea,[45] and, in patients with PD, with or without cognitive impairment, with nocturnal psychotic episodes or nocturnal wandering.

In particular, the diagnostic value of specifically designed RBD questionnaires, such as the RBD-SQ,[109] the RBD single question (RBD1Q),[110] the Innsbruck RBD Inventory,[111] and the RBD questionnaire - Hong Kong,[112] is of limited value if the questionnaires are used outside validation studies[109,113–117]: low sensitivity and/or specificity have been shown for the RBD-SQ in patients with PD[109] and even worse in patients with de novo PD.[113] Epidemiologic studies have revealed that the simultaneous use of different RBD questionnaires gives different prevalences,[114] so, in general, questionnaires only allow the diagnosis of probable RBD. The low value of the questionnaire alone in comparison to video polysomnography in correctly diagnosing RBD also is reflected in the prodromal PD research criteria where video polysomnography proven RBD has a likelihood ratio of 130, whereas RBD as diagnosed by a validated questionnaire with high sensitivity and specificity only has a likelihood ratio of 2.3.[118]

Therefore, video-polysomnography remains at present the single outstanding gold standard for diagnosing RBD. Video polysomnography also is a possible marker of progression and treatment response.[91] Nevertheless, polysomnography is a time-consuming and not always widely available examination. Because of the cumbersomeness of manual quantification of REM sleep without atonia, computerized methods have been used.[119,120]

Therefore, further attempts to develop tools to make an accurate and safe diagnosis of RBD are much needed. Actigraphy has proved useful in raising high suspicion of RBD,[121–124] but this remains to be confirmed in patients with PD. A large study recently has shown that 3-dimensiaonl depth video with time-of-flight measurements of body height maps throughout the night is an extremely useful tool for detecting RBD-related jerks during the night.[125] Further tools have been evaluated in smaller pilot studies but still have not been evaluated in RBD.[126]

Due to different diagnostic criteria and rapid evolution of this field over the past years, with the use of many biomarkers, novel proposed diagnostic methods, and the recent recognition of a prodromal phase, a strong need for a consensus on definitions and research methods in RBD and its prodromal phases has been recognized.[98]

Treatment of Rapid Eye Movement Sleep Behavior Disorder

Treatment of RBD in patients with PD mostly mirrors the treatment of isolated RBD, with the theoretic caveat that a low dose of clonazepam used to treat RBD theoretically could worsen preexisting sleep apnea or daytime sleepiness. The lack of effect of clonazepam in a recent double-blind study[127] probably was due to the underpowered study and inappropriate subjective outcome measures. The same possibly is true for a recent trial with prolonged-release melatonin,[128] where outcomes performed were only with subjective scales and a diary. In addition, previous case reports were based mostly on regular melatonin as opposed to prolonged release.

OTHER PARASOMNIAS

Apart from RBD, non-REM parasomnias, including confusional arousals and sleepwalking, have been reported in PD[129–132] and seem to indicate a risk of cognitive decline.[133]

SLEEP-RELATED MOVEMENT DISORDERS

The category of sleep-related movement disorders has a wide range, including restless legs syndrome (RLS), PLM disorders, sleep-related leg cramps, sleep-related bruxism, sleep-related rhythmic movement disorder, and propriospinal myoclonus of sleep onset. Furthermore, among the subcategory of isolated symptoms and normal variants in sleep-related movement disorders is found excessive fragmentary myoclonus, hypnagogic foot tremor, and alternating leg muscle activation and sleep starts.

Diagnosis of all these disorders is particularly difficult in patients with PD, because (motor and sensory) PD symptoms can interfere with a diagnosis of a sleep-related movement disorder.[134]

Previous studies on the prevalence of RLS in PD have shown percentages ranging between 0 and 52.3% (reviewed by Peralta and colleagues[135] and by Poewe and Högl[136]), which is a clear indicator that there may be some diagnostic difficulties. Confusion of RLS symptoms with motor complications of PD, namely, early morning dystonia, big toe dyskinesia, biphasic dyskinesia, and others, was mentioned as a caveat years ago.[137] Gjerstad and colleagues[138] found that restlessness was frequent but that true RLS did not increase compared with controls in patients with PD, and similar findings were found in another study.[139]

PD patients usually are on dopaminergic treatment. Concerning RLS, dopaminergic-induced augmentation is frequent in patients treated with levodopa[140] and pramipexole.[141] The contribution of dopaminergic-induced augmentation of RLS-like symptoms in patients with PD remains an open question,[142] not always easy to disentangle. Moreover, specifically in patients with PD, RLS also must be differentiated from akathisia.[136]

Periodic leg movements during sleep (PLMSs) are a frequent finding in patients with PD[134,143] and seem to respond to dopaminergic treatment.[29] Because PLMSs are a common finding, the presence of PLMSs during polysomnography is not sufficient to make a diagnosis of PLM disorder. In contrast, when PLMSs occur in PD, specific questioning for symptoms of RLS should follow.[144] In cases of diagnostic difficulties, a suggested immobilization test should be performed.[145]

Several other motor disorders of sleep might be present in patients with PD, including nocturnal akinesia and impaired turning in bed.[146,147] Sleep bruxism also has been reported in PD[121,148,149] and has been suggested as a marker of RBD.[150] Sleep-related leg cramps are a frequent sign in many elderly patients and should be treated adequately.[10] Sleep-related rhythmic movement disorder theoretically could present a differential diagnosis for tremor but it is expected to be infrequent in an elderly population with PD. In contrast, propriospinal myoclonus at sleep onset is characterized by intense whole-body jerks (originating from trunk muscles and spreading to upper and lower extremities with propriospinal propagating speed) and could be a relevant differential diagnosis for intensified PLMs or other types of myoclonus[144]; but, at least for propriospinal myoclonus during wakefulness, a volitional origin has been reported for a large proportion of patients.[151] On the other hand, hypnic jerks seem to be underestimated in PD.[152]

A frequent collateral finding in polysomnography of patients with PD is excessive fragmentary myoclonus, characterized by random occurrence of very brief potentials in the tibial anterior muscles during light sleep, non-REM sleep, and REM sleep.[89,153,154] The occurrence of excessive fragmentary myoclonus has been related to age and the presence of polyneuropathy, benign fasciculation, or lumbar L5 radiculopathy.[155,156] Fragmentary myoclonus also has been observed frequently during non-REM sleep in patients with RBD.[157] Nevertheless, the clinical relevance of the presence of excessive fragmentary myoclonus of sleep still is not known but should prompt further search for peripheral nerve system abnormalities.[156]

Hypnagogic foot tremor and alternating leg movement activation have been described as further random findings during polysomnography and have been added to isolated symptoms and normal variants in the *ICSD-3*. The authors believe that these disorders all belong in the same group of motor phenomena during the transition into sleep[144,158] and can be summarized under the more general and more descriptive name, high-frequency leg movements during sleep (HFLMs).[159] In PD, HFLMs might be a differential diagnosis for tremor before sleep onset (based on their frequency) and also could indicate involuntary movements caused by the medication or voluntary movements to get rid of unpleasant feelings in toes with RLS.[144,158] So the presence of these phenomena (despite the unclear clinical meaningfulness) should prompt further questioning into potential complaints of the patient.

Assessment of Sleep-Related Movement Disorders in Parkinson Disease

Diagnosis of RLS requires a careful history taking and the active exclusion of mimics. The same is true for diagnosis of augmentation, where a detailed clinical interview is essential.[134]

Diagnosis of propriospinal myoclonus never should be made in patients with PD without previously performing a video polysomnography with multiple electromyography channels and averaging of EEG for the jerks (in true propriospinal myoclonus of sleep onset, absence of bereitschaftspotential is expected).[144]

Treatment of Sleep-Related Movement Disorders

Treatment of RLS recently has been the subject of extensive evidence-based reviews.[160,161] There are no specific considerations on treatment of RLS in PD, but the chronic enhancement of the dopaminergic system causes RLS progression or augmentation. Therefore, dopaminergic treatment no longer is recommended as first-line therapy for RLS and alpha-2-delta ligands are a suggested alternative.

SLEEP MOTOR INTERACTION

In PD, sleep benefit (ie, the experience of improvement of motor function upon awakening),[162–166] and a positive effect of sleep deprivation on motor function[167–169] have been reported. Although the concept of sleep benefit has been supported by these studies, there was a significant subjective component in sleep benefit and pharmacodynamic effects, but no relation with specific sleep variables,[162] and other studies did not find any motor improvement at all in PD patients reporting sleep benefit,[170,171] but the definition of sleep benefit always has been a matter of debate and would be worthwhile to consider as an open issue and perhaps be re-evaluated.

CLINICS CARE POINTS

- The spectrum of sleep disorders in PD is large and deserves careful attention.
- A detailed and specific sleep history needs to cover and address all potential categories of sleep disorders to help guide subsequent diagnostic decisions and treatment.
- Movement disorders of sleep, for example, RLS, often are difficult to distinguish from sensory and motor symptoms of PD, unless specific, and deserve careful history taking.
- Parasomnias of non-REM and REM sleep require video polysomnography for differential diagnosis.
- Treatment needs to be tailored individually for each specific sleep disorder and patient and includes nonpharmacological approaches.

DISCLOSURE

The authors have nothing to disclose.

REFERENCES

1. Parkinson J. An essay on the shaking palsy. London: Whittingham and Rowland; 1817.
2. Askenasy JJ. Sleep patterns in extrapyramidal disorders. Int J Neurol 1981;15:62–76.
3. Ferrari E, Puca F, Margherita G. [Anomalies of the spindles during sleep in patients with Parkinson's disease]. Riv Neurol 1964;34:48–55.
4. April RS. Observations on parkinsonian tremor in all-night sleep. Neurology 1966;16:720–4.
5. Matsuoka S, Domino EF, Terada C, et al. The sleep cycle of dyskinetic patients before and after cryothalamotomy. Electroencephalogr Clin Neurophysiol 1967;23:80–1.
6. Stern M, Roffwarg H, Duvoisin R. The parkinsonian tremor in sleep. J Nerv Ment Dis 1968;147:202–10.
7. Puca FM, Bricolo A, Turella G. Effect of L-dopa or amantadine therapy on sleep spindles in Parkinsonism. Electroencephalogr Clin Neurophysiol 1973;35:327–30.
8. Kales A, Ansel RD, Markham CH, et al. Sleep in patients with Parkinson's disease and normal subjects prior to and following levodopa administration. Clin Pharmacol Ther 1971;12:397–406.
9. Hirata K, Hogl B, Tan EK, et al. Sleep problems in Parkinson's disease. Parkinsons Dis 2015;2015:507948.
10. Stefani A, Högl B. Sleep in Parkinson's disease. Neuropsychopharmacology 2020;45:121–8.
11. Vardi J, Glaubman H, Rabey J, et al. EEG sleep patterns in Parkinsonian patients treated with bromocriptine and L-dopa: a comparative study. J Neural Transm 1979;45:307–16.
12. Traczynska-Kubin D, Atzef E, Petre-Quadens O. [Sleep in parkinsonism]. Acta Neurol Psychiatr Belg 1969;69:727–33.
13. Wein A, Golubev V, Yakhno N. Polygraphic analysis of sleep and wakefulness in patients with Parkinson's syndrome. Waking Sleeping 1979;3:31–40.
14. Trenkwalder C, Högl B. Sleep in Parkinson syndromes. In: Handbook of clinical neurology. Elsevier; 2007. p. 365–76.
15. Poewe W, Hogl B. Parkinson's disease and sleep. Curr Opin Neurol 2000;13:423–6.
16. Bhidayasiri R, Sringean J, Trenkwalder C. Mastering nocturnal jigsaws in Parkinson's disease: a dusk-to-dawn review of night-time symptoms. J Neural Transm 2020;127:763–77.
17. Trenkwalder C, Hogl B. Sleep in Parkinson syndromes. Handb Clin Neurol 2007;83:365–76.
18. Tholfsen LK, Larsen JP, Schulz J, et al. Changes in insomnia subtypes in early Parkinson disease. Neurology 2017;88:352–8.
19. Gao J, Huang X, Park Y, et al. Daytime napping, nighttime sleeping, and Parkinson disease. Am J Epidemiol 2011;173:1032–8.
20. Sixel-Doring F, Trautmann E, Mollenhauer B, et al. Age, drugs, or disease: what alters the macrostructure of sleep in Parkinson's disease? Sleep Med 2012;13:1178–83.
21. Schrag A, Horsfall L, Walters K, et al. Prediagnostic presentations of Parkinson's disease in primary care: a case-control study. Lancet Neurol 2015; 14:57–64.
22. Hsiao YH, Chen YT, Tseng CM, et al. Sleep disorders and an increased risk of Parkinson's disease in individuals with non-apnea sleep disorders: a population-based cohort study. J Sleep Res 2017; 26:623–8.
23. Plouvier AO, Hameleers RJ, van den Heuvel EA, et al. Prodromal symptoms and early detection of Parkinson's disease in general practice: a nested case-control study. Fam Pract 2014;31:373–8.
24. Lysen TS, Darweesh SKL, Ikram MK, et al. Sleep and risk of parkinsonism and Parkinson's disease: a population-based study. Brain 2019;142:2013–22.
25. Diederich NJ, Rufra O, Pieri V, et al. Lack of polysomnographic Non-REM sleep changes in early Parkinson's disease. Mov Disord 2013;28:1443–6.
26. Priano L, Bigoni M, Albani G, et al. Sleep microstructure in Parkinson's disease: cycling alternating pattern (CAP) as a sensitive marker of early NREM sleep instability. Sleep Med 2019;61:57–62.
27. Wetter TC, Brunner H, Högl B, et al. Increased alpha activity in REM sleep in de novo patients with Parkinson's disease. Mov Disord 2001;16:928–33.
28. Brunner H, Wetter TC, Hogl B, et al. Microstructure of the non-rapid eye movement sleep electroencephalogram in patients with newly diagnosed Parkinson's disease: effects of dopaminergic treatment. Mov Disord 2002;17:928–33.
29. Högl B, Rothdach A, Wetter TC, et al. The effect of cabergoline on sleep, periodic leg movements in sleep, and early morning motor function in patients with Parkinson's disease. Neuropsychopharmacology 2003;28:1866–70.
30. Sobreira EST, Sobreira-Neto MA, Pena-Pereira MA, et al. Global cognitive performance is associated with sleep efficiency measured by polysomnography in patients with Parkinson's disease. Psychiatry Clin Neurosci 2019;73:248–53.
31. Schreiner SJ, Imbach LL, Werth E, et al. Slow-wave sleep and motor progression in Parkinson disease. Ann Neurol 2019;85:765–70.
32. Amato N, Manconi M, Moller JC, et al. Levodopa-induced dyskinesia in Parkinson disease: sleep matters. Ann Neurol 2018;84:905–17.
33. Hogl B, Arnulf I, Comella C, et al. Scales to assess sleep impairment in Parkinson's disease: critique and recommendations. Mov Disord 2010;25:2704–16.

34. Chaudhuri KR, Pal S, DiMarco A, et al. The Parkinson's disease sleep scale: a new instrument for assessing sleep and nocturnal disability in Parkinson's disease. J Neurol Neurosurg Psychiatry 2002;73:629–35.

35. Trenkwalder C, Kohnen R, Högl B, et al. Parkinson's disease sleep scale – validation of the Revised version PDSS-2. Mov Disord 2011;26(4):644–52.

36. Seppi K, Ray Chaudhuri K, Coelho M, et al. Update on treatments for nonmotor symptoms of Parkinson's disease-an evidence-based medicine review. Mov Disord 2019;34:180–98.

37. Baglioni C, Altena E, Bjorvatn B, et al. The European academy for cognitive behavioural therapy for insomnia: an initiative of the European insomnia Network to promote implementation and dissemination of treatment. J Sleep Res 2020;29:e12967.

38. Park M, Comella CL. Insomnia in Parkinson's disease. In: Videnovic A, Högl B, editors. Disorders of sleep and circadian rhythms in Parkinson's disease. Wien: Springer-Verlag; 2015. p. 79–91.

39. Lebrun C, Gely-Nargeot MC, Rossignol A, et al. Efficacy of cognitive behavioral therapy for insomnia comorbid to Parkinson's disease: a focus on psychological and daytime functioning with a single-case design with multiple baselines. J Clin Psychol 2020;76:356–76.

40. Lebrun C, Gely-Nargeot MC, Maudarbocus KH, et al. Presleep cognitive arousal and insomnia comorbid to Parkinson disease: evidence for a serial Mediation model of sleep-related safety behaviors and dysfunctional Beliefs about sleep. J Clin Sleep Med 2019;15:1217–24.

41. Tandberg E, Larsen JP, Karlsen K. A community-based study of sleep disorders in patients with Parkinson's disease. Mov Disord 1998;13:895–9.

42. Hogl B, Seppi K, Brandauer E, et al. Increased daytime sleepiness in Parkinson's disease: a questionnaire survey. Mov Disord 2003;18:319–23.

43. Djamshidian A, Poewe W, Hogl B. Impact of impulse control disorders on sleep-wake regulation in Parkinson's disease. Parkinsons Dis 2015;2015:970862.

44. Merino-Andreu M, Arnulf I, Konofal E, et al. Unawareness of naps in Parkinson's disease and in disorders with excessive daytime sleepiness. Neurology 2003;60:1553–4.

45. American Psychiatric Association. Diagnostic and statistical manual of mental disorders : DSM-5. 5th edition. Washington, DC: American Psychiatric Association; 2013.

46. Rye DB, Bliwise DL, Dihenia B, et al. Fast TRACK: daytime sleepiness in Parkinson's disease. J Sleep Res 2000;9:63–9.

47. Lal S, Grassino A, Thavundayil JX, et al. A simple method for the study of yawning in man induced by the dopamine receptor agonist, apomorphine. Prog Neuropsychopharmacol Biol Psychiatry 1987;11:223–8.

48. Hogl B, Seppi K, Brandauer E, et al. Irresistible onset of sleep during acute levodopa challenge in a patient with multiple system atrophy (MSA): placebo-controlled, polysomnographic case report. Mov Disord 2001;16:1177–9.

49. Seppi K, Hogl B, Diem A, et al. Levodopa-induced sleepiness in the Parkinson variant of multiple system atrophy. Mov Disord 2006;21:1281–3.

50. Frucht S, Rogers JD, Greene PE, et al. Falling asleep at the wheel: motor vehicle mishaps in persons taking pramipexole and ropinirole. Neurology 1999;52:1908–10.

51. Shprecher DR, Adler CH, Zhang N, et al. Do Parkinson disease subject and caregiver-reported Epworth sleepiness scale reponses correlate? Clin Neurol Neurosurg 2020;192:105728.

52. Abbott RD, Ross GW, Duda JE, et al. Excessive daytime sleepiness and topographic expansion of Lewy pathology. Neurology 2019;93:e1425–32.

53. Simuni T, Caspell-Garcia C, Coffey C, et al. Correlates of excessive daytime sleepiness in de novo Parkinson's disease: a case control study. Mov Disord 2015;30:1371–81.

54. Amara AW, Chahine LM, Caspell-Garcia C, et al. Longitudinal assessment of excessive daytime sleepiness in early Parkinson's disease. J Neurol Neurosurg Psychiatry 2017;88:653–62.

55. Arnulf I, Leu-Semenescu S, Dodet P. Precision medicine for idiopathic Hypersomnia. Sleep Med Clin 2019;14:333–50.

56. Arnulf I, Konofal E, Merino-Andreu M, et al. Parkinson's disease and sleepiness: an integral part of PD. Neurology 2002;58:1019–24.

57. Arnulf I, Neutel D, Herlin B, et al. Sleepiness in idiopathic REM sleep behavior disorder and Parkinson disease. Sleep 2015;38:1529–35.

58. Hogl B, Saletu M, Brandauer E, et al. Modafinil for the treatment of daytime sleepiness in Parkinson's disease: a double-blind, randomized, crossover, placebo-controlled polygraphic trial. Sleep 2002; 25:905–9.

59. Rodrigues TM, Castro Caldas A, Ferreira JJ. Pharmacological interventions for daytime sleepiness and sleep disorders in Parkinson's disease: Systematic review and meta-analysis. Parkinsonism Relat Disord 2016;27:25–34.

60. Adler CH, Caviness JN, Hentz JG, et al. Randomized trial of modafinil for treating subjective daytime sleepiness in patients with Parkinson's disease. Mov Disord 2003;18:287–93.

61. Braga-Neto P, da Silva-Junior FP, Sueli Monte F, et al. Snoring and excessive daytime sleepiness in Parkinson's disease. J Neurol Sci 2004;217:41–5.

62. Suzuki K, Miyamoto M, Miyamoto T, et al. Snoring is associated with an impaired motor function, disease severity and the quality of life but not with

excessive daytime sleepiness in patients with Parkinson's disease. Intern Med 2013;52:863–9.

63. Cochen De Cock V, Abouda M, Leu S, et al. Is obstructive sleep apnea a problem in Parkinson's disease? Sleep Med 2010;11:247–52.

64. Cochen De Cock V, Benard-Serre N, Driss V, et al. Supine sleep and obstructive sleep apnea syndrome in Parkinson's disease. Sleep Med 2015;16:1497–501.

65. Hogl B. Sleep apnea in Parkinson's disease: when is it significant? Sleep Med 2010;11:233–5.

66. Diederich NJ, Vaillant M, Leischen M, et al. Sleep apnea syndrome in Parkinson's disease. A case-control study in 49 patients. Mov Disord 2005;20:1413–8.

67. Trotti LM, Bliwise DL. No increased risk of obstructive sleep apnea in Parkinson's disease. Mov Disord 2010;25:2246–9.

68. Vincken W, Cosio MG. Flow oscillations on the flow-volume loop: a nonspecific indicator of upper airway dysfunction. Bull Eur Physiopathol Respir 1985;21:559–67.

69. Chokroverty S. Sleep disorders medicine : basic science, technical considerations, and clinical aspects. 3rd edition. Philadelphia: Saunders/Elsevier; 2009.

70. Cortelli P, Calandra-Buonaura G, Benarroch EE, et al. Stridor in multiple system atrophy: consensus statement on diagnosis, prognosis, and treatment. Neurology 2019;93:630–9.

71. Harmell AL, Neikrug AB, Palmer BW, et al. Obstructive sleep apnea and cognition in Parkinson's disease. Sleep Med 2016;21:28–34.

72. Videnovic A, Högl B. Disorders of sleep and circadian rhythms in Parkinson's disease. Wien: Springer-Verlag; 2015.

73. Shochat T, Martin J, Marler M, et al. Illumination levels in nursing home patients: effects on sleep and activity rhythms. J Sleep Res 2000;9:373–9.

74. Videnovic A, Golombek D. Circadian and sleep disorders in Parkinson's disease. Exp Neurol 2013;243:45–56.

75. Videnovic A, Lazar AS, Barker RA, et al. 'The clocks that time us'–circadian rhythms in neurodegenerative disorders. Nat Rev Neurol 2014;10:683–93.

76. Fertl E, Auff E, Doppelbauer A, et al. Circadian secretion pattern of melatonin in de novo parkinsonian patients: evidence for phase-shifting properties of l-dopa. J Neural Transm Park Dis Dement Sect 1993;5:227–34.

77. Garcia-Borreguero D, Larrosa O, Granizo JJ, et al. Circadian variation in neuroendocrine response to L-dopa in patients with restless legs syndrome. Sleep 2004;27:669–73.

78. Hogl B. Circadian rhythms and chronotherapeutics-underappreciated approach to improving sleep and wakefulness in Parkinson disease. JAMA Neurol 2017;74:387–8.

79. Gu Z, Wang B, Zhang YB, et al. Association of ARNTL and PER1 genes with Parkinson's disease: a case-control study of han Chinese. Sci Rep 2015;5:15891.

80. Smith MT, McCrae CS, Cheung J, et al. Use of actigraphy for the evaluation of sleep disorders and circadian rhythm sleep-wake disorders: an American Academy of Sleep Medicine Clinical Practice Guideline. J Clin Sleep Med 2018;14:1231–7.

81. Zee PC, Abbott SM. Circadian rhythm sleep-wake disorders. Continuum (Minneap Minn) 2020;26:988–1002.

82. Videnovic A, Klerman EB, Wang W, et al. Timed light therapy for sleep and daytime sleepiness associated with Parkinson's disease: results of a randomized trial. JAMA Neurol 2016;74(4):411–8.

83. Endo T, Matsumura R, Tokuda IT, et al. Bright light improves sleep in patients with Parkinson's disease: possible role of circadian restoration. Sci Rep 2020;10:7982.

84. Videnovic A. Management of sleep disorders in Parkinson's disease and multiple system atrophy. Mov Disord 2017;32:659–68.

85. Pfeffer M, Zimmermann Z, Gispert S, et al. Impaired photic entrainment of spontaneous locomotor activity in mice overexpressing human mutant alpha-synuclein. Int J Mol Sci 2018;19:1651.

86. Delgado-Lara DL, Gonzalez-Enriquez GV, Torres-Mendoza BM, et al. Effect of melatonin administration on the PER1 and BMAL1 clock genes in patients with Parkinson's disease. Biomed Pharmacother 2020;129:110485.

87. Frauscher B, Gschliesser V, Brandauer E, et al. Video analysis of motor events in REM sleep behavior disorder. Mov Disord 2007;22:1464–70.

88. Frauscher B, Gschliesser V, Brandauer E, et al. The relation between abnormal behaviors and REM sleep microstructure in patients with REM sleep behavior disorder. Sleep Med 2009;10:174–81.

89. American Academy of Sleep Medicine. The international classification of sleep disorders : diagnostic & coding manual (ICSD-3). 3rd edition. Westchester (IL): American Academy of Sleep Medicine; 2014.

90. Schenck CH, Montplaisir JY, Frauscher B, et al. Rapid eye movement sleep behavior disorder: devising controlled active treatment studies for symptomatic and neuroprotective therapy–a consensus statement from the International Rapid Eye Movement Sleep Behavior Disorder Study Group. Sleep Med 2013;14:795–806.

91. Hogl B, Stefani A, Videnovic A. Idiopathic REM sleep behaviour disorder and neurodegeneration - an update. Nat Rev Neurol 2018;14:40–55.

92. Postuma RB, Iranzo A, Hu M, et al. Risk and predictors of dementia and parkinsonism in idiopathic REM sleep behaviour disorder: a multicentre study. Brain 2019;142:744–59.

93. Schenck CH, Boeve BF, Mahowald MW. Delayed emergence of a parkinsonian disorder or dementia in 81% of older men initially diagnosed with idiopathic rapid eye movement sleep behavior disorder: a 16-year update on a previously reported series. Sleep Med 2013;14:744–8.

94. Wetter TC, Trenkwalder C, Gershanik O, et al. Polysomnographic measures in Parkinson's disease: a comparison between patients with and without REM sleep disturbances. Wien Klin Wochenschr 2001;113:249–53.

95. Sixel-Doring F, Zimmermann J, Wegener A, et al. The Evolution of REM sleep behavior disorder in early Parkinson disease. Sleep 2016;39:1737–42.

96. Braak H, Del Tredici K, Rub U, et al. Staging of brain pathology related to sporadic Parkinson's disease. Neurobiol Aging 2003;24:197–211.

97. Lai YY, Siegel JM. Physiological and anatomical link between Parkinson-like disease and REM sleep behavior disorder. Mol Neurobiol 2003;27:137–52.

98. Stefani A, Iranzo A, Sixel-Doring F, et al. Need for a consensus on definitions and on research methods in RBD and its prodromal phases. Sleep 2019;42: zsz057.

99. Mahlknecht P, Iranzo A, Hogl B, et al. Olfactory dysfunction predicts early transition to a Lewy body disease in idiopathic RBD. Neurology 2015; 84:654–8.

100. Stiasny-Kolster K, Doerr Y, Moller JC, et al. Combination of 'idiopathic' REM sleep behaviour disorder and olfactory dysfunction as possible indicator for alpha-synucleinopathy demonstrated by dopamine transporter FP-CIT-SPECT. Brain 2005;128:126–37.

101. Videnovic A, Ju YS, Arnulf I, et al. Clinical trials in REM sleep behavioural disorder: challenges and opportunities. J Neurol Neurosurg Psychiatry 2020;91:740–9.

102. Iranzo A, Molinuevo JL, Santamaria J, et al. Rapid-eye-movement sleep behaviour disorder as an early marker for a neurodegenerative disorder: a descriptive study. Lancet Neurol 2006;5:572–7.

103. Lai YY, Hsieh KC, Nguyen D, et al. Neurotoxic lesions at the ventral mesopontine junction change sleep time and muscle activity during sleep: an animal model of motor disorders in sleep. Neuroscience 2008;154:431–43.

104. Horsager J, Andersen KB, Knudsen K, et al. Brain-first versus body-first Parkinson's disease: a multimodal imaging case-control study. Brain 2020; 143(10):3077–88.

105. Valli K, Frauscher B, Peltomaa T, et al. Dreaming furiously? A sleep laboratory study on the dream content of people with Parkinson's disease and with or without rapid eye movement sleep behavior disorder. Sleep Med 2015;16:419–27.

106. Iranzo A, Stefani A, Ninerola-Baizan A, et al. Left-hemispheric predominance of nigrostriatal deficit in isolated REM sleep behavior disorder. Neurology 2020;94:e1605–13.

107. Iranzo A, Santamaria J, Valldeoriola F, et al. Dopamine transporter imaging deficit predicts early transition to synucleinopathy in idiopathic REM sleep behavior disorder. Ann Neurol 2017;82: 419–28.

108. Iranzo A, Stefani A, Serradell M, et al. Characterization of patients with longstanding idiopathic REM sleep behavior disorder. Neurology 2017;89:242–8.

109. Stiasny-Kolster K, Sixel-Doring F, Trenkwalder C, et al. Diagnostic value of the REM sleep behavior disorder screening questionnaire in Parkinson's disease. Sleep Med 2015;16:186–9.

110. Postuma RB, Arnulf I, Hogl B, et al. A single-question screen for rapid eye movement sleep behavior disorder: a multicenter validation study. Mov Disord 2012;27:913–6.

111. Frauscher B, Ehrmann L, Zamarian L, et al. Validation of the Innsbruck REM sleep behavior disorder inventory. Mov Disord 2012;27:1673–8.

112. Li SX, Wing YK, Lam SP, et al. Validation of a new REM sleep behavior disorder questionnaire (RBDQ-HK). Sleep Med 2010;11:43–8.

113. Halsband C, Zapf A, Sixel-Doring F, et al. The REM sleep behavior disorder screening questionnaire is not Valid in de novo Parkinson's disease. Mov Disord Clin Pract 2018;5:171–6.

114. Mahlknecht P, Seppi K, Frauscher B, et al. Probable RBD and association with neurodegenerative disease markers: a population-based study. Mov Disord 2015;30:1417–21.

115. Stefani A, Mahlknecht P, Seppi K, et al. Consistency of "probable RBD" diagnosis with the RBD screening questionnaire: a follow-up study. Mov Disord Clin Pract 2017;4:403–5.

116. Frauscher B, Mitterling T, Bode A, et al. A prospective questionnaire study in 100 healthy sleepers: non-bothersome forms of recognizable sleep disorders are still present. JCSM 2014.

117. Pujol M, Pujol J, Alonso T, et al. Idiopathic REM sleep behavior disorder in the elderly Spanish community: a primary care center study with a two-stage design using video-polysomnography. Sleep Med 2017;40:116–21.

118. Berg D, Postuma RB, Adler CH, et al. MDS research criteria for prodromal Parkinson's disease. Mov Disord 2015;30:1600–11.

119. Frauscher B, Gabelia D, Biermayr M, et al. Validation of an integrated software for the detection of rapid eye movement sleep behavior disorder. Sleep 2014;37:1663–71.

120. Cesari M, Christensen JAE, Muntean M-L, et al. A data-driven system to identify REM sleep behavior disorder and to predict its progression from the prodromal stage in Parkinson's disease. Sleep Med 2021;77:238–48.

121. Stefani A, Heidbreder A, Brandauer E, et al. Screening for idiopathic REM sleep behavior disorder: usefulness of actigraphy. Sleep 2018;41: zsy053.

122. Filardi M, Stefani A, Holzknecht E, et al. Objective rest-activity cycle analysis by actigraphy identifies isolated rapid eye movement sleep behavior disorder. Eur J Neurol 2020;27(10):1848–55.

123. Louter M, Arends JB, Bloem BR, et al. Actigraphy as a diagnostic aid for REM sleep behavior disorder in Parkinson's disease. BMC Neurol 2014;14:76.

124. Feng H, Chen L, Liu Y, et al. Rest-activity pattern alterations in idiopathic REM sleep behavior disorder. Ann Neurol 2020;88(4):817–29.

125. Waser M, Stefani A, Holzknecht E, et al. Automated 3D video analysis of lower limb movements during REM sleep: a new diagnostic tool for isolated REM sleep behavior disorder. Sleep 2020;43(11): zsaa100.

126. Shustak S, Inzelberg L, Steinberg S, et al. Home monitoring of sleep with a temporary-tattoo EEG, EOG and EMG electrode array: a feasibility study. J Neural Eng 2019;16:026024.

127. Shin C, Park H, Lee WW, et al. Clonazepam for probable REM sleep behavior disorder in Parkinson's disease: a randomized placebo-controlled trial. J Neurol Sci 2019;401:81–6.

128. Jun JS, Kim R, Byun JI, et al. Prolonged-release melatonin in patients with idiopathic REM sleep behavior disorder. Ann Clin Transl Neurol 2019;6: 716–22.

129. Fernandez-Arcos A, Iranzo A, Serradell M, et al. The clinical phenotype of idiopathic rapid eye movement sleep behavior disorder at presentation: a study in 203 consecutive patients. Sleep 2016; 39:121–32.

130. Oberholzer M, Poryazova R, Bassetti CL. Sleepwalking in Parkinson's disease: a questionnaire-based survey. J Neurol 2011;258:1261–7.

131. Di Fabio N, Poryazova R, Oberholzer M, et al. Sleepwalking, REM sleep behaviour disorder and overlap parasomnia in patients with Parkinson's disease. Eur Neurol 2013;70:297–303.

132. Poryazova R, Waldvogel D, Bassetti CL. Sleepwalking in patients with Parkinson disease. Arch Neurol 2007;64:1524–7.

133. Terzaghi M, Minafra B, Zangaglia R, et al. NREM sleep arousal-related disorders reflect cognitive impairment in Q5 Parkinson's disease. Sleep Med 2020;75:491–6.

134. Hogl B, Stefani A. Restless legs syndrome and periodic leg movements in patients with movement disorders: specific considerations. Mov Disord 2017;32:669–81.

135. Peralta CM, Frauscher B, Seppi K, et al. Restless legs syndrome in Parkinson's disease. Mov Disord 2009;24:2076–80.

136. Poewe W, Högl B. Akathisia, restless legs and periodic limb movements in sleep in Parkinson's disease. Neurology 2004;63:S12–6.

137. Comella CL. Sleep disturbances in Parkinson's disease. Curr Neurol Neurosci Rep 2003;3:173–80.

138. Gjerstad MD, Tysnes OB, Larsen JP. Increased risk of leg motor restlessness but not RLS in early Parkinson disease. Neurology 2011;77:1941–6.

139. Verbaan D, van Rooden SM, van Hilten JJ, et al. Prevalence and clinical profile of restless legs syndrome in Parkinson's disease. Mov Disord 2010;25:2142–7.

140. Hogl B, Garcia-Borreguero D, Kohnen R, et al. Progressive development of augmentation during long-term treatment with levodopa in restless legs syndrome: results of a prospective multi-center study. J Neurol 2010;257:230–7.

141. Hogl B, Garcia-Borreguero D, Trenkwalder C, et al. Efficacy and augmentation during 6 months of double-blind pramipexole for restless legs syndrome. Sleep Med 2011;12:351–60.

142. Ferini-Strambi L, Carli G, Casoni F, et al. Restless legs syndrome and Parkinson disease: a causal relationship between the two disorders? Front Neurol 2018;9:551.

143. Wetter TC, Collado-Seidel V, Pollmacher T, et al. Sleep and periodic leg movement patterns in drug-free patients with Parkinson's disease and multiple system atrophy. Sleep 2000;23:361–7.

144. Stefani A, Högl B. Diagnostic criteria, differential diagnosis, and treatment of minor motor activity and less well-known movement disorders of sleep. Curr Treat Options Neurol 2019;21:1.

145. De Cock VC, Bayard S, Yu H, et al. Suggested immobilization test for diagnosis of restless legs syndrome in Parkinson's disease. Mov Disord 2012;27:743–9.

146. Sringean J, Taechalertpaisarn P, Thanawattano C, et al. How well do Parkinson's disease patients turn in bed? Quantitative analysis of nocturnal hypokinesia using multisite wearable inertial sensors. Parkinsonism Relat Disord 2016;23:10–6.

147. Louter M, van Sloun RJ, Pevernagie DA, et al. Subjectively impaired bed mobility in Parkinson disease affects sleep efficiency. Sleep Med 2013;14: 668–74.

148. Verhoeff MC, Lobbezoo F, Wetselaar P, et al. Parkinson's disease, temporomandibular disorders and bruxism: a pilot study. J Oral Rehabil 2018; 45:854–63.

149. Ylikoski A, Martikainen K, Partinen M. Parasomnias and isolated sleep symptoms in Parkinson's disease: a questionnaire study on 661 patients. J Neurol Sci 2014;346:204–8.

150. Abe S, Gagnon JF, Montplaisir JY, et al. Sleep bruxism and oromandibular myoclonus in rapid eye movement sleep behavior disorder: a preliminary report. Sleep Med 2013;14:1024–30.

151. van der Salm SM, Erro R, Cordivari C, et al. Proprio-spinal myoclonus: clinical reappraisal and review of literature. Neurology 2014;83:1862–70.

152. Chiaro G, Maestri M, Riccardi S, et al. Sleep-related rhythmic movement disorder and obstructive sleep apnea in five Adult patients. J Clin Sleep Med 2017;13:1213–7.

153. Vetrugno R, Plazzi G, Provini F, et al. Excessive fragmentary hypnic myoclonus: clinical and neuro-physiological findings. Sleep Med 2002;3:73–6.

154. Montagna P, Liguori R, Zucconi M, et al. Physiological hypnic myoclonus. Electroencephalogr Clin Neurophysiol 1988;70:172–6.

155. Frauscher B, Kunz A, Brandauer E, et al. Fragmentary myoclonus in sleep revisited: a polysomnographic study in 62 patients. Sleep Med 2011;12:410–5.

156. Raccagni C, Loscher WN, Stefani A, et al. Peripheral nerve function in patients with excessive fragmentary myoclonus during sleep. Sleep Med 2016;22:61–4.

157. Nepozitek J, Dostalova S, Kemlink D, et al. Fragmentary myoclonus in idiopathic rapid eye movement sleep behaviour disorder. J Sleep Res 2019;28:e12819.

158. Bergmann M, Stefani A, Brandauer E, et al. Hypnagogic foot tremor, alternating leg muscle activation or high frequency leg movements: clinical and phenomenological considerations in two cousins. Sleep Med 2018;54:177–80.

159. Yang C, Winkelman JW. Clinical and polysomnographic characteristics of high frequency leg movements. J Clin Sleep Med 2010;6:431–8.

160. Winkelmann J, Allen RP, Hogl B, et al. Treatment of restless legs syndrome: evidence-based review and implications for clinical practice (Revised 2017)(section sign). Mov Disord 2018;33:1077–91.

161. Winkelman JW, Armstrong MJ, Allen RP, et al. Practice guideline summary: treatment of restless legs syndrome in adults: report of the guideline development, dissemination, and implementation subcommittee of the american academy of neurology. Neurology 2016;87(24):2585–93.

162. Högl B, Gomez-Arevalo G, Garcia S, et al. A clinical, pharmacologic, and polysomnographic study of sleep benefit in Parkinson's disease. Neurology 1998;50:1332–9.

163. Hogl B, Gershanik O. Sleep benefit in Parkinson's disease. J Neurol Neurosurg Psychiatry 2000;68:798–9.

164. Tandberg E, Larsen JP, Karlsen K. Excessive daytime sleepiness and sleep benefit in Parkinson's disease: a community-based study. Mov Disord 1999;14:922–7.

165. Merello M, Hughes A, Colosimo C, et al. Sleep benefit in Parkinson's disease. Mov Disord 1997;12:506–8.

166. Currie LJ, Bennett JP Jr, Harrison MB, et al. Clinical correlates of sleep benefit in Parkinson's disease. Neurology 1997;48:1115–7.

167. Reist C, Sokolski KN, Chen CC, et al. The effect of sleep deprivation on motor impairment and retinal adaptation in Parkinson's disease. Prog Neuropsychopharmacol Biol Psychiatry 1995;19:445–54.

168. Bertolucci PH, Andrade LA, Lima JG, et al. Total sleep deprivation and Parkinson disease. Arq Neuropsiquiatr 1987;45:224–30.

169. Hogl B, Peralta C, Wetter TC, et al. Effect of sleep deprivation on motor performance in patients with Parkinson's disease. Mov Disord 2001;16:616–21.

170. van Gilst MM, Bloem BR, Overeem S. Prospective assessment of subjective sleep benefit in Parkinson's disease. BMC Neurol 2015;15:2.

171. van Gilst MM, van Mierlo P, Bloem BR, et al. Quantitative motor performance and sleep benefit in Parkinson disease. Sleep 2015;38:1567–73.

The Isolated Form of Rapid Eye Movement Sleep Behavior Disorder
The Upcoming Challenges

Alex Iranzo, MD[a,*], Lina Agudelo Ramos, MD[b], Sabela Novo, MD[c,d]

KEYWORDS

- REM sleep behavior disorder • Synucleinopathy • Parkinson disease • Dementia with Lewy bodies
- Multiple system atrophy • Neuroprotection

KEY POINTS

- The first upcoming challenge is to provide a reliable, accurate, easy, and fast diagnostic methodology for the diagnosis of rapid eye movement (REM) sleep behavior disorder.
- The second upcoming challenge is the implementation of a neuroprotective clinical trial in isolated REM sleep behavior disorder to prevent the onset of parkinsonism and dementia.
- The third upcoming challenge is to identify an effective symptomatic therapy for REM sleep behavior disorder symptoms in patients in whom clonazepam and melatonin are not effective or are associated with side effects.

DEFINITION

Rapid eye movement (REM) sleep behavior disorder (RBD) is an REM sleep parasomnia characterized by loss of muscular atonia during healthy REM sleep that is linked to vigorous movements and vocalizations and fearful dreams.[1,2]

CLINICAL FINDINGS

Patients with RBD have a wide range of manifestations, ranging from small jerky hand movements to violent elaborate and complex activities such as punching, kicking, screaming, shouting, or even leaping out of bed, having a risk to hurt themselves and their bedpartners.[3] Typically, if patients wake up after one of the RBD events, they might recall a nightmare where the dreamer is attacked by an unknown person for unknown reason, acting vigorously in self-defense by fighting back against the attacker or escaping.[3] However, some patients do not recall having an unpleasant dream when awakened. These activities are more often found in the second half of the night, where REM sleep predominates. In a study involving 203 patients with well-characterized isolated RBD (IRBD), 80% were men with a median age at IRBD diagnosis of 68 years (range, 50–85 years).[3] The most frequent reported sleep behaviors were talking (96%), screaming (90%), punching (87%), kicking (82%), and falling out of bed (77%). Sleep-related injuries occurred in 59% of patients and 21% of bed partners. The most frequent nightmare was being attacked (77%). Seventy percent of the patients reported good sleep quality despite showing vigorous dream-enacting behaviors; 44% were unaware of their sleep behaviors, and in these cases bed partners were essential to report the patients' dream-enacting behaviors

---

[a] Neurology Service, Sleep Disorders Center, Hospital Clinic de Barcelona, CIBERNED, IDIBAPS, University of Barcelona, Spain; [b] Neurology Service, Instituto Neurológico de Colombia (INDEC), Calle 55, 46-36, Medellín 050012, Colombia; [c] Instituto de Investigaciones del Sueño, Calle Padre Damián, 44, Madrid 28036, Spain; [d] Hospital Universitario Puerta de Hierro, Majadahonda, Spain
* Corresponding author. Neurology Service, Hospital Clínic de Barcelona, Villarroel 170, Barcelona 08036, Spain.
E-mail address: airanzo@clinic.cat

Sleep Med Clin 16 (2021) 335–348
https://doi.org/10.1016/j.jsmc.2021.03.002

and to convince them to seek medical help. RBD was elicited in 11% only after specific questioning when patients consulted for other reasons. Getting out of bed occurred in 24%, although this happened only on a few nights and 7% did not recall nightmares.[3]

PATHOPHYSIOLOGY

The key structures that generate REM sleep muscle paralysis are the subcoeruleus nucleus in the mesopontine tegmentum and the gigantocellularis nucleus in the ventral medial medulla. Using glutamatergic, GABAergic, and glycinergic inputs, direct and indirect projections from these 2 areas inhibit the motoneurons of the spinal cord, resulting in skeletal paralysis during normal REM sleep.[4] Experimental studies in cats and rodents where the subcoeruleus nucleus and ventral medial medulla were impaired by electrolytic, pharmacologic, and genetic manipulations have repeatedly produced increased electromyography (EMG) activity during REM sleep associated with abnormal motor behaviors (eg, prominent twitching, attack-like behaviors). These animal models represent the pathophysiologic model of RBD indicating that this parasomnia is the result of direct or indirect dysfunction of the lower brainstem.[5]

CLASSIFICATION

RBD may be (1) isolated (also known as idiopathic), when the disorder is primary not linked to any manifest condition or medication, or (2) secondary to a condition such as neurodegenerative diseases (eg, spinocerebellar ataxias, the synucleinopathies Parkinson disease [PD], dementia with Lewy bodies [DLB], and multiple system atrophy [MSA]), lesions that damage the structures in the brainstem that modulate REM sleep atonia (eg, stroke, plaque of multiple sclerosis, neoplasm), autoimmune diseases (eg, anti-IgLON5 disease, paraneoplastic encephalitis, narcolepsy) and diseases related to the introduction of some medications (eg, antidepressants, β-blockers) and withdrawal of alcohol and barbiturates (**Fig. 1**, **Box 1**).[5] This article focuses on IRBD because, in most patients, this parasomnia constitutes the first manifestation of those neurodegenerative diseases characterized by abnormal deposition of the protein alpha-synuclein within the neuron and glial cells, namely the synucleinopathies PD, DLB, and MSA.

EPIDEMIOLOGY

IRBD very rarely occurs in people less than the age of 50 years. IRBD has a prevalence of 0.5% to 1%

in people more than the age of 60 years.[6,7] Most individuals with IRBD do not seek medical consultation because they are unaware of their RBD symptoms or they (and their bed partners) think that they are a normal phenomenon and not a disorder.[6,7] About half of the patients with IRBD are unaware of having dream-enacting behaviors, indicating that the sleep history has to be taken with the bed partner or a reliable informant of the patient's sleep.[3] For unknown reasons, 75% to 85% of the patients with IRBD diagnosed in sleep disorder centers are male. Sex hormone levels are normal in male patients with IRBD.

DIAGNOSIS

A correct diagnosis of IRBD is crucial because it carries a high risk of an eventual evolving synucleinopathy. The diagnosis of IRBD requires (1) chronic history of vigorous behaviors during sleep, (2) videopolysomnographic demonstration of REM sleep with increased EMG activity, (3) absence of motor and cognitive complaints, (4) unremarkable neurologic examination, and (5) normal brain MRI.[2]

The American Academy of Sleep Medicine has established the following diagnostic criteria for RBD that must be met[1]:

A. Repeated episodes of sleep-related vocalization and/or complex motor behaviors
B. Behaviors are documented by polysomnography to occur during REM sleep or, based on a clinical history of dream enactment, are presumed to occur during REM sleep
C. Polysomnography shows REM sleep without atonia
D. The disturbance is not better explained by another sleep disorder, mental disorder, medication, or substance abuse

However, in point C (Polysomnography shows REM sleep without atonia) it was not stated where the EMG has to be measured, and neither it was the exact meaning of REM sleep without atonia defined. There was no indication when the EMG activity in REM sleep is considered excessive or increased for RBD to be diagnosed, because no cutoffs of EMG activity were provided to define what is normal and what is abnormal. The Sleep Innsbruck Barcelona (SINBAR) group using visual/manual quantification of the EMG activity in 3-second miniepochs of REM sleep concluded that the diagnosis of RBD can be made with very high accuracy and sensitivity when the phasic and tonic EMG activity in REM sleep is greater than 32% of the entire REM sleep period measured simultaneously in the mentalis in the chin and both flexor digitorum superficialis

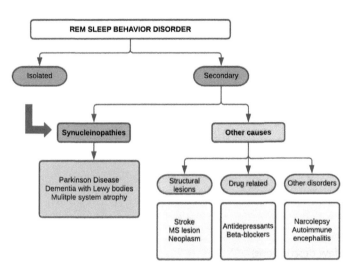

Fig. 1. Isolated (primary) and secondary RBD classification. MS, multiple sclerosis.

muscles in the forearms.[8] A study compared 2 currently used EMG montages, isolated mentalis versus mentalis plus bilateral upper limb muscles in the baseline videopolysomnogram (V-PSG) of patients with IRBD who later developed a synucleinopathy. The montage of mentalis combined with upper limbs best identified the occurrence of RBD. However, videorecording of abnormal behaviors in REM sleep was essential to diagnose RBD in a small subset of patients with EMG values within the normal range.[9] Moreover, in 1 study, V-PSG had to be repeated in 16% of cases for the diagnosis of RBD because of insufficient REM sleep or EMG artifacts from coexistent apneas.[3] Absent or insufficient REM sleep usually occurs in patients treated with antidepressants, because these medications reduce the amount of REM sleep and increase its latency onset.

It is accepted that current diagnosis of RBD requires documentation of excessive EMG activity using V-PSG (**Figs. 2** and **3**). However, V-PSG is expensive, not available in all centers, in some cases it has to be repeated, and the manual/visual quantification of EMG activity is time consuming and requires training and expertise. Thus, one of the current challenges is to find out an easier, faster, and more reliable diagnostic methodology, which may be delayed because of the difficult access and high cost of this type of study in some populations. Experts have proposed several alternatives, namely automatic analysis of the EMG activity, actigraphy, analysis of audiovisual recordings, actigraphy, and questionnaires.

Automatic analysis of the V-PSG studies in RBD is necessary, allowing quantitative measurements in a much easier way. These systems analyze the amount of EMG activity in REM sleep and they include the evaluation of the mentalis plus the flexor digitorum superficialis muscles in both upper extremities.[10,11] The automatic analysis systems need expert human supervision to identify each REM episode and exclude EMG artifacts from the analysis. A recent study proposes an automated method for detecting RBD that consists of automatic sleep staging and subsequently the identification of RBD.[12]

Another option is to study the patients outside the sleep laboratory in their own home environments. One approach is to evaluate visually with a camera the movements the patients display, assuming they correspond with REM sleep. A recent study evaluated the automated three-dimensional video analysis of leg movements during REM sleep as an objective diagnostic tool for the diagnosis of IRBD using specific software.[12] Another diagnostic method is actigraphy on the dominant hand during several weeks to obtain a specific motor pattern during the night in RBD. One study with actigraphy assessed the identification of IRBD against controls and patients with obstructive sleep apnea and restless legs syndrome, and this showed (in the hands of sleep experts) sensitivity of 85% to 95% and specificity of 79% to 91% to identify the typical pattern of RBD.[13]

Available validated questionnaires and single questions for the diagnosis of RBD are sensitive but their specificity is moderate because of misidentification of individuals with IRBD mimics (false-positives), particularly those affected with severe obstructive sleep apnea, periodic leg movements in sleep, sleep terrors, and sleep walking.[14] These questionnaires and single questions have not been validated in persons seeking

---

Box 1
Conditions associated with REM sleep behavior disorder

A. Neurodegenerative diseases

   PD

   Parkinsonism linked to Parkin 2 gene mutations

   Parkinsonism linked to LRRK2 gene mutations

   Parkinsonism linked to GABA gene mutations

   DLB

   MSA

   Mild cognitive impairment

   Pure autonomic failure

   Alzheimer disease (anecdotal cases)

   Progressive supranuclear palsy (a few descriptions)

   Guadalupean parkinsonism (a few descriptions)

   Frontotemporal dementia (anecdotal descriptions)

   Corticobasal syndrome (anecdotal descriptions)

   DJ-1 mutations and parkinsonism-dementia-amyotrophic lateral sclerosis complex (anecdotal descriptions)

   Amyotrophic lateral sclerosis (anecdotal descriptions)

   Neurodegeneration with brain accumulation type 1 (anecdotal descriptions)

   Dentatorubropallidoluysian atrophy (a few descriptions)

   Huntington disease (a few descriptions)

   Spinocerebellar ataxia type 2 (a few descriptions)

   Spinocerebellar ataxia type 3 (a few descriptions)

   Spinocerebellar ataxia type 31 (a few descriptions)

   Wilson disease (a few descriptions)

B. Autoimmune disorders

   Narcolepsy with cataplexy

   Limbic encephalitis associated with antibodies to voltage-gated potassium channels/LIG-1

   Anti-NMDAR encephalitis

   Anti-Ma1 and anti-Ma2 encephalitis

   Guillain-Barré syndrome

C. Other neurologic conditions

   Myotonic dystrophy type 2 (anecdotal descriptions)

   Autism (anecdotal descriptions)

   Tourette syndrome (anecdotal descriptions)

   Arnold-Chiari malformation (anecdotal description)

   Smith-Magenis syndrome (anecdotal description)

   Moebius syndrome (anecdotal description)

   Attention-deficit/hyperactive disorder (anecdotal description)

   Essential tremor (few descriptions)

   Focal brainstem lesions (stroke, cavernoma, tumor, multiple sclerosis plaques) (few descriptions)

D. Medications

   Antidepressants

   β-Blockers

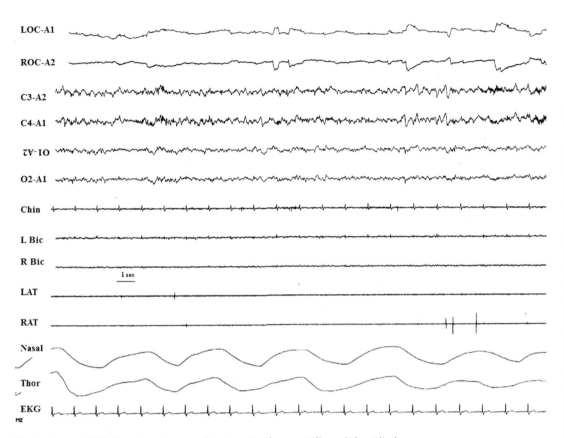

Fig. 2. Normal REM sleep showing muscle atonia in the mentalis and the 4 limbs.

medical advice at their first visits with the complaint of abnormal sleep behaviors but rather in patients diagnosed with RBD and other sleep disorders and followed in routine visits for years.

These diagnostic options need to be better studied to verify their usefulness with respect to V-PSG, which still is the gold standard for the diagnosis of RBD. They can be used in the general population in big cohorts as a first diagnostic step before the implementation of V-PSG in positive cases. In conclusion, current challenges include the validation of accessible methods compared with the gold standard V-PSG with high sensitivity and specificity to distinguish RBD from healthy people and from patients with other conditions that represent the so-called RBD mimics.

RELEVANCE

It is accepted that IRBD is in most, if not all, cases a manifestation of the prodromal stages of the synucleinopathies PD and DLB, and less commonly of MSA.[2] This article review the accumulative data indicating that IRBD represents an early stage of a synucleinopathy before the onset of parkinsonism and cognitive impairment.

Patients with IRBD show clinical and subclinical abnormalities that are characteristic of the synucleinopathies (**Boxes 2** and **3**) (for review, see Ref.[15–17]). Some of the risk factors for IRBD are shared with PD, such as male sex, older age, pesticide exposure, and head injury. The clinical abnormalities typical of the synucleinopathies are seen in patients with IRBD and include soft parkinsonian signs (eg, reduced arm swinging, hypomimia, and upper limb mild bradykinesia), asymptomatic cognitive deficits detected in neuropsychological tests (mainly in the memory, visuospatial, and executive domains), hyposmia (particularly the smell identification function), constipation orthostatic hypotension, erectile dysfunction, and depression. Neurophysiologic evaluation may disclose dysautonomia, abnormalities in heart rate variability, reduced sleep cyclic alternating pattern, and subtle electroencephalographic slowing during wakefulness and REM sleep. Neuroimaging performed while the patient is awake reveals cerebellar atrophy and the hot-cross-bun sign in conventional brain MRI in those

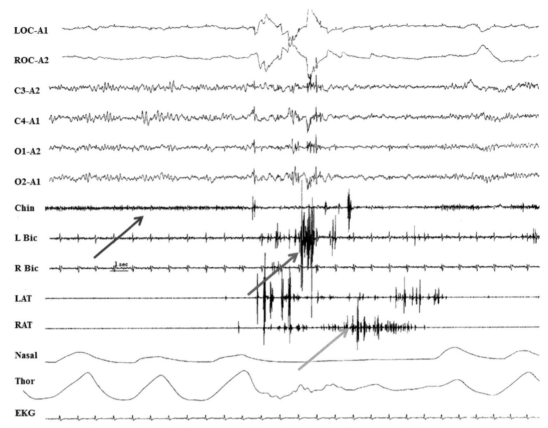

Fig. 3. RBD showing increased tonic electromyographic in the mentalis (*blue arrow*) and increased phasic electromyographic in the left flexor digitorum superficialis (*red arrow*) and in the right anterior tibialis (*green arrow*).

IRBD individuals who will develop MSA with time, decreased diffusion in the brainstem nuclei that modulate REM sleep, loss of dorsolateral hyperintensity in the substantia nigra, reduction in the neuromelanin-sensitive intensity sequences at the locus coeruleus/subcoeruleus complex, hyperechogenicity of the substantia nigra and hypoechogenicity of the brainstem raphe on transcranial sonography, decreased dopamine transporter uptake in the striatum (particularly in the putamen of the dominant hemisphere), increased microglia activation within the substantia nigra, abnormal cardiac scintigraphy, neocortical cholinergic denervation, cortical and right hippocampal atrophy, and reduced cortical perfusion.

These observations indicate that, in IRBD, the neurodegenerative process is not restricted to the brainstem nuclei that regulate REM sleep but extends to other structures, such as the olfactory system, the nigrostriatal system, the autonomic system, and the cortex, which are typically damaged in the synucleinopathies.

Importantly, at the time of diagnosis of IRBD, several abnormalities are able to identify the patients with a high short-term risk to be diagnosed with a clinically defined synucleinopathy. They include dysfunction of the nigrostriatal dopaminergic system disclosed by dopamine transporter single-photon emission computed tomography (DAT-SPECT),[18] abnormal quantitative motor test, hyposmia,[19] color vision abnormalities, and the severity of REM sleep without atonia detected in the mentalis muscle in V-PSG.

Some serial tests are able to monitor the degenerative process, showing progression of baseline deficits. Dopamine transporter imaging shows progressive dopamine content decline in the striatum, particularly in the putamen.[20] Longitudinal neuropsychological testing shows progressive worsening until mild cognitive impairment and subsequent dementia develop. Similarly, motor function declines with time until bradykinesia and rigidity are discernible and the diagnosis of parkinsonism can be made (resting tremor only occurs in a few cases because the rigid-akinetic motor subtype is the most common form of presentation). In contrast, serial midbrain transcranial sonography and smell tests show that the echogenic size of

Box 2
Coexisting abnormalities in isolated rapid eye movement sleep behavior disorder

1. Clinical symptoms and signs
    1.1. Subtle parkinsonian signs
    1.2. Olfactory impairment
    1.3. Color vision impairment
    1.4. Autonomic abnormalities (constipation, orthostatic hypotension, sudomotor abnormalities, urinary symptoms, and erectile dysfunction)
    1.5. Depression
    1.6. Pareidolic responses
    1.7. Deficits in dual tasking
    1.8. Impaired rhythm skills
    1.9. Emotion dysregulation
    1.10. Apathy
2. Neuropsychological deficits in the visuospatial, executive, and memory domains
3. Electrophysiologic abnormalities
    3.1. Electroencephalographic slowing in frontal, temporal, and occipital regions during wakefulness and REM sleep
    3.2. Decreased sleep cyclic alternating pattern
    3.3. Reduced heart rate variability during wakefulness and sleep
    3.4. Esophageal motor impairment
    3.5. Retinal nerve fiber layer thinning
    3.6. Abnormal vestibular evoked myogenic potentials
    3.7. Reduced P300 amplitude
4. Neuroimaging abnormalities
    4.1. Reduced putamen and caudate dopaminergic uptake
    4.2. Substantia nigra hyperechogenicity
    4.3. Brainstem raphe hypoechogenicity
    4.4. Substantia nigra loss of dorsolateral nigral hyperintensity
    4.5. Substantia nigra microglia activation
    4.6. Basal ganglia connectivity dysfunction
    4.7. Altered connectivity between the left substantia nigra with the left putamen and the right occipital lobe
    4.8. Decreased fractional anisotropy and increased mean diffusivity in the midbrain and pontine nuclei that regulate REM sleep
    4.9. Reduced neuromelanin signal intensity in the coeruleus/subcoeruleus area
    4.10. Decreased metaiodobenzylguanidine uptake
    4.11. Hyperperfusion in the pons and right hippocampus, and hypoperfusion in the frontal lobe
    4.12. Abnormal metabolic network characterized by increased activity in the pons and hippocampus and decreased activity in occipital and temporal areas
    4.13. Disrupted posterior functional brain connectivity
    4.14. Increased gray matter density in the hippocampus
    4.15. Decreased gray matter volume in the frontal, temporal, parietal, and occipital cortices as well as increased gray matter volume in cerebellum posterior lobe, putamen, and thalamus
    4.16. Neocortical cholinergic denervation
    4.17. Altered sensorimotor cortex noradrenergic function

4.18. Noradrenergic thalamic denervation

4.19. Cerebellar atrophy and the hot-cross-bun sign in conventional brain MRI

4.20. Small pineal gland volume

5. Biological abnormalities

5.1. Misfolded alpha-synuclein in the cerebrospinal fluid

5.2. Misfolded alpha-synuclein in the olfactory mucosa

5.3. Aggregates of phosphorylated alpha-synuclein in the autonomic nerve fibers that innervate the colon, salivary glands, and skin

5.4. Reduced intraepidermal nerve fiber density

5.5. The microRNA 19b is downregulated in the serum

5.6. Presence of single nucleotide polymorphisms SCARB2 and MAPT

5.7. Presence of GBA gene mutations

5.8. Genetic variants of the 3' and 5' untranslated region (UTR) of alpha-synuclein

5.9. Altered expression of the clock genes (Per2 and 3, Bmal1, and Nr1d1)

5.10. Increased tumor necrosis factor alpha and interleukin (IL)-10 and reduced IL-6/IL-10 and IL-8/IL-10 in the plasma

5.11. CD4+ T-cell dysregulation characterized by lower TBX21, STAT3, and STAT4, and higher FOXP3 transcription factors expression

5.12. Abnormal proteomic expression in the serum

5.13. Abnormal gut microbiota in stool samples

the substantia nigra and hyposmia do not change with time and remain stable.

Patients with IRBD show genetic abnormalities that are seen in the synucleinopathies (for review see Gan-Or and Rouleau[21]). The most common genetic abnormalities linked to PD, namely mutations in the GABA and LRRK2 genes, are associated with RBD. In 1 study, 7 missense GBA variants (E326K, L444P, A446T, A318G, R329C, T369M, and N370S) were identified in 8 of 69 (11.6%) patients and in 1 of 89 (1.2%) controls.[22] The GBA variants were more frequent compared with controls, associated with impending PD and DLB but not indicating a short-term risk for PD and DLB after IRBD diagnosis. In a larger study involving 1061 patients with IRBD and 3086 controls, GBA variants were found in 9.5% of patients and 4.1% of controls.[23] LRRK2 mutations are not identified in patients with IRBD[24] but they are seen in patients with mutations of these genes that developed RBD years after the onset of parkinsonism.[25] Likewise, RBD occurs after parkinsonism onset in patients with PD linked to PARK mutations.[26]

Single nucleotide polymorphisms in the 3' UTR of several alpha-synuclein (SNCA)–specific genetic variants (KP876057, KP876056, NM_000345.3:c*860T>A, NM_000345.3:c*2320A>T)[27] and in the 5'-region SNCA variant (rs10005233) have been associated with IRBD.[28] The

TMEM175/GAK/DGKQ p.M393T locus variant has also been associated with IRBD[29] as well as dysregulation of the microRNA miR-19b.[30] In contrast, MAPT H2/H1 haplotypes are not associated with IRBD.[31] Mutations in the sphingomyelin phosphodiesterase 1 (SMPD1) gene[32] and the APOE ε4 allele are not risk factors for IRBD either.[33]

A study showed lack of circadian rhythmicity in the clock genes Per2 and Per3, Bmal1, and Nr1d1 and an abnormal delayed secretion of melatonin in patients with IRBD compared with healthy individuals.[34] This finding is interesting because melatonin may improve RBD symptoms.

Overall, these genetic observations imply that patients with IRBD share some of the genetic substrates seen in manifest PD and provide another clue that this parasomnia in its idiopathic form is an early manifestation of a neurodegenerative disorder.

Patients with IRBD are eventually diagnosed with a clinically defined synucleinopathy. In a seminal study, Schenck and colleagues[35] in Minneapolis, Minnesota, reported that parkinsonism developed in 11 of 29 (38%) patients with IRBD 4 years after the diagnosis of the parasomnia. After 16 additional years, 81% of patients from this original cohort were diagnosed with PD, DLB, and MSA.[36] In a second series from Barcelona, Spain, 36 of 44 (82%) patients with IRBD were diagnosed

Box 3

Relevance of biomarkers in isolated rapid eye movement sleep behavior disorder

1. Biomarkers that predict short-term risk of conversion
   1.1. Subtle signs of parkinsonism
   1.2. Olfactory loss
   1.3. Abnormal color vision
   1.4. Combination of hyperechogenicity of the substantia nigra with reduced nigrostriatal dopaminergic binding in the striatum
   1.5. Reduced nigrostriatal dopaminergic binding in the putamen alone
   1.6. Impaired neuropsychological tests
   1.7. Increased delta and theta activity in occipital and central regions in electroencephalography
   1.8. Severity of REM sleep without atonia in the mentalis muscle
2. Biomarkers that progress over time
   2.1. Signs of parkinsonism
   2.2. Neuropsychological deficits
   2.3. Tonic and phasic muscle activity during REM sleep
   2.4. Reduced striatal dopaminergic uptake in the striatum
3. Biomarkers that remain stable over time
   3.1. Smell loss
   3.2. Dysautonomic features
   3.3. Hyperechogenicity of the substantia nigra

with PD, DLB, MSA, and mild cognitive impairment. The risk of a defined neurodegenerative syndrome from IRBD diagnosis was 35% at 5 years, 73% at 10 years, and 92% at 14 years. Patients who remained disease free had markers of the synucleinopathies such as decreased striatal dopamine transporter uptake and hyposmia.[37] A multicenter study involving 1280 patients with IRBD using the Kaplan-Meier method estimated that the risk of conversion was 10.6% at 2 years, 18% at 3 years, 32% at 5 years, 51% at 8 years, 60% at 10 years, and 74% at 12 years.[38] A recent systematic review and meta-analysis of longitudinal studies concluded that the risk of developing neurodegenerative diseases was 33.5% at 5 years' follow-up, 82.5% at 10.5 years, and 96.6% at 14 years.[39]

The risk for conversion from IRBD diagnosis increases with the duration of follow-up. Patients with long-standing IRBD of more than 10 years of follow-up frequently show markers of PD such as abnormal DAT-SPECT, hyperechogenicity of the substantia nigra, and hyposmia.[40]

Emerging diagnoses are PD and DLB in a similar magnitude, and much less frequently MSA of both parkinsonian and cerebellar subtypes. Very rarely, other neurodegenerative disorders emerge. The median age at disease diagnosis is advanced, around 75 years. It is difficult to predict which IRBD patient will evolve to PD, to DLB, or to MSA. However, the coexistence of nocturnal stridor and cerebellar atrophy in brain MRI indicates underlying MSA. Normal olfaction also indicates MSA but is not exclusive because it is present in about 40% of patients with IRBD that develop PD and DLB.[19] The development of mild cognitive impairment predicts evolution to dementia in only 2 to 3 years.[2] Orthostatic hypotension may also precede PD, DLB, and MSA. When parkinsonism manifests (in the setting of PD, DLB, or MSA), the akinetic-rigid subtype is much more frequent than tremor dominant, and the first signs to appear are usually hypomimia, hypophonia, and reduced arm swing.

Pathologic alpha-synuclein is found in IRBD. The neuropathologic hallmarks of PD and DLB are neuronal cell loss and deposits of Lewy bodies containing aggregates of misfolded alpha-synuclein in the surviving neurons.[41] The very few patients with IRBD who underwent neuropathologic examination showed the same neuropathologic changes seen in PD and DLB within the brainstem sparing the cortex.[42–44] One multicenter postmortem study examined the brain of 80 patients with PSG-confirmed RBD who had comorbid parkinsonism or dementia and found alpha-synuclein pathology in 78 (98%) of them.[45]

Several studies using the anti-serine 129–phosphorylated alpha-synuclein antibody have shown that phosphorylated alpha-synuclein (pAS) can be detected in living patients with IRBD undergoing biopsies of peripheral tissues. These studies have shown variable sensitivity to detect pAS but very high specificity because it is a rare feature in healthy controls. In the first study, aggregates of pAS were found in the submucosal nerve fibers of the colon in 4 of 17 (24%) living patients with IRBD and in none of the 14 healthy controls.[46] In another study, 21 patients with IRBD and 7 healthy controls underwent submandibular gland biopsy with ultrasonography guidance.[47] Adequate sample containing parenchymal tissue was obtained only in 9 patients with IRBD, and pAS was seen in 8 (89%) of these, whereas none of the 7 controls showed pAS. In a study performed in patients undergoing biopsy of the salivary glands in the inner part of the lower lip, pAS aggregates were observed in 31 of 62 (50%) patients and in 1 of 33 (3%) controls.[48] Also, pAS was detected in the parotid gland of a patient with IRBD undergoing parotid surgery for cancer and in 2 of 9 controls undergoing elective parotid gland for different diseases of this gland.[49] There are 2 works that have evaluated the presence of pAS in the skin of patients with IRBD, showing pAS in 56% to 75% of the patients and in none of the controls.[50,51] The sensitivity to detect pAS in these 2 biopsy skin studies varied depending on the location of the sampling site, the number of sites examined, and the thickness of the sections analyzed. These 2 skin studies used different methodological protocols. One study biopsied bilateral sites at the cervical area (C8) and distal leg, punches were 3 mm of diameter, and 2 different sections per site were analyzed.[50] The other study biopsied unilateral sites (right side) at the cervical area (C7), thoracic area (Th10), proximal leg, and distal leg; punches were 5 mm in diameter; and 5 different sections per site were evaluated.[51] These 2 studies showed that the sensitivity to detect pAS depended on the site were the biopsy was performed showing heterogeneous data; sensitivity of 72% in C8, of 28% in C7, of 44% in Th10, of 17% in proximal leg, and of 28% to 31% in the distal leg. The sensitivity to detect pAS in the skin also depends on the occurrence of small fiber neuropathy, a feature that has been described in IRBD.[52] Thus, no methodological consensus exists on skin biopsy performance in IRBD. Overall, the variable diagnostic accuracy, invasiveness of the procedures, number of slides screened, and limited amount of adequate material obtained limit the applicability of these peripheral biopsies using immunohistochemical methodology. It still remains to be determined what peripheral tissue and methodology are the best to detect pAS disorder in IRBD.

The cerebrospinal fluid (CSF) is another option for the search of pathologic alpha-synuclein in living individuals with IRBD. The CSF levels of biomarkers of Alzheimer disease (beta-amyloid, total tau, and phosphorylated tau) are normal in IRBD. Total and oligomeric levels of alpha-synuclein determined by the ELISA (enzyme-linked immunosorbent assay) technique are not different between patients with IRBD and controls.[53] In contrast, real-time quaking-induced conversion (RT-QuIC) is an essay that, in the CSF, is able to detect misfolded alpha-synuclein in 90% to 100% of patients with IRBD and manifest PD and DLB, whereas this is also found in about 10% of the healthy controls 70 years of age.[54–56] This 10% of RT-QuIC positivity in the CSF of healthy controls is similar to the 10% to 20% of incidental Lewy bodies found in the brains of individuals who died without antemortem parkinsonism and dementias.[57] In 1 study, alpha-synuclein in the CSF was detected by RT-QuIC in 47 out of 52 (90%) patients with IRBD and in 4 out of 40 (10%) controls.[56] During follow-up, 32 (62%) patients were diagnosed with PD or DLB and 31 (97%) of these were positive for CSF alpha-synuclein RT-QuIC. Patients with IRBD who were CSF alpha-synuclein RT-QuIC positive had higher risk for developing PD or DLB than those patients with IRBD who were CSF alpha-synuclein RT-QuIC negative. Six patients who were CSF alpha-synuclein RT-QuIC positive died, and postmortem brain examination showed widespread alpha-synuclein immunoreactive pathology in each case. Serial determination of CSF alpha-synuclein RT-QuIC was positive in 13 of 14 patients, and, in the remaining patient, the alpha-synuclein positivity was found in a fourth CSF determination. Overall, detection of pathologic alpha-synuclein in the CSF of patients with IRBD by the RT-QuIC assay obtained by lumbar puncture seems to be the most reliable procedure.

Detection of abnormal alpha-synuclein may also be found in the olfactory mucosa using R-QuIC in PD and IRBD. In 1 study with 63 patients with IRBD, 41 patients with PD and 59 controls, alpha-synuclein was detected in the olfactory mucosa by RT-QuIC in 44% of patients with IRBD, in 46% of patients with PD, and in 10% of controls. The presence of alpha-synuclein in the olfactory mucosa in IRBD was associated with poor smell in patients with IRBD.[58]

NEUROPROTECTION

Early intervention is a key point in preventing the onset of parkinsonism and cognitive impairment in the synucleinopathies.[59,60] At present, no effective neuroprotective therapies have been found to slow the neurodegenerative process in individuals already diagnosed with PD, DLB, and MSA. One of the possible reasons for failure is that the neurodegenerative process is too advanced for intervention at the time of diagnosis of PD, DLB, and MSA.[2] IRBD seems to be an optimal target population to test neuroprotective agents aiming to delay or stop the emergence of parkinsonism and cognitive impairment. Development of a neuroprotective strategy is an unmet need in IRBD, but this task carries important caveats and challenges that need to be considered. The target IRBD population can be enriched for hyposmia, abnormal DAT-SPECT, and subtle parkinsonian

Table 1
Therapeutic strategies against synuclein

Phase	Study	Mechanism	Intervention/ Treatment	Population	Status
1	AFF008	Vaccine	Affitope PD01A	Early PD (≤4 y), H&Y 1–2	Completed
1	AFF011	Vaccine	Affitope PD03A	Early PD (≤4 y), H&Y 1–2	Completed
1	NCT03272165	Monoclonal antibody	MEDI1341	Healthy patients	Recruiting
1	NCT02606682	Neuropore therapies	NPT200–11	Healthy patients	Completed
1	NCT04208152	α-Syn aggregation modulator	ANLE 138b	Healthy patients	Completed
1	NCT03611569	Monoclonal antibody	Lu AF82422	Healthy patients	Recruiting
2	NCT03100149 (PASADENA)	Monoclonal antibody	Prasinezumab (RO7046015/ PRX002)	Early PD (<2 y) H&Y 1 or 2	Active, not recruiting
2	NCT03318523 (SPARK)	Monoclonal antibody	BIIB054	Early PD (<3 y) H&Y ≤ 2.5	Recruiting
2	NCT02954978 NCT03205488	Protein c-ABL inhibitor	Nilotinib	Cohort 1: PD duration >5 y H&Y stage >2 and <4. Cohort 2: PD duration <3. H&Y ≤ 2	Completed
2	NCT02906020	G-case enhancer	GZ/SAR4027671	PD and who are heterozygous carriers of a GBA mutation associated with PD. Variants associated with GBA-PD (such as E326K) must have RBD confirmed	Active, not recruiting
2	NCT02941822	G-case Enhancer chaperone	Ambroxol	PD and H&Y stage 1–3	Completed

Abbreviation: H&Y, Hoehn and Yahr.

signs. In IRBD, the neuroprotective effect can be monitored using serial DAT-SPECT, motor function evaluations, and cognitive tests that are known to deteriorate spontaneously with time. In contrast, serial smell tests and transcranial sonography are not useful to monitor the disease process because the damage is stable with time. Sample sizes can also be calculated per arm as part of the design of a future double-blind placebo-controlled randomized trial. There are plenty of drug candidates to be tested in the IRBD population. One option is to implement immunotherapy against alpha-synuclein, which is a strategy currently being evaluated in manifest early PD in phase 1 and 2 clinical trials (**Table 1**).[60] This option is particularly promising in the IRBD population because pathologic alpha-synuclein can be detected in living patients with IRBD in the CSF with high sensitivity and specificity by the RT-QuIC method.

MANAGEMENT

Once RBD has been diagnosed, one of the goals is to reduce the frequency and intensity of the vigorous motor manifestations and the unpleasant dreams. RBD manifestations can be violent and potentially dangerous for the patient and the bed partner. Thus, one of the main recommendations is to establish a safe environment for sleeping. The treatment of concomitant sleep disorders such as obstructive sleep apnea, and avoiding therapy with β-blockers and antidepressants, may produce some benefit.[2]

Symptomatic treatment with medications for RBD symptoms is based on expert recommendations and data from few studies of short duration involving small sample sizes. Clonazepam and melatonin are usually recommended based on expert recommendations rather than on robust and strong clinical and pharmacologic data. With level of evidence A, the use of clonazepam (0.25−2 mg) is recommended with special attention in the elderly, patients with coexistent obstructive sleep apnea, and gait disorders. With level B, melatonin (3–12 mg) is recommended.[61] Prolonged-release melatonin and the melatonin receptor agonist ramelteon seem not to improve RBD symptoms.

There are patients with IRBD in whom clonazepam and melatonin are not effective or cannot be administrated because of side effects. In these cases, it seems that there are no other pharmacologic options. For the treatment of RBD, there is little or no evidence supporting the use of dopaminergics such as pramipexol or rotigotine, zopiclone, benzodiazepines other than clonazepam, Yi-Gan San, clozapine, gabapentin, carbamazepine, paroxetine, rivastigmine, and bupropion. Thus, there is a need to find alternative therapies for the RBD symptoms. One strategy is the administration of antidepressants because these medications reduce the amount of REM sleep and increase the REM sleep latency. However, antidepressants may increase the percentage of EMG activity in REM sleep.

Because IRBD is an early manifestation of a synucleinopathy, the question raised is how to inform individuals that sought medical advice for dream-enacting behaviors while their daily lives are pleasant and the individuals are healthy. A practical approach could include taking into account the desire of knowing, and also the cultural and education background and the personality of the patient. A recommendation is to provide a general disclosure of prognostic risk rather than giving specific information.[62] In addition, clinicians should make patients feel welcome for any care they need as well as send a message of hope for future neuroprotective therapies.

CLINICS CARE POINTS

- IRBD is a parasomnia occurring in adulthood and earlier that is characterized by unpleasant dreams and vigorous movement during REM sleep.
- Because other sleep disorders may also be characterized by nightmares and abnormal movements and behaviors during REM sleep, the diagnosis of IRBD requires polysomnography.
- Most patients with IRBD develop cognitive problems, parkinsonism, dysautonomia, and cerebellar syndrome fulfilling diagnostic criteria for the synucleinopathies PD, MSA, and DLB.
- Patients with IRBD show abnormal synuclein in the CSF and peripheral organs.
- Patients with IRBD are candidates to test neuroprotective medication to halt the neurodegenerative process.

DISCLOSURE

The authors have nothing to disclosure regarding the current article and have no conflicts of interest.

REFERENCES

1. American Academy of Sleep Medicine. International classification of sleep disorders. 3rd edition. Darien, IL: American Academy of Sleep Medicine; 2014.
2. Iranzo A, Santamaria J, Tolosa E. Idiopathic rapid eye movement sleep behaviour disorder: diagnosis, management, and the need for neuroprotective interventions. Lancet Neurol 2016;15:405–19.
3. Fernández-Arcos A, Iranzo A, Serradell M, et al. The clinical phenotype of idiopathic REM sleep behavior disorder at presentation: a study in 203 consecutive patients. Sleep 2016;39:121–32.
4. Iranzo A. The REM sleep circuit and how its impairment leads to REM sleep behavior disorder. Cell Tissue Res 2018;73:245–66.
5. Högl B, Santamaria J, Iranzo A, et al. Precision medicine in rapid eye movement sleep behavior disorder. Sleep Med Clin 2019;14:351–62.
6. Pujol M, Pujol J, Alonso T, et al. Idiopathic REM sleep behavior disorder in the elderly Spanish community: a primary care center study with a two-stage design using video-polysomnography. Sleep Med 2017;40:116–21.

7. Haba-Rubio J, Frauscher B, Marques-Vidal P, et al. Prevalence and determinants of rapid eye movement sleep behavior disorder in the general population. Sleep 2018;41(2):zsx197.

8. Frauscher B, Iranzo A, Gaig C, et al. Normative EMG values during REM sleep for the diagnosis of REM sleep behavior disorder. Sleep 2012;35:835–47.

9. Fernández-Arcos A, Iranzo A, Serradell M, et al. Diagnostic value of isolated mentalis versus mentalis plus upper limb electromyography in idiopathic REM sleep behavior disorder patients eventually developing a neurodegenerative syndrome. Sleep 2017;40(4).

10. Frauscher B, Gabelia D, Biermayr M, et al. Validation of an integrated software for the detection of rapid eye movement sleep behavior disorder. Sleep 2014;37:1663–71.

11. Cooray N, Andreotti F, Lo C, et al. Detection of REM sleep behaviour disorder by automated polysomnography analysis. Clin Neurophysiol 2019;130:505–14.

12. Waser M, Stefani A, Holzknecht E, et al. Automated 3D video analysis of lower limb movements during REM sleep: a new diagnostic tool for isolated REM sleep behavior disorder. Sleep 2020;43(11):zsaa100.

13. Stefani A, Heidbreder A, Brandauer E, et al. Screening for idiopathic REM sleep behavior disorder: usefulness of actigraphy. Sleep 2018;41(6):zsy053.

14. Lam SP, Li SX, Zhang J, et al. Development of scales for assessment of rapid eye movement sleep behavior disorder (RBD). Sleep Med 2013;14:734–8.

15. Pérez-Carbonell L, Iranzo A. Clinical aspects of idiopathic RBD. In: Schenck CH, Högl B, Videnovic A, editors. Rapid-eye-movement sleep behavior disorder. Cham: Springer; 2019. p. 33–52.

16. Kogan RV, Meles SK, Leenders KL, et al. Brain imaging in RBD. In: Schenck CH, Högl B, Videnovic A, editors. Rapid-eye-movement sleep behavior disorder. Cham: Springer; 2019. p. 403–46.

17. Gagnon JF, Bourgouin PA, De Roy J, et al. Neuropsychological aspects: cognition in RBD. In: Schenck CH, Högl B, Videnovic A, editors. Rapid-eye-movement sleep behavior disorder. Springer; 2019. p. 491–508.

18. Iranzo A, Santamaría J, Valldeoriola F, et al. Dopamine transporter imaging deficit predicts early transition to synucleinopathy in idiopathic rapid eye movement sleep behavior disorder. Ann Neurol 2017;82:419–28.

19. Iranzo A, Marrero-González P, Serradell M, et al. Significance of hyposmia in isolated REM sleep behavior disorder. J Neurol 2021;268(3):963–6.

20. Iranzo A, Valldeoriola F, Lomeña F, et al. Serial dopamine transporter imaging of nigrostriatal function in patients with idiopathic rapid-eye-movement sleep behaviour disorder: a prospective study. Lancet Neurol 2011;10:797–805.

21. Gan-Or Z, Rouleau GA. Genetics of REM sleep behavior disorder. RBD. In: Schenck CH, Högl B, Videnovic A, editors. Rapid-eye-movement sleep behavior disorder. Springer; 2019. p. 589–610.

22. Gámez-Valero A, Iranzo A, Serradell M, et al. Glucocerebrosidase gene variants are accumulated in idiopathic REM sleep behavior disorder. Parkinsonism Relat Disord 2018;50:94–8.

23. Krohn L, Ruskey JA, Rudakou U, et al. GBA variants in REM sleep behavior disorder: a multicenter study. Neurology 2020;95(8):e1008–16.

24. Fernández-Santiago R, Iranzo A, Gaig C, et al. Absence of LRRK2 mutations in a cohort of patients with idiopathic REM sleep behavior disorder. Neurology 2016;86:1072–3.

25. Pont-Sunyer C, Iranzo A, Gaig C, et al. Sleep disorders in parkinsonian and Nonparkinsonian LRRK2 mutation Carriers. PLoS One 2015;10(7):e0132368.

26. Kumru H, Santamaria J, Tolosa E, et al. Rapid eye movement sleep behavior disorder in parkinsonism with parkin mutations. Ann Neurol 2004;56:599–603.

27. Toffoli M, Dreussi E, Cecchin E, et al. SNCA 3'UTR genetic variants in patients with Parkinson's disease and REM sleep behavior disorder. Neurol Sci 2017;38:1233–40.

28. Krohn L, Wu RYJ, Heilbron K, et al. Fine-mapping of SNCA in rapid eye movement sleep behavior disorder and overt synucleinopathies. Ann Neurol 2020;87:584–98.

29. Krohn L, Öztürk TN, Vanderperre B, et al. Genetic, structural, and functional evidence link TMEM175 to synucleinopathies. Ann Neurol 2020;87:139–53.

30. Fernández-Santiago R, Iranzo A, Gaig C, et al. MicroRNA association with synucleinopathy conversion in rapid eye movement behavior disorder. Ann Neurol 2015;77:895–901.

31. Li J, Ruskey JA, Arnulf I, et al. Full sequencing and haplotype analysis of MAPT in Parkinson's disease and rapid eye movement sleep behavior disorder. Mov Disord 2018;33:1016–20.

32. Rudakou U, Futhey NC, Krohn L, et al. SMPD1 variants do not have a major role in rapid eye movement sleep behavior disorder. Neurobiol Aging 2020;93:142.e5–7.

33. Gan-Or Z, Montplaisir JY, Ross JP, et al. The dementia-associated APOE ε4 allele is not associated with rapid eye movement sleep behavior disorder. Neurobiol Aging 2017;49:218.e13–5.

34. Weissová K, Škrabalová J, Skálová K, et al. Circadian rhythms of melatonin and peripheral clock gene expression in idiopathic REM sleep behavior disorder. Sleep Med 2018;52:1–6.

35. Schenck CH, Bundlie SR, Mahowald MW. Delayed emergence of a parkinsonian disorder in 38% of 29 older men initially diagnosed with idiopathic

rapid eye movement sleep behavior disorder. Neurology 1996;46:388–92.

36. Schenck C, Boeve B, Mahowald M. Delayed emergence of a parkinsonian disorder or dementia in 81% of older men initially diagnosed with idiopathic rapid eye movement sleep behaviour disorder: a 16-year update on a previously reported series. Sleep Med 2013;14:744–8.

37. Iranzo A, Tolosa E, Gelpi E. Neurodegenerative disease status and post-mortem pathology in idiopathic rapid-eye-movement sleep behavior disorder: an observational cohort study. Lancet Neurol 2013;12:443–53.

38. Postuma R, Iranzo A, Hu M. REM sleep behaviour disorder: an early window for prevention in neurodegeneration? Brain 2019;142:498–501.

39. Galbiati A, Verga L, Giora E, et al. The risk of neurodegeneration in REM sleep behavior disorder: a systematic review and meta-analysis of longitudinal studies. Sleep Med Rev 2019;43:37–46.

40. Iranzo A, Stefani A, Serradell M, et al. Characterization of patients with longstanding idiopathic REM sleep behavior disorder. Neurology 2017;89:242–8.

41. Dickson DW, Braak H, Duda JE, et al. Neuropathological assessment of Parkinson's disease: refining the diagnostic criteria. Lancet Neurol 2009;8:1150–7.

42. Uchiyama M, Isse K, Tanaka K, et al. Incidental Lewy body disease in a patient with REM sleep behaviour disorder. Neurology 1999;45:709–12.

43. Boeve BF, Dickson DW, Olson EJ, et al. Insights into REM sleep behaviour disorder pathophysiology in brainstem-predominant Lewy body disease. Sleep Med 2007;8:60–4.

44. Iranzo A, Gelpi E, Tolosa E, et al. Neuropathology of prodromal Lewy body disease. Mov Disord 2014;29:410–5.

45. Boeve BF, Silber MH, Ferman TJ, et al. Clinicopathologic correlations in 172 cases of rapid eye movement sleep behavior disorder with or without a coexisting neurologic disorder. Sleep Med 2013;14:754–62.

46. Sprenger FS, Stefanova N, Gelpi E, et al. Enteric nervous system α-synuclein immunoreactivity in idiopathic REM sleep behavior disorder. Neurology 2015;85:1761–8.

47. Vilas D, Iranzo A, Tolosa E, et al. Assessment of α-synuclein in submandibular glands of patients with idiopathic rapid-eye-movement sleep behaviour disorder: a case-control study. Lancet Neurol 2016;15:708–18.

48. Iranzo A, Borrego S, Vilaseca I, et al. α-Synuclein aggregates in labial salivary glands of idiopathic rapid eye movement sleep behavior disorder. Sleep 2018;41(8).

49. Fernández-Arcos A, Vilaseca I, Aldecoa I, et al. Alpha-synuclein aggregates in the parotid gland of idiopathic REM sleep behavior disorder. Sleep Med 2018;52:14–7.

50. Antelmi E, Donadio V, Incensi A, et al. Skin nerve phosphorylated α-synuclein deposits in idiopathic REM sleep behavior disorder. Neurology 2017;88:2128–31.

51. Doppler K, Jentschke HM, Schulmeyer L, et al. Dermal phospho-alpha-synuclein deposits confirm REM sleep behaviour disorder as prodromal Parkinson's disease. Acta Neuropathol 2017;133:535–45.

52. Schrempf W, Katona I, Dogan I, et al. Reduced intra-epidermal nerve fiber density in patients with REM sleep behavior disorder. Parkinsonism Relat Disord 2016;29:10–6.

53. Compta Y, Valente T, Saura J, et al. Correlates of cerebrospinal fluid levels of oligomeric and total α-synuclein in premotor, motor and dementia stages of Parkinson's disease. J Neurol 2015;262:294–306.

54. Fairfoul G, McGuire LI, Pal S, et al. Alpha-synuclein RT-QuIC in the CSF of patients with alpha-synucleinopathies. Ann Clin Transl Neurol 2016;3:812–8.

55. Rossi M, Candelise N, Baiardi S, et al. Ultrasensitive RT-QuIC assay with high sensitivity and specificity for Lewy body-associated synucleinopathy. Acta Neuropathol 2020;140:49–62.

56. Iranzo A, Fairfoul G, Ayudhay N, et al. Cerebrospinal fluid α-synuclein detection by RT-QuIC in patients with isolated REM sleep behavior disorder. Lancet Neurol 2021;20(3):203–12.

57. Beach TG, Adler CH, Lue L, et al. Unified staging system for Lewy body disorders: correlation with nigrostriatal degeneration, cognitive impairment and motor dysfunction. Acta Neuropathol 2009;117:613–34.

58. Stefani A, Iranzo A, Holzknecht E, et al. Alpha-synuclein seeds in olfactory mucosa of patients with isolated rapid-eye-movement sleep behaviour disorder. Brain 2020 [in press].

59. Espay AJ, Kalia LV, Gan-Or Z, et al. Disease modification and biomarker development in Parkinson disease. Neuroloy 2020;94:481–94.

60. Fernández-Valle T, Gabilondo I, Gómez-Esteban JC. New therapeutic approaches to target alpha-synuclein in Parkinson's disease: the role of immunotherapy. Int Rev Neurobiol 2019;146:281–95.

61. Aurora RN, Zak RS, Maganti RK, et al. Best practice guide for the treatment of REM sleep behavior disorder (RBD). J Clin Sleep M 2010;6:85–95.

62. Arnaldi D, Antelmi E, St Louis EK, et al. Idiopathic REM sleep behavior disorder and neurodegenerative risk: to tell or not to tell to the patient? How to minimize the risk? Sleep Med Rev 2017;36:82–95.

Fragmentary Hypnic Myoclonus and Other Isolated Motor Phenomena of Sleep

Luca Baldelli, MD[a], Federica Provini, MD, PhD[a,b],*

KEYWORDS

- Sleep-related movement disorders • Excessive fragmentary hypnic myoclonus • Hypnic jerks
- Hypnagogic foot tremor • Alternating leg muscle activation • Sleep-related leg cramps
- Differential diagnosis

KEY POINTS

- Excessive fragmentary hypnic myoclonus, hypnic jerks, hypnagogic foot tremor, alternating leg muscle activation, and sleep-related cramps are less known sleep-related motor disorders (SRMDs).
- Less known SRMDs are frequently missed or misidentified as the more frequent ones.
- Less known SRMDs can present as isolated motor symptoms or incidental polygraphic findings, but also be the cause of otherwise cryptogenic insomnias and somnolence.
- Acknowledging the existence and features of these manifestations can increase the diagnostic accuracy.

INTRODUCTION

Sleep-related movement disorders (SRMDs) are relatively simple, usually stereotyped, involuntary movements that disturb sleep or its onset.[1] Motor manifestations are usually positive (hyperkinesias), and their simple nature distinguishes them from the complex movements associated with parasomnias (eg, sleepwalking).[2] Many physicians associate SRMDs with restless legs syndrome (RLS) or periodic limb movements during sleep (PLMS), while the other SRMDs are often considered less frequent, less important, or not clinically relevant. This leads to the fact that some of them are frequently missed or misinterpreted in their meaning and implications or confounded in differential diagnosis.[3] SRMDs are usually benign variants, but they are classified as movement disorders when they are frequent or lead to consequences during night-time (eg, insomnia and sleep fragmentation) and/or daytime

(eg, somnolence). SRMDs can also be associated with other sleep disorders.

This article will focus on the isolated SRMDs or isolated variants, including excessive fragmentary myoclonus (EFHM), hypnagogic foot tremor (HFT), alternating leg muscle activation (ALMA), and sleep starts (or hypnic jerks – HJs). EFHM, HJs, HFT, and ALMA are listed within the SRMD chapter in the International Classification of Sleep Disorders, 3rd edition[1] (ICSD-3) subcategory of "isolated symptoms and normal variants." Sleep-related leg cramps will be also briefly taken into consideration as a common but often underestimated condition. The discussion will focus on SRMDs clinical presentation and pathophysiology, prevalence and diagnosis, giving correct hints to avoid misinterpretation with the better known SRMDs, and, when appropriate, their treatment.

[a] Department of Biomedical and NeuroMotor Sciences (DiBiNeM), University of Bologna, Ospedale Bellaria, Via Altura 3, Bologna 40139, Italy; [b] IRCCS Istituto delle Scienze Neurologiche di Bologna, Bologna, Italy
* Corresponding author. Department of Biomedical and NeuroMotor Sciences, University of Bologna, Via Altura 3, Bologna 40139, Italy.
E-mail address: federica.provini@unibo.it

Sleep Med Clin 16 (2021) 349–361
https://doi.org/10.1016/j.jsmc.2021.02.008
1556-407X/21/© 2021 Elsevier Inc. All rights reserved.

PHYSIOLOGICAL AND EXCESSIVE FRAGMENTAR HYPNIC MYOCLONUS
Historic Overview and Definition

Fragmentary hypnic myoclonus (FHM) was first described by De Lisi in 1932 as physiologic sudden, arrhythmic, asynchronous, and asymmetrical brief twitches involving various body areas, in particular distal limb and facial muscles, occurring during sleep in a large population of children.[4] The phenomenon was subsequently studied in detail also in adults and in animals.[5,6] Half a century later, Broughton and colleagues characterized and defined the entity of EFHM as the "presence of electromyographic activity consisting of brief, usually less than 150 milliseconds, hypersynchronous potentials exceeding 50 μV in amplitude" recorded during at least 20 consecutive minutes of stage 2, 3, or 4 sleep, with a rate of at least 5/min.[7,8] Eventually, Montagna demonstrated that the brief electromyography (EMG) activities of FHM could also be part of physiologic sleep, highlighting physiologic fragmentary (hypnic) myoclonus (PFHM) as a "simple" sleep-related motor phenomenon, variably present also during relaxed wakefulness.[9] FHM activity, in its simplest form, displaying the characteristics of fasciculation potentials, represents PFHM, while when increased in frequency and persistent throughout the sleeping time, gives origin to EFHM.[8,9]

Clinical Relevance

Patients presenting with EFHM can suffer from sleep fragmentation and insomnia or can report excessive daytime sleepiness, not primarily explained by other sleep disturbances.[7,10] On the other hand, EFHM has also been described in combination with other sleep disorders such as obstructive sleep apnea, primary central sleep apnea, sleep-related hypoxemic and hypoventilation syndromes, periodic limb movement disorder, and narcolepsy.[8,11] Moreover, a few works have reported the occurrence of EFHM in some neurodegenerative diseases such as Parkinson disease,[12] multiple system atrophy,[13] amyotrophic lateral sclerosis,[14] Machado-Joseph disease,[15] and Niemann-Pick disease type C.[16] Because of the occurrence of EFHM in relation to such sleep and neurologic comorbidities, it can be hypothesized that EFHM could be an epiphenomenon of a specific pathophysiological etiology.

Diagnosis and Assessment

FHM is a largely incidental polysomnographic finding on EMG; often no movement at all is documented by video recordings. When visible, it consists of small movements of the corners of the mouth, fingers, or toes; large limb movements across large joint spaces are not characteristic and should rule out the diagnosis (**Fig. 1**).[1] According to the American Academy of Sleep Medicine (AASM) scoring manual,[17] several criteria define EFHM:

1. The presence of FHM as EMG potentials with maximal duration of 150 milliseconds (more frequently 75–150 millisecomds)
2. At least 20 minutes of nonrapid eye movement (NREM) sleep with FHM must be recorded
3. At least 5 EMG potentials per minute must be recorded
4. The disorder is not better explained by another current sleep disorder, medical or neurologic disorder, medication use, or substance use disorder

It should be noted that the minimum required time of 20 minutes of EFHM resides in the caveat that the current criteria are based exclusively on the ad hoc definition by Broughton, who had reviewed 20-minute segments of NREM sleep PSG in a series of 38 patients.[8]

An EMG potential cut-off of 50 μV (rarely rising above 200 μV to several hundred μV) is internationally accepted to define FHM.[3] In 2013, Hoque and colleagues, studying 8 patients with EFHM, proposed a different amplitude criterion to assess FHM activities, reducing the minimum required potential to 25 μV,[18] justified by newer technologies and better skin preparation techniques. However, to date, no accepted minimum amplitude criterion has been specified by the AASM.[1]

Quantitative assessment
Montagna was the first to suggest a quantification method for PFHM, obtained by dividing the percentage of FHM occurring during each sleep stage by the percentage of total recording time taken by that sleep stage.[9] Later on, in 1993, Lins and colleagues presented the fragmentary myoclonus index (FMI) to assess EFHM intensity, where the presence of EFHM potentials is evaluated among 3-second miniepochs and then referenced to the hours of night or to the duration of individual sleep stages.[19] However, a quantitative cut-off of FMI to define the presence of EFHM is lacking.[20]

Sleep stage distribution
FHM activity in people shows an inverse relationship with the degree of sleep electroencephalogram (EEG) synchronization,[21] prevailing equally during sleep-wake transition and N1 sleep and during REM sleep (Montagna and colleagues, 1988).[9] FHM potentials can also extend into

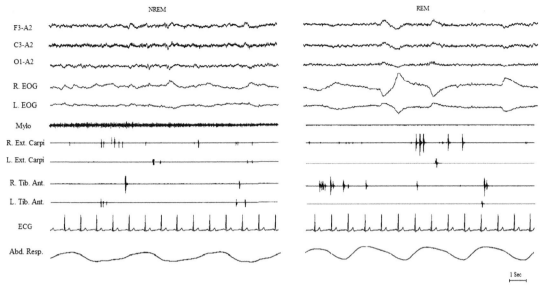

Fig. 1. Excerpts of polygraphic recordings of excessive fragmentary hypnic myoclonus in NREM and REM sleep. Brief, asymmetrical, asynchronous potentials are visible in the explored muscles, sometimes without any associated visible movement. Abd. Resp., abdominal respirogram; ECG, electrocardiogram; EOG, electrooculogram; Ext. Carpi, extensor carpi muscle; L., left; Mylo., mylohyoideus muscle; R., right; Tib. Ant., tibialis anterior muscle.

wakefulness.[9,22,23] The excessive intensity of EFHM in contrast to PFHM is kept among the sleep stages as the highest amounts occurring in REM and the lowest in N3.[19,24,25] The time of night distribution has been studied also; the number of potentials rises sharply after the initial lower level in the first hour of sleep and remains unchanged across the rest of the night.[19]

Differential diagnosis

Differential diagnosis of EFHM includes PLMS, whose periodicity is in contrast with EFHM, and it is represented by longer movements (0.5–10 seconds) than FHM potentials. Epileptic myoclonus in sleep is often associated with an EEG discharge; episodes are stereotyped and isolated, with possible but less frequent recurrence during the night; they also involve a greater variety of body areas.[19,26] Sleep-related leg cramps unlike FHM potentials last much longer (for a few seconds up to several minutes) and are associated with painful sensations, muscle spasm, and hardness.[1] HFT presents in contrast with EFHM a rhythmic character and a predominant occurrence in N1-N2 stages. Moreover, EFHM lacks the alternating pattern, the rhythmicity and the periodic occurrence of ALMA.[20] Propriospinal myoclonus (PM) (**Fig. 2**) is characterized by irregularly recurring sudden jerks, arising from different muscles, especially in the trunk. From the polygraphic point of view, longer potentials than EFHM are documented (100–300 milliseconds); the peculiar propagation starts from midthoracic segments and then slowly propagates up and down into the spinal cord, resulting in repetitive and irregular jerky flexion of distant muscles.[27,28] PM occurs at the wake-sleep transition when alpha activity is present on the EEG, disappearing with EEG desynchronization and the occurrence of sleep spindles and K-complexes, while EFHM is present throughout sleep.[29] Finally, EFHM must also be differentiated from normal physiologic phasic REM twitches, which have a similar burst duration but are limited to the REM state and tend to occur in clusters within an epoch, as opposed to EFHM, in which bursts tend not to cluster within a particular epoch.[1] However, the differential diagnosis is not always easy as EFHM may be more intense during REM sleep, compared with NREM sleep.[3]

Epidemiology

The Innsbruck group produced the most evidence on PFHM and EFHM prevalence. In 2011, Frauscher and colleagues demonstrated that PFHM is ubiquitous among adults both in men and in women;[22] the same result was replicated in a larger cohort of 100 healthy subjects.[25] The median FMI was 25.5/h, and few patients had very high rates. FMI was higher in men and increased with age.[25] EFHM showed a prevalence of 9%, as recently confirmed by Trimmel and colleagues in a group of 200 patients with various sleep disturbances referring to a sleep clinic.[11]

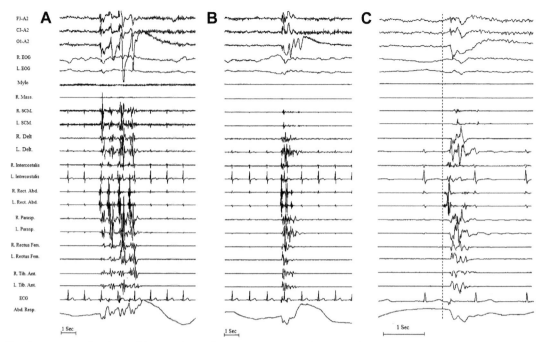

Fig. 2. Excerpts of polygraphic recording of propriospinal myoclonus (PM) at sleep onset. PSG recording shows spontaneous PM jerks (*A*) in brief clusters or (*B*) isolated during relaxed wakefulness preceding sleep onset. (*C*) The recording of a PM jerk shows a slow rostro-caudal propagation of muscular activity. At high paper speed, it is evident that the onset of the EMG activity is in the recti abdominis muscles with ordered spreading to more rostral and caudal muscles (*dotted line*). Abd. Resp., abdominal respirogram; Delt., deltoideus muscle; ECG, electrocardiogram; EOG, electrooculogram; Intercostalis, intercostalis muscle; L., left; Mass, masseter muscle; Mylo, mylohyoideus muscle; Parasp., paraspinalis muscles; R., right; Rect. Abd., rectus abdominis muscle; Rectus Fem., rectus femoralis muscle; SCM., sternocleidomastoid muscle; Tib. Ant., tibialis anterior muscle.

Etiophysiology

Montagna first postulated that FHM potentials originate in the muscle endplate but are modulated by brainstem regions implicated in motor control during sleep.[9,21] The motor inhibition typical of REM sleep is related to state-dependent activity of the pontine nucleus pontis oralis, which, by exciting cells of the medullary nucleus reticularis gigantocellularis, inhibits the alpha motoneurons.[30] A physiologic escape from this state-related motor inhibition hypothetically accounts for the PFHM, which is probably caused by descending volleys within the reticulospinal system impinging on the spinal alpha motoneurons during REM sleep.[21] Abnormal but selective impairment of motor control during sleep could cause the intensity of PFHM to increase, giving rise to EFHM. A subcortical origin of EFHM is suggested also by the absence of cortical potentials at EEG–EMG back-averaging[31] and by anecdotal association of EFHM with brainstem lesions.[32]

Performing an EMG analysis in 98 patients with EFHM, Raccagni and colleagues[23] found that 50% of them had electrophysiological asymptomatic abnormalities (namely polyneuropathy, nerve

root lesions, and benign fasciculations) different from the normal EMG findings of the 2 patients evaluated by Vetrugno and colleagues[31] in a seminal work. These results, apparently in contrast, do not disprove Montagna's brainstem hypothesis,[33] but simply add evidence of how a peripheral disorder can coexist with, and possibly exacerbate, a motor manifestation of central origin.

Treatment

Accepting that severe forms of EHFM might cause sleep fragmentation and daytime somnolence, even if the patient is unaware of the movements, implies, in the absence of other sleep disorders, the necessity of a treatment that is solely based on personal experience and scarce case reports.[34] Successful therapies with pramipexole (0.125 mg), carbamazepine (200 mg), and clonazepam (2 mg) at bedtime have been reported.[31,34]

HYPNIC JERKS (SLEEP STARTS)
Historic Overview and Definition

Mitchell is credited with the earliest description of HJs[35] in 1890. He also mentioned the possibility of insomnia as a result of their starts. Seventy years later, Ostwald (1959) first described the EEG correlates of the HJs;[36] subsequently Gastaut and Broughton (1965) made the first polygraphic observation of HJs.[37] Later, in 1988, Broughton coined the term "intensified hypnic jerks" to describe enhanced HJs in 2 patients causing sleep-onset insomnia.[38]

HJs, or sleep starts, are normal physiologic events, primarily occurring at the transition from wakefulness to sleep, often associated with sensory phenomena, such as a feeling of falling into the void, unexplained alarm or fear, inner electric shock, or light flash.[21] HJs may be either spontaneous or induced by stimuli.[33] Jerks consist of nonrepetitive, nonstereotyped, abrupt, and brief flexion or extension movements, generalized, or, more frequently, segmental, and asymmetrical with neck and/or limb muscles involvement. A noisy gasp can occasionally accompany the jerks, which are usually associated with autonomic activation (tachycardia, irregular breathing, and pseudomotor activation).[39] Sensory phenomena can also occur alone, in the absence of any muscular activation.[21]

Clinical Relevance

As HJs are physiologic events, physical and neurologic examinations and routine laboratory tests are otherwise normal. However, as HJs intensify, sleep may be disturbed, resulting in sleep-onset insomnia.[40] This condition in turn may worsen the occurrence of HJs. The bedpartner may also be bothered with the jerks, resulting in sleep problems for the partner also. Stressful conditions including fatigue, stress, sleep deprivation, and vigorous exercise may cause an intensification of HJs, as do stimulants like caffeine and nicotine.[41]

Polygraphic Assessment

HJs typically appear during drowsiness or stage N1 sleep, sometimes associated with a negative vertex sharp wave; occurrence during N2 sleep is also possible, when they are associated with K-complexes. An EEG arousal or an awakening usually follows the jerk. Recently, in a series of parkinsonian patients, HJs have been documented during N3 and REM sleep.[42]

Superficial EMG recordings of the involved muscles show brief (generally 75–250 milliseconds) high-amplitude potentials, either singly or in succession. Over the last years, the neurophysiological characteristics of HJ have been studied in detail (**Fig. 3**). Chokroverty and colleagues recognized 4 recurring motor patterns of muscle propagation among 10 patients with an intensified form of HJ.[43] The first pattern consisted of synchronous and symmetric muscle bursts between the 2 sides and agonist-antagonist muscles similar to those noted in audiogenic startle reflex. The reticular reflex myoclonus pattern sees a bidirectional propagation up the brainstem and down the spinal cord. A mixture of myoclonic and dystonic synchronous EMG bursts defines the extrapyramidal type. Finally a rostrocaudal propagation defines the pyramidal type.[43] Soon after, the authors' group identified a new motor pattern originating from intracranial muscles then spreading to the rostral and caudal muscles without any ordered pattern of propagation.[44] The authors later confirmed the same pattern with a lack of recurring HJ patterns in a group of parkinsonian patients.[42]

Differential Diagnosis

HJs must be differentiated from several physiologic or pathologic movements that occur at sleep onset or during sleep. Fragmentary hypnic myoclonus, contrarily to the massive jerks of HJ, consist of small muscular twitches, often representing only an EMG finding not associated with overt movements at the joints. Moreover, although HJs occur at sleep onset, EFHM is present throughout all stages. Different from HJs, PM is characterized by a specific motor pattern; the contraction usually arises first in spinal innervated axial muscles of the trunk and then slowly propagates up and down into the spinal cord to distant muscles. PM at sleep onset is usually a chronic condition associated with sleep-onset insomnia. Epileptic myoclonus can be differentiated by possible coexistent EEG discharges, the presence of other features of epileptic seizures, and the occurrence of the myoclonus in both wakefulness and during sleep. Finally, HJs associated with excessive startling may occur as part of the genetically based hyperekplexia syndrome, the major form of this condition being also characterized by stiffness and falls.

Epidemiology

Sleep starts affect all ages and both sexes. A prevalence of 60% to 70% has been reported, but with a highly sporadic occurrence,[1] as in a quantitative PSG study on normal sleep motor events, the authors did not report any HJ among a population of 100 healthy sleepers.[25] Surprisingly, HJ occurrence has been found much higher in parkinsonian patients (16 out of 62 patients recorded), opening speculations as to whether jerks may be more frequent in these subjects,[42] as outlined in a seminal case report.[45] Higher prevalence has also

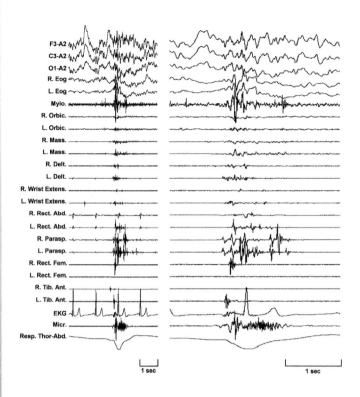

Fig. 3. Excerpt of a polygraphic recording of HJ during stage 2 NREM. The EMG activity originates in the left paraspinalis muscle and then spreads to the more cranial and rostral axial and limb muscles, without any rostrocaudal order as better visible at high paper speed (right part). Delt., deltoideus muscle; ECG, electrocardiogram; EOG, electrooculogram; L., left; Mass, masseter muscle; Mylo, mylohyoideus muscle; Orbic., orbicularis muscle; Parasp., paraspinalis muscle; R., right; Rect. Abd., rectus abdominis muscle; Rectus Fem., rectus femoralis muscle; Resp. Thor-Abd., thoraco-abdominal respirogram; Tib. Ant., tibialis anterior muscle; Wrist Extens., wrist extensor muscle.

been found in patients with postpolio syndrome,[46] in children with migraine[47] and epilepsy,[48] and in snorers, both adult[49] and juvenile.[50]

Etiophysiology

It is not known what causes HJs; however, some evidence seems to support its subcortical origin, both in animals[51] and in people as outlined in symptomatic or lesional case reports.[48,52] HJs presumably arise from sudden descending volleys that originate in the brainstem reticular formation and are activated mostly at the transition between wake and sleep.[33] The variability in motor recruitment and pattern during HJ may be related to variable spinal motor neuron excitability in the spinal cord during sleep, indicating the engagement of different and sometimes unsynchronized pools of spinal motor neurons at different times for each HJ.[53]

Treatment

Although sporadic and benign in almost the totality of cases, HJs can cause apprehension to the patients referred to the sleep clinic, for whom reassurance and counseling are often enough to prevent the development of sleep-onset insomnia. Although an adequate explanation and reassurance may be sufficient, some patients may require

a small dose of clonazepam (0.5–1 mg at bedtime) to ameliorate symptoms on a short-term basis.

Sensory Sleep Starts and Its Variants

First anecdotally described by Mahowald and Schenck[54] and better evaluated by Sander and colleagues,[55] HJs can also present without an actual jerk, but only with purely sensory phenomena restricted to the onset of sleep. They can vary from electric shock-like sensation, sense of suffocation, numbness, to tactile sensations such as itch or puncture.[55] Exploding head syndrome (EHS) and blip syndrome could be also considered different manifestations of this same phenomenon.

Exploding head syndrome

Classified among "other parasomnias" in ICSD-3,[1] EHS may actually represent a variety of purely sensory sleep starts. First described by Armstrong-Jones in 1920 as a "snapping of the brain",[56] it is characterized by the sensation lasting some seconds that an explosive noise has occurred in the head, which wakes the individual from sleep. Patients describe this sensation variously as a terrifying loud bang or a shotgun- or bomb-like explosion. Polysomnographic studies have documented the occurrence of these manifestations during all sleep stages, including REM sleep,[57] and during the passage from wakefulness to sleep.[58] More frequently a cause of insomnia, treatment can be fulfilled with tricyclics such as clomipramine, calcium channel blockers (nifedipine), and also carbamazepine.[59]

Blip syndrome

Described only once by Lance in 1996,[60] blip syndrome probably represents a variant of sensory sleep starts. Blip syndrome defines a condition when momentary sensations of impending loss of consciousness are perceived, particularly when relaxed, without any obvious cardiac, cerebral vascular, or epileptic basis.[60]

HYPNAGOGIC FOOT TREMOR, ALTERNATING LEG MUSCLE ACTIVATION, AND HIGH-FREQUENCY LEG MOVEMENT SPECTRUM
Hypnagogic Foot Tremor

The term hypnagogic foot tremor (HFT) was originally introduced by Broughton in 1988[38] documenting 2 patients with severe head injury presenting "grouped phasic tremor potentials at varying frequencies between 0.5 and 1.5/s, from both anterior tibialis muscles," occurring during presleep wakefulness and sleep stages N1 and N2. Wichniak and colleagues later described[61] a similar phenomenon of "rhythmic oscillating movements of the whole foot or toes with a frequency of 1 to 2 per second and a single movement duration between 300 and 700 milliseconds" in 28 of 375 adult patients (more frequently males) referred to his sleep disorders center, coining the term rhythmic feet movements (RFMs).

According to ICSD-3,[1] both entities are classified as HFT, which is now defined as "rhythmic movement of the feet or toes that occurs at the transition between wake and sleep or during light NREM sleep." In HFT, the patient typically presents with foot movements (directly experienced or observed by others)[38,62] or, occasionally, movements are not observed and HFT is seen as an incidental finding on sleep study conducted for other indications[61] (Fig. 4). International scoring criteria[17] include: a pattern of brief, repeated activation of the anterior tibialis in 1 leg, with a minimum number of 4 HFT bursts on EMG needed to make a train of bursts in an HFT series; a range of frequency of 0.3 to 4.0 Hz; and a range of duration of 250 to 1000 milliseconds. The typical duration of trains is 10 to 15 seconds, although longer bursts and trains have been reported.[1]

The etiophysiology of HFT is unknown, although HFT has been associated with head injuries[38] and with other SRMDs, namely rhythmic movement disorder (RMD).[62] Clinical consequences of HFT

alone have never been reported; thus, treatment is not needed outside of patient education on the diagnosis and the benign nature of this movement.[2] When associated with RMD, pramipexole has been proven effective.[62]

Alternating Leg Muscle Activation

In 2003, Chervin and colleagues named ALMA for the first time,[63] documenting in 16 patients a brief activation of the anterior tibialis in one leg alternated with similar activation contralaterally, in the absence of any visible movement. The phenomenon was particularly frequent during arousals and presented with a movement duration of 0.1 to 0.5 second, a frequency of 1 to 2 Hz and with sequences lasting from a few seconds to 20 seconds. Twelve of the original 16 patients were taking antidepressants; later case reports did not confirm this association.[64,65]

ICSD-3 defines ALMA as "brief activation of the anterior tibialis in one leg in alternation with similar activation in the other leg during sleep or arousals from sleep." Usually found as an isolated polygraphic finding[1] (Fig. 5), in the original case series, patients with ALMA complained of sleepiness, insomnia, or restless of the legs, but only 1 patient reported more specific complaints of sudden nocturnal muscle contractions in his legs and a sensation that his legs "were vibrating".[63] Polygraphic scoring criteria[17] consist of: the presence of discrete and alternating EMG bursts of leg muscle activity events with a minimum number of 4 ALMAs needed to score an ALMA series; a range of frequency of 0.5 to 3.0 Hz; and a range of duration of 100 to 50 milliseconds. An ALMA series can begin with one to several lengthier activations (1–2 seconds) in one or both legs. The patient may report foot movements, but frequently no observation of movement is reported.[34]

Although the pathophysiologic mechanism of ALMA is currently unknown, the association with antidepressants suggested a relation with serotoninergic and dopaminergic pathways in the spinal network. In the seminal case series, ALMA was evaluated in patients with concurrent obstructive sleep apnea and with proved PLMS, but it can be present also as an isolated symptom.[21,63] ALMA alone usually does not need any treatment; however, when described in a patient with concurrent insomnia and daytime sleepiness not caused by any other disorder, pramipexole has been administered with efficacy.[64]

High-Frequency Leg Movements

In 2010 Yang and Winkelman defined and documented high-frequency leg movements (HFLMs)[66]

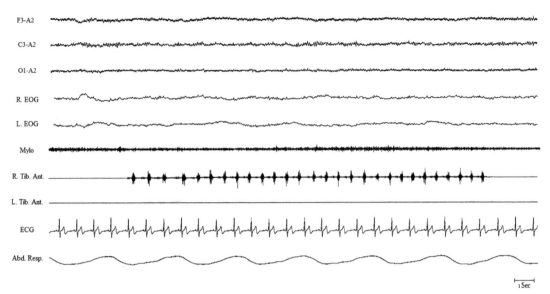

Fig. 4. Excerpt of a polygraphic recording of HFT. Brief sequence of repeated activation of the right anterior tibialis can be seen during relaxed wakefulness, at a frequency of about 1 Hz. Abd. Resp., abdominal respirogram; ECG, electrocardiogram; EOG, electrooculogram; L., left; Mylo, mylohyoideus muscle; R., right; Tib. Ant., tibialis anterior muscle.

in a group of 486 patients referred to their sleep center. These phenomena were described as overlapping but distinct from HFT and ALMA, in an effort to clarify the nature and the scoring criteria of rhythmic leg movements sensu stricto. HFLMs were defined as at least 4 consecutive discrete EMG bursts of leg muscle activity (unilateral, bilateral, or alternating) with a duration between 0.1 and 0.5 second and a frequency of 0.3

to 4 Hz.[66] Thirty-seven patients (7.6%) with equal sex distribution presented with HFLM, mostly occurring during relaxed wakefulness and light sleep. Notably, patients with HFLM complained of RLS symptoms significantly more often than subjects without HFLM.[66]

More recently, Frauscher and colleagues verified these criteria in a population of 100 healthy sleepers,[25] observing a prevalence of HFLMs of

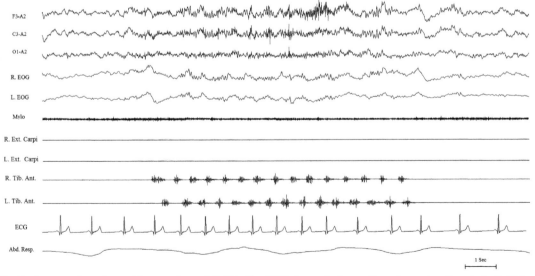

Fig. 5. Excerpt of a polygraphic recording of ALMA. The EMG channels show alternate contractions in both tibialis anterior muscles at about 1 to 2 Hz. Abd. Resp., abdominal respirogram; ECG, electrocardiogram; EOG, electrooculogram; Ext. Carpi., extensor carpi muscle; L., left.; Mylo, mylohyoideus muscle; R., right; Tib. Ant., tibialis anterior muscle.

33%, with a low median number of episodes per night (2 episodes), a short mean duration of 3.4 second, and a median frequency of 2.1 Hz. These results confirmed HFLMs as greatly overlapping with HFT and ALMA. In addition, a moderate correlation between the number of HFLMs and PLMS index was found.[25]

Are Hypnagogic Foot Tremor, Alternating Leg Muscle Activation, and High-Frequency Leg Movements Different Entities? The High-Frequency Leg Movement Spectrum

In light of this evidence, the Innsbruck group further hypothesized that HFT, ALMA, and HFLM (sensu stricto - HFLMs), overlapping minor motor activity during relaxed wakefulness and sleep, should all fall under the most comprehensive descriptive and neutral term of HFLM (sensu lato - HFLMs). In support of this, both HFT and ALMA have been recently described in a pair of cousins,[65] suggesting a common etiophysiology.

In addition, the relationship between ALMA and HFLMs with PLMS[25,63] and the association between HFLMs and RLS symptoms suggests that HFLMs might be abortive PLMS and hence be part of the broad PLMS spectrum.[25,65] In light of this, in case of polygraphic findings of HFLMs, it could be helpful to investigate RLS symptoms as a potential underlying condition causing these phenomena.[3]

SLEEP-RELATED LEG CRAMPS
Definition and Essential Features

Sleep-related leg cramps (SLCs) are involuntary forceful contractions of muscles, especially affecting the lower limbs and in particular the muscles of the posterior compartment of the leg and the small muscles of the foot, usually 1 leg at a time.[21] The triceps surae (calf muscle) is the muscle most frequently affected. During the cramps, the muscles involved become firm and tender, and feet and toes are held in extreme plantar flexion.[33] The contraction is painful and can last from few seconds up to 10 minutes, but the soreness may linger for the whole night.[21] The patient can usually relieve the soaring pain by stretching the affected muscle and sometimes also by local massage, application of heat, or movement of the affected limb.[1]

Clinical Relevance

The frequency of SLCs varies considerably from less than yearly to multiple episodes every night. However, in almost one-half of patients with leg cramps, symptoms are reported several times per week or daily.[67] Twenty-one percent of cramp sufferers described their symptoms as distressing.[68] In addition, nocturnal sleep may be impaired with difficulty in falling asleep and/or frequent awakening at night; persisting discomfort after the cramps often delays subsequent return to sleep.

Diagnosis and Assessment
Diagnostic criteria

According to the ICSD-3,[1] several criteria define SLC:

- A painful sensation in the leg or foot associated with sudden, involuntary muscle hardness or tightness, indicating a strong muscle contraction
- The painful muscle contractions occur during the time in bed, although they may arise from either wakefulness or sleep
- The pain is relieved by forceful stretching of the affected muscles, thus releasing the contraction

Polygraphic evaluation

SLCs reveal nonperiodic bursts of gastrocnemius EMG activity that arise without any specific preceding physiologic changes during sleep.[2] Electrophysiologic recordings show that the cramps typically start with spontaneous firing of anterior horn cells followed by motor unit discharges for contractions at rates up to 300 Hz (considerably more than with voluntary muscle contractions).[69,70] Moreover, SLC are attended by contractions of a slowly moving fraction of muscle fibers, with very short EMG potentials, again, unlike maximal voluntary contractions.[71]

Sleep-related leg cramps may be observed during relaxed wakefulness and throughout all sleep stages, which further demonstrates that they cannot be attributed to physiologic changes during particular stages.[2]

Differential diagnosis

SLCs must be distinguished from RLS as the leg discomfort could be easily confused. The leg discomfort of RLS, although it can consist of cramping sensations, does not typically involve actual spasm or hardening of the muscle that occurs during the cramp. Furthermore, leg cramp events tend to be much briefer compared with the typical symptoms of RLS, which can persist for hours.[1] SLC can also be confused with other organic disorders, such as chronic myelopathy, peripheral neuropathy, and dystonias; clinical history, physical examination, and EMG examination help to discriminate between these conditions.[2]

Unlike SLC, peripheral neuropathy tends to be associated with sensory or motor findings, whereas focal dystonias of the feet can be distinguished demonstrating the co-contraction of agonist and antagonist muscles.[72]

Epidemiology and Associated Conditions

SLCs occur in about 7% of children and adolescents, 33% of adults older than 60 years, and 50% of adults older than 80 years, with both older groups reporting a symptom frequency of at least once every 2 months.[67,68,73] Pregnancy has also been associated with sleep-related leg cramps; about 33% to 50% of pregnant women experience leg cramps that also tend to become worse.[74,75] Heavy physical exercise, medications (eg, naproxen, intravenous iron sucrose, estrogens, and teriparatide) and fluid and electrolyte disturbances can trigger nocturnal cramps.[2] In addition, individuals with certain medical disorders, such as diabetes, sleep apnea,[76] blood vessel disease, and nerve or muscle diseases, may be more likely to have sleep-related cramps.[34]

Etiophysiology

The mechanism of SLCs is still debated. Muscle cramps may be brought about by repetitive stimulation of homonymous fusal afferents and the after discharges typically found following M and F waves suggest impaired motor neuron excitability.[77] Other pathophysiological hypotheses attribute muscle cramps to abnormal central nervous drive on the lower motor neuron or still, to enhanced fusal with decreased Golgi tendon organ activity.[78] Studies aimed at answering this question have used several methods to elicit cramps, such as direct electrical stimulation of nerves, which has demonstrated a lower threshold of intensity necessary to trigger cramps in cramp-prone individuals compared with those without history of cramps.[79,80]

Treatment

Quinine is the only drug with proved Class 1 efficacy for the prevention and reduction in intensity of sleep-related leg cramps,[69] but after the alert launched by the US Food and Drug Administration in 2012, it is no longer a recommended treatment because of its unfavorable risk-benefit profile.[81] Oral magnesium supplements, calcium channel blockers, gabapentin, complex B vitamins, and vitamin E have also been used, however, with little or no evidence.[69]

SUMMARY

Isolated motor symptoms are frequently missed or misinterpreted polygraphic findings that can be frequently confused with the more frequent SRMDs. Expanding the knowledge on these isolated symptoms and defining their polygraphic and clinical features are therefore essential for their identification. As a matter of fact, these symptoms can also be the cause of otherwise cryptogenic insomnias and somnolence, and by acknowledging their existence and features, diagnostic accuracy can be increased. However, up-to-date clear cut-offs to discern between the isolated phenomenon and the disorder are not available. Hence, it is necessary to perform multicenter and multimodal observations on larger groups, which will allow also better defining their pathophysiological origins, understanding the fine mechanisms of motor regulation during (and outside) sleep.

CLINICS CARE POINTS

- Fragmentary Hypnic Myoclonus and many others Isolated Motor Phenomena of Sleep can be paraphysiological and are frequently incidental polygraphic findings.
- Accurate history taking with the help of the patient's sleep partner, if present, is mandatory for a correct differential diagnosis.
- Definite diagnosis is frequently only achieved by means of videopolysomnography.
- Treatment is appropriate only when sleep-related motor phenomena become intense and/or frequent, impacting nocturnal sleep and causing diurnal symptoms.

ACKNOWLEDGMENTS

The authors thank Annagrazia Cecere, Francesco Mignani, and Rosalia Cilea for providing figures and Cecilia Baroncini for English revision.

DISCLOSURE

F. Provini received fees for consultancy and speaking engagements from Vanda Pharmaceutical, Sanofi, Zambon, Italfarmaco, Fidia, Bial, Eisai Japan. L. Baldelli has nothing to disclose.

REFERENCES

1. American Academy of Sleep Medicine. International classification of sleep disorders. 3rd edition. Darien (IL): American Academy of Sleep Medicine; 2014.

2. Salas R, Gulyani S, Kwan A, Gamaldo C. Sleep-related movement disorders and their unique motor manifestations. In: Kryger M, Roth T, Dement WC, editors. Principles and practice of sleep medicine, Sixth Edition, Elsevier; Philadelfia (USA); 2017. p.1020-9.

3. Stefani A, Högl B. Diagnostic criteria, differential diagnosis, and treatment of minor motor activity and less well-known movement disorders of sleep. Curr Treat Options Neurol 2019;21(1):1.

4. De Lisi L. Su di un fenomeno motorio costante del sonno normale: le mioclonie ipniche fisiologiche. Riv Pat Nerv Ment 1932;39:481–96.

5. Gassel MM, Marchiafava PL, Pompeiano O. Phasic changes in muscular activity during desynchronized sleep in unrestrained cats. An analysis of the pattern and organization of myoclonic twitches. Arch Ital Biol 1964;102:449–70.

6. Dagnino N, Loeb C, Massazza G, et al. Hypnic physiological myoclonias in man: an EEG-EMG study in normals and neurological patients. Eur Neurol 1969;2(1):47–58.

7. Broughton R, Tolentino MA. Fragmentary pathological myoclonus in NREM sleep. Electroencephalography Clin Neurophysiol 1984;57(4):303–9.

8. Broughton R, Tolentino MA, Krelina M. Excessive fragmentary myoclonus in NREM sleep: a report of 38 cases. Electroencephalogr Clin Neurophysiol 1985;61(2):123–33.

9. Montagna P, Liguori R, Zucconi M, et al. Physiological hypnic myoclonus. Electroencephalography Clin Neurophysiol 1988;70(2):172–6.

10. Kumar Goyal M, Kumar G, Sivaraman M, et al. Teaching neuroimages: excessive fragmentary hypnic myoclonus. Neurology 2011;77(10):e59–60.

11. Trimmel K, Lindinger G, Böck M, et al. It twitches without kicking - an association between fragmentary myoclonus and arousal? Clin Neurophysiol 2019;130(8):1358–63.

12. Sobreira-Neto MA, Pena-Pereira MA, Sobreira ES, et al. Excessive fragmentary myoclonus in patients with Parkinson's disease: prevalence and clinico-polysomnographic profile. Sleep & breathing 2015; 19(3):997–1002.

13. Vetrugno R, Liguori R, Cortelli P, et al. Sleep-related stridor due to dystonic vocal cord motion and neurogenic tachypnea/tachycardia in multiple system atrophy. Mov Disord 2007;22(5):673–8.

14. Šonka K, Fiksa J, Horváth E, et al. Sleep and fasciculations in amyotrophic lateral sclerosis. Somnologie - Schlafforschung und Schlafmedizin 2004;8(1): 25–30.

15. dos Santos DF, Pedroso JL, Braga-Neto P, et al. Excessive fragmentary myoclonus in Machado-Joseph disease. Sleep Med 2014;15(3):355–8.

16. Vankova J, Stepanova I, Jech R, et al. Sleep disturbances and hypocretin deficiency in Niemann-Pick disease type C. Sleep 2003;26(4):427–30.

17. Berry R, Brooks R, Gamaldo C, et al. The AASM manual for the scoring of sleep and associated events: rules, terminology and technical specifications, version 2.6. American Academy of Sleep Medicine, Darien, Illinois. Darien (IL): American Academy of Sleep Medicine; 2020.

18. Hoque R, McCarty DE, Chesson AL. Manual quantitative assessment of amplitude and sleep stage distribution of excessive fragmentary myoclonus. J Clin Sleep Med 2013;09(01):39–45.

19. Lins O, Castonguay M, Dunham W, et al. Excessive fragmentary myoclonus: time of night and sleep stage distributions. Can J Neurol Sci 1993;20(2): 142–6.

20. Nepožitek J, Šonka K. Excessive fragmentary myoclonus: what do we know? Prague Med Rep 2017; 118(1):5–13.

21. Vetrugno R, Provini F, Montagna P. Chapter 54 - isolated motor phenomena and symptoms of sleep. In: Montagna P, Chokroverty S, editors. Handbook of clinical neurology, vol. 99. Amsterdam: Elsevier; 2011. p. 883–99.

22. Frauscher B, Kunz A, Brandauer E, et al. Fragmentary myoclonus in sleep revisited: a polysomnographic study in 62 patients. Sleep Med 2011;12(4):410–5.

23. Raccagni C, Löscher WN, Stefani A, et al. Peripheral nerve function in patients with excessive fragmentary myoclonus during sleep. Sleep Med 2016;22: 61–4.

24. Mizuma H, Sakamoto T. Excessive twitch movements in rapid eye movement sleep with daytime sleepiness. Psychiatry Clin Neurosciences 1997; 51(6):393–6.

25. Frauscher B, Gabelia D, Mitterling T, et al. Motor events during healthy sleep: a quantitative polysomnographic study. Sleep 2014;37(4):763–73, 773a-773b.

26. Tinuper P, Provini F, Bisulli F, et al. Movement disorders in sleep: guidelines for differentiating epileptic from non-epileptic motor phenomena arising from sleep. Sleep Med Rev 2007;11(4):255–67.

27. Montagna P, Provini F, Vetrugno R. Propriospinal myoclonus at sleep onset. Neurophysiol Clin 2006; 36(5–6):351–5.

28. Montagna P, Provini F, Plazzi G, et al. Propriospinal myoclonus upon relaxation and drowsiness: a cause of severe insomnia. Mov Disord 1997;12(1):66–72.

29. Antelmi E, Provini F. Propriospinal myoclonus: the spectrum of clinical and neurophysiological phenotypes. Sleep Med Rev 2015;22:54–63.

30. Moruzzi G. The sleep-waking cycle. Ergebnisse Physiol 1972;64:1–165.

31. Vetrugno R, Plazzi G, Provini F, et al. Excessive fragmentary hypnic myoclonus: clinical and neurophysiological findings. Sleep Med 2002;3(1):73–6.

32. Pincherle A, Mantoani L, Villani F, et al. Excessive fragmentary hypnic myoclonus in a patient affected

by a mitochondrial encephalomyopathy. Sleep Med 2006;7(8):663.

33. Montagna P. Sleep-related non epileptic motor disorders. J Neurol 2004;251(7):781–94.

34. Merlino G, Gigli GL. Sleep-related movement disorders. Neurol Sci 2012;33(3):491–513.

35. Mitchell SW. Some disorders of sleep. 1. Am J Med Sci 1890;100(2):109.

36. Oswald I. Sudden bodily jerks on falling asleep. Brain 1959;82(1):92–103.

37. Gastatut H, Broughton R. A clinical and polygraphic study of episodic phenomena during sleep. In: Wortis J, editor. Recent advances in biology and psychiatry, vol. 7. New York: Plenum Press; 1965. p. 197–222.

38. Broughton R. Pathological fragmentary myoclonus, intensified hypnic jerks and hypnagogic foot tremor: three unusual sleep-related movement disorders. In: Koella W, editor. Sleep '86. Proceedings of the eighth european congress on sleep research, vol. 86. Gustav Fischer; 1988. p. 240–3.

39. Vetrugno R, Montagna P. Sleep-to-wake transition movement disorders. Sleep Med 2011;12(Suppl 2):S11–6.

40. Walters AS. Clinical identification of the simple sleep-related movement disorders. Chest 2007; 131(4):1260–6.

41. Cuellar NG, Whisenant D, Stanton MP. Hypnic jerks: a scoping literature review. Sleep Med Clin 2015; 10(3):393–401, xvi.

42. Chiaro G, Calandra-Buonaura G, Sambati L, et al. Hypnic jerks are an underestimated sleep motor phenomenon in patients with parkinsonism. A video-polysomnographic and neurophysiological study. Sleep Med 2016;26:37–44.

43. Chokroverty S, Bhat S, Gupta D. Intensified hypnic jerks: a polysomnographic and polymyographic analysis. J Clin Neurophysiol 2013;30(4):403–10.

44. Calandra-Buonaura G, Alessandria M, Liguori R, et al. Hypnic jerks: neurophysiological characterization of a new motor pattern. Sleep Med 2014;15(6): 725–7.

45. Clouston PD, Lim CL, Fung V, et al. Brainstem myoclonus in a patient with non-dopa-responsive parkinsonism. Mov Disord 1996;11(4):404–10.

46. Bruno RL. Abnormal movements in sleep as a post-polio sequelae. Am J Phys Med Rehabil 1998;77(4): 339–43.

47. Bruni O, Galli F, Guidetti V. Sleep hygiene and migraine in children and adolescents. Cephalalgia 1999;19(Suppl 25):57–9.

48. Fusco L, Pachatz C, Cusmai R, et al. Repetitive sleep starts in neurologically impaired children: an unusual non-epileptic manifestation in otherwise epileptic subjects. Epileptic Disord 1999;1(1):63–7.

49. Iyer S, Iyer R. Sleep disordered breathing in Dombivli and Mumbai (India): interesting observations. Sleep 2014;37. Abstract Supplement.

50. Eitner S, Urschitz MS, Guenther A, et al. Sleep problems and daytime somnolence in a German population-based sample of snoring school-aged children. J Sleep Res 2007;16(1):96–101.

51. Lai YY, Siegel JM. Brainstem-mediated locomotion and myoclonic jerks. I. Neural substrates. Brain Res 1997;745(1):257–64.

52. Salih F, Klingebiel R, Zschenderlein R, et al. Acoustic sleep starts with sleep-onset insomnia related to a brainstem lesion. Neurology 2008;70(20):1935–7.

53. Provini F, Vetrugno R, Meletti S, et al. Motor pattern of periodic limb movements during sleep. Neurology 2001;57(2):300–4.

54. Mahowald MW, Schenck CH. NREM sleep parasomnias. Neurol Clin 1996;14(4):675–96.

55. Sander HW, Geisse H, Quinto C, et al. Sensory sleep starts. J Neurol Neurosurg Psychiatry 1998;64(5):690.

56. Armstrong-Jones R. Snapping of the brain. Lancet 1920;196(5066):720.

57. Sachs C, Svanborg E. The exploding head syndrome: polysomnographic recordings and therapeutic suggestions. Sleep 1991;14(3):263–6.

58. Pearce JM. Clinical features of the exploding head syndrome. J Neurol Neurosurg Psychiatry 1989; 52(7):907–10.

59. Sharpless BA. Exploding head syndrome. Sleep Med Rev 2014;18(6):489–93.

60. Lance JW. Transient sensations of impending loss of consciousness: the "blip" syndrome. J Neurol Neurosurg Psychiatry 1996;60(4):437–8.

61. Wichniak A, Tracik F, Geisler P, et al. Rhythmic feet movements while falling asleep. Mov Disord 2001; 16(6):1164–70.

62. Merlino G, Serafini A, Dolso P, et al. Association of body rolling, leg rolling, and rhythmic feet movements in a young adult: a video-polysomnographic study performed before and after one night of clonazepam. Mov Disord 2008;23(4):602–7.

63. Chervin RD, Consens FB, Kutluay E. Alternating leg muscle activation during sleep and arousals: a new sleep-related motor phenomenon? Mov Disord 2003;18(5):551–9.

64. Cosentino FI, Iero I, Lanuzza B, et al. The neurophysiology of the alternating leg muscle activation (ALMA) during sleep: study of one patient before and after treatment with pramipexole. Sleep Med 2006;7(1):63–71.

65. Bergmann M, Stefani A, Brandauer E, et al. Hypnagogic foot tremor, alternating leg muscle activation or high frequency leg movements: clinical and phenomenological considerations in two cousins. Sleep Med 2019;54:177–80.

66. Yang C, Winkelman JW. Clinical and polysomnographic characteristics of high frequency leg movements. J Clin Sleep Med 2010;6(5):431–8.

67. Abdulla AJ, Jones PW, Pearce VR. Leg cramps in the elderly: prevalence, drug and disease associations. Int J Clin Pract 1999;53(7):494–6.

68. Naylor JR, Young JB. A general population survey of rest cramps. Age Ageing 1994;23(5):418–20.
69. Tipton PW, Wszołek ZK. Restless legs syndrome and nocturnal leg cramps: a review and guide to diagnosis and treatment. Polish Arch Intern Med 2017;127(12):865–72.
70. Minetto MA, Holobar A, Botter A, et al. Origin and development of muscle cramps. Exerc Sport Sci Rev 2013;41(1):3–10.
71. Roeleveld K, Engelen BGMv, Stegeman DF. Possible mechanisms of muscle cramp from temporal and spatial surface EMG characteristics. J Appl Physiol 2000;88(5):1698–706.
72. Monderer RS, Wu WP, Thorpy MJ. Nocturnal leg cramps. Curr Neurol Neurosci Rep 2010;10(1):53–9.
73. Oboler SK, Prochazka AV, Meyer TJ. Leg symptoms in outpatient veterans. West J Med 1991;155(3):256–9.
74. Zhou K, West HM, Zhang J, et al. Interventions for leg cramps in pregnancy. Cochrane Database Syst Rev 2015;(8):Cd010655.
75. Hensley JG. Leg cramps and restless legs syndrome during pregnancy. J Midwifery Women Health 2009;54(3):211–8.
76. Westwood AJ, Spector AR, Auerbach SH. CPAP treats muscle cramps in patients with obstructive sleep apnea. J Clin Sleep Med 2014;10(6):691–2.
77. Baldissera F, Cavallari P, Dworzak F. Motor neuron 'bistability'. A pathogenetic mechanism for cramps and myokymia. Brain 1994;117(Pt 5):929–39.
78. Schwellnus MP, Derman EW, Noakes TD. Aetiology of skeletal muscle 'cramps' during exercise: a novel hypothesis. J Sports Sci 1997;15(3):277–85.
79. Miller KC, Knight KL. Electrical stimulation cramp threshold frequency correlates well with the occurrence of skeletal muscle cramps. Muscle Nerve 2009;39(3):364–8.
80. Minetto MA, Botter A. Elicitability of muscle cramps in different leg and foot muscles. Muscle Nerve 2009;40(4):535–44.
81. Garcia-Malo C, Peralta SR, Garcia-Borreguero D. Restless legs syndrome and other common sleep-related movement disorders. Continuum: Lifelong Learn Neurol 2020;26(4):963–87.

Propriospinal Myoclonus

Marco Zucconi, MD[a,*], Francesca Casoni, MD, PhD[a], Andrea Galbiati, PhD[a,b,c]

KEYWORDS

- Propriospinal myoclonus • Sleep-related movement disorder • Sleep and myoclonus
- Sleep onset insomnia

KEY POINTS

- Propriospinal myoclonus consists of paroxysmal and sudden jerks involving axial flexion trunk and hip muscles typically arising during the transition between wake and sleep.
- Propriospinal myoclonus originates from a thoracic myelomere and spreads caudally and rostrally, provoking flexion and/or extension movements, leading to jumps or trunk jerks.
- The main consequences are difficulties in sleep start and the reappearance during period of wakefulness after sleep onset.

INTRODUCTION

Myoclonus as a neurologic sign may originate at different central nervous system (CNS) levels: when it starts within the spinal cord, it is called "spinal myoclonus" (SM), and it is of segmental origin and without propagation. Whereas, when it arises from the spinal cord and it does not remain restricted to one or a few segmental innervated muscles but propagates up and down the spinal cord, provoking repetitive and arrhythmic jerks, in flexions or extension, of the trunks, neck, and less often arms and legs, it is defined as "propriospinal myoclonus" (PSM). The PSM usually originates from thoracoabdominal paraspinal muscles, rarer from the neck and cervical ones, with diffuse jerks different from the focal ones because of the SM. Generally, the jerks are spontaneous and can appear in any body position, but they may be evoked by external stimuli or sensory inputs, frequently when the subject is sitting or lying. It is more frequent and triggered by the relaxed wakefulness preceding sleep onset and during transition from wake to sleep, and it propagates along a propriospinal pathway intrinsic to the spinal cord, with a slow conduction velocity through a multisynaptic slow-conduction pathway, as first described by Brown and colleagues.[1,2] The cause is to search in a spinal generator, physiologically involved in locomotor activity, exposed to a dysfacilitation of supraspinal motor pattern generator.[3]

CLINICAL PICTURE

The initial case described by Brown and colleagues[1] was a 55-year-old man complaining of paroxysmal jerks involving axial flexion trunk and hip muscles, conditioning sudden myoclonic movement of the trunk and arms/limbs, both spontaneous and triggered by external sensory stimulations of the abdominal wall. The jerks last up to 3 hours, and they repeat periodically every minute, spontaneously or evoked by taps of the abdominal wall.[4]

Generally, the jerks originate in the muscles of a particular thoracic myelomere, and they progressively and synchronously spread to the other trunk muscles, both rostrally and caudally. This myoclonic activity provokes flexion and/or extension movements, leading sometimes to sudden movements, jumps, or simply trunk jerks. Cranial and limb muscles are generally less involved. The jerks and the movements appear to be position dependent, triggered by the lying-down position and disappearing when the

[a] Sleep Disorders Centre, Department of Clinical Neurosciences, San Raffaele Hospital, Via Stamira d'Ancona, 20, Milan 20127, Italy; [b] School of Psychology, Vita-Salute San Raffaele University, Milan, Italy; [c] Division of Neuroscience, Neurologic Unit, Sleep Disorders Center, IRCCS San Raffaele Scientific Institute, IRCCS San Raffaele Hospital, Università Vita-Salute San Raffaele, Milan, Italy
* Corresponding author.
E-mail address: zucconi.marco@hsr.it

Sleep Med Clin 16 (2021) 363–371
https://doi.org/10.1016/j.jsmc.2021.02.009
1556-407X/21/© 2021 Elsevier Inc. All rights reserved.

subject stands up and walks.[4,5] More frequently, the PSM starts during a period of quiet wakefulness and relaxation preceding the sleep onset, with a clear periodicity, and sometimes accompanied by strange sensations of something shocklike or electrical-like in the chest, neck, head, or other trunk portions before the start of the myoclonic jerks.[6] With the mental activity or the volition, the patients report that they can partially control but not completely suppress the jerks. PSM is much more frequent when the subject tries to fall asleep, provoking a rapid reappraisal of wake state, therefore preventing sleep onset and determining a sleep-onset insomnia.[7,8] This characteristic seems a peculiar feature of PSM even though it is not reported in some of the descriptions.[4,6] However, when the patients present to a sleep medicine physician and electroencephalogram (EEG) or polysomnographic recordings are carried out, the start of myoclonic jerks coincides with the diffusion of posterior alpha-wave activity, spreading to anterior leads and intermittently mixed with slow theta activity, typical of non–rapid eye movement sleep (NREM) stage N1, but making the sleep onset very difficult and sometimes unsuccessful.[6,7,9,10] Once the sleep onset is reached, with difficulty, and the stable sleep starts with an NREM stage N2 (K-complexes and spindles), the jerks disappear and the PSM ceases. The movements may reappear during arousals or awakenings with similar features, and generally, they may be more segmental than completely involving the trunk.[8,11–14] PSM during sleep is very rare, and the jerks are subtle and nonperiodic.[7,15,16]

PSM originates in the thoracoabdominal paraspinal muscles and less frequently in the cervical muscles. It is not age related but is typical of middle-aged subjects, more frequent in men (symptomatic forms more frequent in women), and rare in children.[3,17] Most of the cases described in the literature are considered idiopathic because no clear organic lesions of the spinal cord or of other CNS levels have been demonstrated. However, also in the "symptomatic" forms, the causal link between the organic lesions and PSM is unclear also because the temporal link between lesions and onset of PSM remains uncertain. The medical conditions include neoplastic and paraneoplastic lesions, cervical and thoracic herniations, lumbar disc protrusion, thoracic herpes zoster, neuropathy and demyelinating lesions, Lyme disease, myasthenia gravis, HIV infection, breast cancer, drug abuse, vitamin B12 deficiency, and celiac disease.[2,12,13,18–24] Associated back trauma was also reported[3,4,17,25]

as well as administered medications, such as interferon, ciprofloxacin, bupivacaine, and others.[16,26–28]

The clinical observations with the support of neurophysiology indicate the involvement of muscles with segmental innervation representing virtually the entire length of the spinal cord. Therefore, the spinal generator theory with propagation caudally and rostrally via propriospinal pathways remains the best shown cause, considering also the lack of any cortical premovement EEG activity (documented by the back-averaging studies) of the myoclonic jerks.[5,29,30] The spreading of the motor volleys is slow, around 5 to 6 m/s, confirming the propriospinal conduction.[4]

It is rare that patients refer to possible suppression of the jerks on volition, whereas sometimes they refer to some "need" to do the movements, as a compulsion. For the former, the differential diagnosis with a functional movement is necessary, and for the latter, some differentiation from a tic disorder may be useful to confirm the diagnosis.[5,30]

The age of onset is variable, with case reports of a wide range of ages between pediatric and old age, without gender prevalence. The characteristics of the movements are also variable: in most of the cases, the jerks start and involve the axial muscles, and at least 50% are considered position dependent, with worsening in the supine position. In at least one-third of the cases, the movements are stimulus sensitive, sometimes periodic or rhythmic, generally in flexion more than in extension, and, in the authors' experience, they are triggered mostly by falling asleep.[6,7,15]

Different clinical and neurophysiologic phenotypes have been described. The most frequent PSM is the form at sleep onset, where the movement disorder occurs when the subject is recumbent but is falling asleep, starting or increasing when there is a diffusion of the EEG alpha activity not only to the occipital leads but also to the central and frontal ones[7,9,11,15] (Figs. 1–4). PSM continues during stage N1 (presence of theta activity for >50% of the 30-second epoch of sleep scoring) and stops when a stage N2 is reached, with the appearance of K-complexes and spindles.[8,11,14,17] Rarely, the myoclonic jerks appear during stable sleep.[1,7,16] They may reappear when an arousal or an awakening interrupts sleep continuity, mainly from stage N1 and N2, but are less diffuse to the other muscles and may affect only the segments where the PSM originated.

Other clinical phenotypes might be the "tic-like characteristics" with some premonitory sensations as an urgency to move or to jerk that cannot be voluntarily controlled.[5] The functional

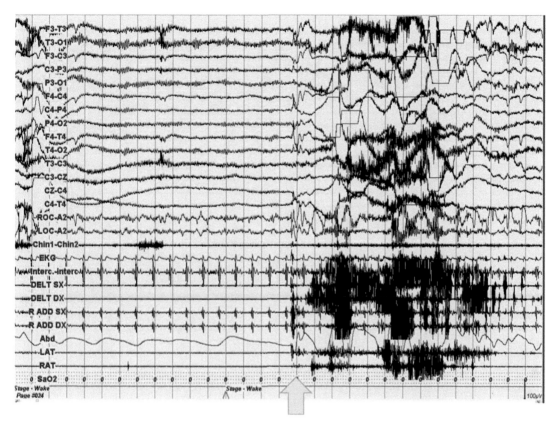

Fig. 1. Propriospinal myoclonus in a patient, with some episodes in wakefulness at different speeds of the screen. EEG leads: LOG-A2 and ROC-A2, eye movements; Chin 1-Chin 2, submental EMG; EKG: Interc-interc, EMG of intercostal (right IV space); Delt dx and Delt sx, EMG of deltoid muscles; R ADD sx and R ADD dx, EMG of the rectus abdominal muscles; Abd, abdominal effort; RAT, EMG of the right tibialis anterior muscle; LAT, EMG of the left tibialis anterior muscle; Sao₂, o₂ saturation (not working in wakefulness). A single episode (*arrow*) of PSM with spread at the different muscles (speed velocity, 30 seconds per epoch).

movement disorder is consistent with abnormal movements with a supposed psychogenic origin and a different pattern in respect to the typical organic movement disorder: intra-individual variability also over time, distractibility, involvement of facial and cranial muscles, and associated emotional components with psychological or psychiatric disturbances. In these cases, electrophysiologic and eventual video-polysomnographic examinations may clarify the different behaviors and phenotype.[29,30]

CAUSE AND ETIOPATHOGENESIS

The main differentiation of PSM, according to the cause, is primary and secondary forms. The first descriptions indicated cervical spinal cord lesions as the cause of the PSM, where the propriospinal system has been considered responsible for the rhythmic myoclonic movements of the trunk and lower limbs.[1,3,31] Intrinsic spinal cord lesions, mainly at the thoracic level, have been associated

with PSM, but in a minority of the cases (not >30%) include myelopathy, myelitis, cervical tumors, and syringomyelia.[4,5,7,13,19,22,25,32,33] However, sometimes the putative lesion, that is, disc protrusion evidenced by MRI, might not be the cause of the myoclonic jerks because there is not clear evidence of structural lesions at the spinal cord level.[7] No structural lesions have been found also for cervical disc herniation, lumbar disc protrusion, or back trauma. Some other cases have been reported as isolated PSM associated with herpes zoster, Lyme disease, hepatitis C, anti-MAG antibodies, myasthenia gravis, breast cancer, *Escherichia coli* infection, and also in association (however, with no proved causality) with drug exposure to interferon, antibiotics (as ciprofloxacin), or bupivacaine.[3,11,12,16,18,21,23,26,27,34] In many of these cases, the direct relationship between the lesion or the supposed drug action, because of the lack of a temporary causality between the PSM and the hypothetical responsible factor, remains to be proved.

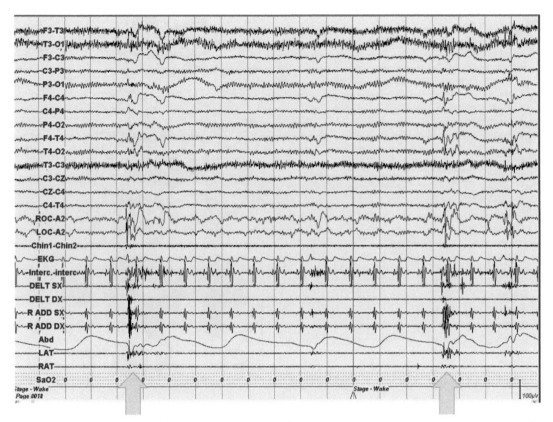

Fig. 2. Two episodes (*arrows*) of PSM with spread at the different muscles (speed velocity, 30 seconds per epoch).

Most of the cases have been considered primary or idiopathic: these might be for the functional abnormalities of the spinal generator with hyperexcitability of the myoclonic volleys triggered by afferent stimuli coming from the distal part of the spinal cord.[6] As an alternative, PSM might be provoked by lesions undetectable from the current MRI.[4] The start of the jerks in the lying-down position and the persistence with increasing frequency, when the subject is falling asleep, are possibly explained by the different response of propriospinal stimuli to the different body positions (with more intensive hyperexcitability in the supine position than in the standing position).[35] The loss of the supraspinal inhibition and control of the spinal generator, with relaxation and sleep onset, may be an alternative pathophysiologic explanation.

NEUROPHYSIOLOGY AND IMAGING

Polymyography is essential for the diagnosis of PSM,[1,18] although formal criteria do not exist. PSM consists of single or repetitive jerks of a duration less than 1000 milliseconds.[3] Electrophysiology reveals recruitment or simultaneous spread of ascending and descending segments typically from a thoracic or abdominal spinal source (myoclonic generator) with a slow spinal cord conduction velocity (5–15 m/s), suggesting a polysynaptic transmission in the ventrolateral funiculus.[1,3] The pattern of muscle activation is constant, with synchronous activation of agonist and antagonist muscles and with no involvement of facial muscles.[1] An inconsistent pattern of muscle activation may be supportive for a functional spinal myoclonus (FMD).[30,36] In FMD cases, jerks are not rhythmic and do not persist during sleep.

Patients with suspected PSM should be recorded with a full polysomnography and polymyography using surface electrodes from masseter, mentalis, sternocleidomastoideus, deltoid, biceps, triceps, paraspinal muscles, intercostal muscles, rectus abdominis, lumbar paraspinal, rectus femoris, tibialis anterior, and gastrocnemius muscles to study the typical pattern. It is also useful as a jerk-locked back-averaging of simultaneous EEG-electromyography (EMG) recording that can demonstrate a Bereitschaftspotential (BP). This premovement potential consists of a negative electrical shift over the central cortical areas that increases over time with

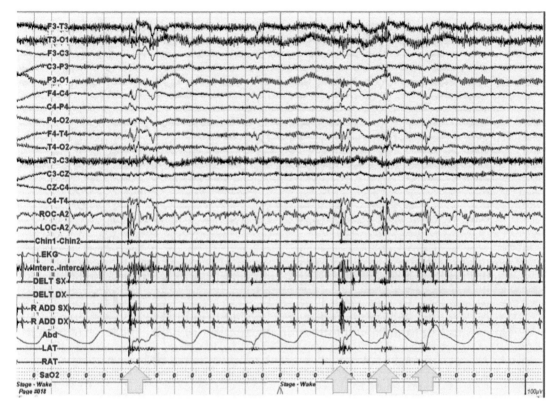

Fig. 3. A series of 4 episodes (*arrows*) of PSM with spread at the different muscles (speed velocity, 60 seconds per epoch).

amplitudes of at least 5 mV,[37] usually recorded before self-paced voluntary movement, indicating a probable functional origin of the disorder (FMD).[38]

The BP can be considered a specific marker to exclude a frontal origin of the jerks and is essential in supporting a presumed FMD cause; however, an absence of BP does not exclude FMD.[39] Indeed, not all functional movements showed a BP, that is, for technical limitations or artifacts due to head movements, its absence does not exclude a cortical origin.

Also, healthy volunteers can mimic the typical EMG pattern of PSM,[40] questioning the role of polymyography in the diagnosis of idiopathic and functional spinal myoclonus.

A recent review of the literature demonstrates that the identification of PSM with electrophysiologic study is difficult because the criteria described by Brown and colleagues[1] are not always respected.[5]

A large cohort of patients with a clinical diagnosis of PSM was evaluated with complete polymyography and jerk-locked back-averaging searching for BP. An incongruent electromyographic pattern was found in 84.6% of patients and the presence of the BP in 86.1% of the entire cohort. The investigators suggest that the clinical distinction of PSM from psychogenic axial jerks is unreliable and that most of the patients with a clinical picture that clinically resembles PSM are likely to be psychogenic.[30]

Neuroimaging should be performed to exclude spinal abnormalities, especially in symptomatic form of PSM.

MRI with diffusion tensor imaging and fiber tracking can reveal spinal tract disorganization and thinning of the spinal fibers, mainly seen in the lemniscal posterior or corticospinal posterolateral tracts.[4,41] These abnormalities did not always match with the myoclonus generator segments as found on electrophysiologic studies, arguing the possibility that these microstructural abnormalities in the spinal cord are consequential rather than causative of the PSM.[4]

DIFFERENTIAL DIAGNOSIS

Different movement disorders may have some clinical similarities with PSM, during both wake and sleep conditions. In general, all spinal segmental myoclonias originating from spinal cord lesions, such as traumatic, inflammatory,

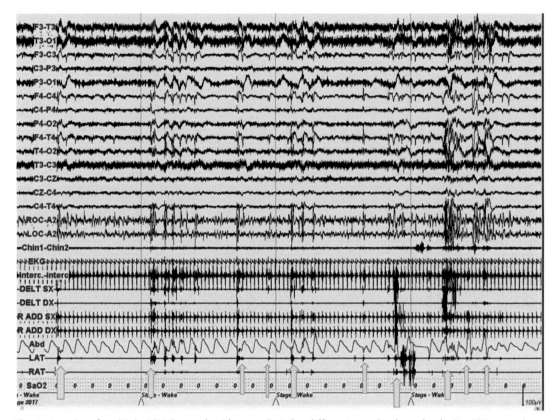

Fig. 4. A series of multiple PSM (*arrows*) with spread at the different muscles (speed velocity, 120 seconds per epoch).

vascular, or neoplastic, may have the neurophysiologic characteristics of PSM, but they show major duration and frequency, with constant and repetitive time sequences. The pathophysiologic condition and trigger, symptoms of lesions, are probably similar, with increasing bursts of the anterior horns and loss of the inhibition coming from supraspinal volleys. The EMG recordings of the different muscular activity with the slow propagation velocity rostrally and caudally may differentiate the 2 phenomena.

Some trunk dystonias may be associated with spasms or jerks involving limbs and trunk but generally are triggered by movements or action and are less represented in relaxation or falling asleep.[42] Similarities are also found with dyskinesia of the diaphragm, often associated with dystonia, characterized by myoclonus and less violent jerks and less associated with axial jump or movements, but more frequently associated with a multidirectional displacement of the abdominal fat and skin similar to a dance.[43] There is variation with position or relaxation, as is well known in PSM.

Some differentiations should be also taken into account with tic disorders, in which myoclonus

with jerks, involving the trunk and arms, is present.[5] When there is a premonitory sensation and supposed voluntary control, the search of the characteristic features of PSM (positional triggering, limit of the myoclonus mostly to trunk and arms with respect of the cranial and facial districts) may help to distinguish the 2 movement disorders.

The more intriguing differentiation is, however, with jerks, movements, and myoclonias arising during the transition from wake to sleep, and during sleep.

Sleep starts or sleep jerks are brief, and simultaneous sudden contractions of some body segments occur almost exclusively at sleep onset. They may be induced by stimuli but generally are spontaneous and not in sequence but isolated. Rarely, they may be particularly frequent and in sequence, causing difficulties to reach a stable stage of sleep.[6] Otherwise, they show a physiologic variation and are considered in the more recent International Classification of Sleep Disorders (Third Edition) as "[i]solated symptoms and normal variants."[44] Sometimes, they are associated with a sensorial component, somesthetic or auditory/visual, with an unpleasant sensation. The polysomnographic recording shows single or repetitive brief muscle jerks (from 75 to 250 milliseconds) with high amplitude at sleep onset and during stage N1, with vertex sharp waves associated with autonomic activation and recruitment.[45] The similarity to PSM might be the propagation from cervical-facial district to caudal muscles, but without a particular order and sequence. The pathophysiology is not completely understood, and with different components: reticulospinal or reticulobulbar volleys, extrapyramidal-type motor component with dystonic and myoclonic features.[45,46] The periodicity or repetitiveness of the myoclonus, the slower velocity of propagation starting in the thoracic segment of spinal cord, and the chronic condition associated with sleep onset insomnia in almost all patients are some distinct features of PSM.

Periodic leg movements during sleep (PLMS), also known by an ancient definition of "nocturnal myoclonus," consist of muscle jerks with dorsiflexion of the anterior leg or feet muscles, sometimes extended to the knee and thigh, and more rarely, to the arms, are frequent in restless legs syndrome (RLS) but recorded in different other sleep disorders, or in healthy elderly subjects.[44] The neurophysiologic characteristics of these periodic movements derived by the EMG analysis of each candidate or leg movement: during sleep with a duration between 0.5 and 10 seconds, separated by an intermovement interval between 10 and 90 seconds, occurring in at least 4 in sequence.[47] Similar but not identical characteristics resulted during wake.[48] PLMS in RLS are mainly in NREM stage N1 and N2 (but not infrequently also in N3 in severe patients) and with a circadian variation and a representation mainly during the first third of the night or with a decrease in frequency going from the beginning to the end of the sleep period.[49]

TREATMENT

Up to now, no official guideline is provided for the treatment of PSM. The mainstay for the management of this disorder is the treatment of the underlying or primary condition, if present. Follow-up of 126 patients reported a resolution of the disorder in 23% of patients treated mostly with clonazepam, and with botulin toxin.[5] Other treatments have been anecdotally reported in the literature. A case study reported that selective serotonin reuptake inhibitors might be effective.[50] Valproate has been suggested as an optional choice.[4] A study described the effectiveness of surgical interventions, such as anterior cervical discectomy

with fusion, that led to a resolution of PSM.[51] Obstructive sleep apnea can aggravate PSM; indeed, a case study reported that continuous positive airway pressure decreased the frequency of the events.[52] Other unconventional therapy, such as biofeedback training and transcutaneous electrical nerve stimulation, showed benefit for PSM.[53,54] In conclusion, future studies should test the efficacy of treatment in randomized controlled trials and in a large cohort of patients.

CLINICS CARE POINTS

- Propriospinal myoclonus is frequently triggered by the relaxed wakefulness preceding sleep onset and can disrupt the transition from wake to sleep.
- Patients with suspected propriospinal myoclonus should be recorded with a full polysomnography and polymyography to reveal the spread of ascending and descending segments typically from a thoracic or abdominal spinal source.
- Differential diagnosis between primary and secondary forms is essential for proper treatment.
- The mainstay for the management of this disorder is the treatment of the underlying or primary condition if present.
- Pharmacologic (clonazepam, selective serotonin reuptake inhibitors, valproate) and nonpharmacologic (biofeedback training and transcutaneous electrical nerve stimulation) treatments might be considered.

DISCLOSURE

The authors have nothing to disclose.

REFERENCES

1. Brown P, Thompson PD, Rothwell JC, et al. Axial myoclonus of propriospinal origin. Brain 1991. https://doi.org/10.1093/oxfordjournals.brain.a101857.
2. Brown P, Thompson PD, Rothwell JC, et al. Paroxysmal axial spasms of spinal origin. Mov Disord 1991. https://doi.org/10.1002/mds.870060108.
3. Brown P, Rothwell JC, Thompson PD, et al. Propriospinal myoclonus: evidence for spinal "pattern" generators in humans. Mov Disord 1994. https://doi.org/10.1002/mds.870090511.
4. Roze E, Bounolleau P, Ducreux D, et al. Propriospinal myoclonus revisited: clinical, neurophysiologic,

and neuroradiologic findings. Neurology 2009. https://doi.org/10.1212/WNL.0b013e3181a0fd50.

5. van der Salm SMA, Erro R, Cordivari C, et al. Propriospinal myoclonus: clinical reappraisal and review of literature. Neurology 2014;83(20):1862–70.

6. Antelmi E, Provini F. Propriospinal myoclonus: the spectrum of clinical and neurophysiological phenotypes. Sleep Med Rev 2015. https://doi.org/10.1016/j.smrv.2014.10.007.

7. Manconi M, Sferraza B, Iannaccone S, et al. Case of symptomatic propriospinal myoclonus evolving toward acute "myoclonic status". Mov Disord 2005. https://doi.org/10.1002/mds.20645.

8. Khoo SM, Tan JH, Shi DX, et al. Propriospinal myoclonus at sleep onset causing severe insomnia: a polysomnographic and electromyographic analysis. Sleep Med 2009. https://doi.org/10.1016/j.sleep.2008.09.012.

9. Vetrugno R, Provini F, Plazzi G, et al. Propriospinal myoclonus: a motor phenomenon found in restless legs syndrome different from periodic limb movements during sleep. Mov Disord 2005. https://doi.org/10.1002/mds.20599.

10. Montagna P, Provini F, Vetrugno R. Propriospinal myoclonus at sleep onset. Neurophysiol Clin 2006. https://doi.org/10.1016/j.neucli.2006.12.004.

11. Vetrugno R, Provini F, Meletti S, et al. Propriospinal myoclonus at the sleep-wake transition: a new type of parasomnia. Sleep 2001. https://doi.org/10.1093/sleep/24.7.835.

12. Vetrugno R, Liguori R, D'Alessandro R, et al. Axial myoclonus in paraproteinemic polyneuropathy. Muscle Nerve 2008. https://doi.org/10.1002/mus.21095.

13. Vetrugno R, D'Angelo R, Alessandria M, et al. Axial myoclonus in devic neuromyelitis optica. Mov Disord 2009. https://doi.org/10.1002/mds.22654.

14. Oguri T, Hisatomi K, Kawashima S, et al. Postsurgical propriospinal myoclonus emerging at wake to sleep transition. Sleep Med 2014. https://doi.org/10.1016/j.sleep.2013.07.020.

15. Montagna P, Provini F, Plazzi G, et al. Propriospinal myoclonus upon relaxation and drowsiness: a cause of severe insomnia. Mov Disord 1997. https://doi.org/10.1002/mds.870120112.

16. Zamidei L, Bandini M, Michelagnoli G, et al. Propriospinal myoclonus following intrathecal bupivacaine in hip surgery: a case report. Minerva Anestesiol 2010;76(4):290–3.

17. Aydin ÖF, Temuçin ÇM, Kayacik ÖE, et al. Propriospinal myoclonus in a child. J Child Neurol 2010. https://doi.org/10.1177/0883073809343610.

18. Chokroverty S, Walters A, Zimmerman T, et al. Propriospinal myoclonus: a neurophysiologic analysis. Neurology 1992. https://doi.org/10.1212/wnl.42.8.1591.

19. Kapoor R, Brown P, Thompson PD, et al. Propriospinal myoclonus in multiple sclerosis. J Neurol Neurosurg Psychiatry 1992. https://doi.org/10.1136/jnnp.55.11.1086.

20. Lubetzki C, Vidailhet M, Jedynak CP, et al. Propriospinal myoclonus in a patient seropositive for human immunodeficiency virus. Rev Neurol (Paris) 1994.

21. De la Sayette V, Schaeffer S, Queruel C, et al. Lyme neuroborreliosis presenting with propriospinal myoclonus. J Neurol Neurosurg Psychiatry 1996. https://doi.org/10.1136/jnnp.61.4.420.

22. Nogués MA, Leiguarda RC, Rivero AD, et al. Involuntary movements and abnormal spontaneous EMG activity in syringomyelia and syringobulbia. Neurology 1999. https://doi.org/10.1212/wnl.52.4.823.

23. Salsano E, Ciano C, Romano S, et al. Propriospinal myoclonus with life threatening tonic spasms as paraneoplastic presentation of breast cancer. J Neurol Neurosurg Psychiatry 2006. https://doi.org/10.1136/jnnp.2005.072066.

24. Zhang Y, Menkes DL, Silvers DS. Propriospinal myoclonus associated with gluten sensitivity in a young woman. J Neurol Sci 2012. https://doi.org/10.1016/j.jns.2011.12.004.

25. Fouillet N, Wiart L, Arné P, et al. Propriospinal myoclonus in tetraplegic patients: clinical, electrophysiological and therapeutic aspects. Paraplegia 1995. https://doi.org/10.1038/sc.1995.142.

26. Benatru I, Thobois S, Andre-Obadia N, et al. Atypical propriospinal myoclonus with possible relationship to alpha interferon therapy. Mov Disord 2003. https://doi.org/10.1002/mds.10614.

27. Post B, Koelman JHTM, de Koning-Tijssen MAJ. Propriospinal myoclonus after treatment with ciprofloxacin. Mov Disord 2004. https://doi.org/10.1002/mds.10717.

28. Lev A, Korn-Lubezki I, Steiner-Birmanns B, et al. Prolonged propriospinal myoclonus following spinal anesthesia for cesarean section: case report and literature review. Arch Gynecol Obstet 2012. https://doi.org/10.1007/s00404-012-2246-1.

29. Esposito M, Edwards MJ, Bhatia KP, et al. Idiopathic spinal myoclonus: a clinical and neurophysiological assessment of a movement disorder of uncertain origin. Mov Disord 2009. https://doi.org/10.1002/mds.22812.

30. Erro R, Bhatia KP, Edwards MJ, et al. Clinical diagnosis of propriospinal myoclonus is unreliable: an electrophysiologic study. Mov Disord 2013. https://doi.org/10.1002/mds.25627.

31. Bussel B, Roby-brami A, Azouvi PH, et al. Myoclonus in a patient with spinal cord transection: possible involvement of the spinal stepping generator. Brain 1988. https://doi.org/10.1093/brain/111.5.1235.

32. Nogués M, Cammarota A, Solá C, et al. Propriospinal myoclonus in ischemic myelopathy secondary to a spinal dural arteriovenous fistula. Mov Disord 2000. https://doi.org/10.1002/1531-8257(200003)15:2<355::AID-MDS1031>3.0.CO;2-R.

33. Jang W, Kim JS, Ahn JY, et al. Reversible propriospinal myoclonus due to thoracic disc herniation: long-term follow-up. J Neurol Sci 2012. https://doi.org/10.1016/j.jns.2011.09.036.

34. Espay AJ, Ashby P, Hanajima R, et al. Unique form of propriospinal myoclonus as a possible complication of an enteropathogenic toxin. Mov Disord 2003. https://doi.org/10.1002/mds.10453.

35. Schulze-Bonhage A, Knott H, Ferbert A. Pure stimulus-sensitive truncal myoclonus of propriospinal origin. Mov Disord 1996. https://doi.org/10.1002/mds.870110116.

36. Edwards MJ, Bhatia KP. Functional (psychogenic) movement disorders: merging mind and brain. Lancet Neurol 2012. https://doi.org/10.1016/S1474-4422(11)70310-6.

37. Van Der Salm SMA, Koelman JHTM, Henneke S, et al. Axial jerks: a clinical spectrum ranging from propriospinal to psychogenic myoclonus. J Neurol 2010. https://doi.org/10.1007/s00415-010-5531-6.

38. Terada K, Ikeda A, Van Ness PC, et al. Presence of Bereitschaftspotential preceding psychogenic myoclonus: clinical application of jerk-locked back averaging. J Neurol Neurosurg Psychiatry 1995. https://doi.org/10.1136/jnnp.58.6.745.

39. Van Der Salm SMA, Tijssen MAJ, Koelman JHTM, et al. The bereitschaftspotential in jerky movement disorders. J Neurol Neurosurg Psychiatry 2012. https://doi.org/10.1136/jnnp-2012-303081.

40. Kang SY, Sohn YH. Electromyography patterns of propriospinal myoclonus can be mimicked voluntarily. Mov Disord 2006. https://doi.org/10.1002/mds.20927.

41. Roze E, Apartis E, Vidailhet M, et al. Propriospinal myoclonus: utility of magnetic resonance diffusion tensor imaging and fiber tracking. Mov Disord 2007. https://doi.org/10.1002/mds.21562.

42. Albanese A, Bhatia K, Bressman SB, et al. Phenomenology and classification of dystonia: a consensus update. Mov Disord 2013. https://doi.org/10.1002/mds.25475.

43. Roggendorf J, Burghaus L, Liu WC, et al. Belly dancer's syndrome following central pontine and extrapontine myelinolysis. Mov Disord 2007. https://doi.org/10.1002/mds.21394.

44. American Academy of Sleep Medicine. The International Classification of Sleep Disorders (ICSD-3). 3rd edition. Darien, (IL): American Academy of Sleep Medicine; 2014.

45. Calandra-Buonaura G, Alessandria M, Liguori R, et al. Hypnic jerks: neurophysiological characterization of a new motor pattern. Sleep Med 2014. https://doi.org/10.1016/j.sleep.2014.01.024.

46. Chokroverty S, Bhat S, Gupta D. Intensified hypnic jerks: a polysomnographic and polymyographic analysis. J Clin Neurophysiol 2013. https://doi.org/10.1097/WNP.0b013e31829dde98.

47. Zucconi M, Ferri R, Allen R, et al. The official World Association of Sleep Medicine (WASM) standards for recording and scoring periodic leg movements in sleep (PLMS) and wakefulness (PLMW) developed in collaboration with a task force from the International Restless Legs Syndrome Study Group. Sleep Med 2006. https://doi.org/10.1016/j.sleep.2006.01.001.

48. Ferri R, Manconi M, Plazzi G, et al. Leg movements during wakefulness in restless legs syndrome: time structure and relationships with periodic leg movements during sleep. Sleep Med 2012. https://doi.org/10.1016/j.sleep.2011.08.007.

49. Ferri R. The time structure of leg movement activity during sleep: the theory behind the practice. Sleep Med 2012. https://doi.org/10.1016/j.sleep.2011.10.027.

50. Wong SH, Selvan A, White RP. Propriospinal myoclonus associated with fragile-X-premutation and response to selective serotonin reuptake inhibitor. Parkinsonism Relat Disord 2011. https://doi.org/10.1016/j.parkreldis.2011.04.009.

51. Shprecher D, Silberstein H, Kurlan R. Propriospinal myoclonus due to cord compression in the absence of myelopathy. Mov Disord 2010. https://doi.org/10.1002/mds.23049.

52. Okura M, Tanaka M, Sugita H, et al. Obstructive sleep apnea syndrome aggravated propriospinal myoclonus at sleep onset. Sleep Med 2012. https://doi.org/10.1016/j.sleep.2011.06.012.

53. Sugimoto K, Theoharides TC, Kempuraj D, et al. Response of spinal myoclonus to a combination therapy of autogenic training and biofeedback. Biopsychosoc Med 2007. https://doi.org/10.1186/1751-0759-1-18.

54. Maltête D, Verdure P, Roze E, et al. TENS for the treatment of propriospinal myoclonus. Mov Disord 2008. https://doi.org/10.1002/mds.22315.

Sleep Bruxism
An Integrated Clinical View

Thomas Bornhardt, DDS, MSc*, Veronica Iturriaga, DDS, MSc, PhD

KEYWORDS

- Bruxism • Sleep bruxism • Obstructive sleep apnea • Gastroesophageal reflux • Sleep arousal

KEY POINTS

- Clinically, sleep bruxism presents mainly as teeth grinding associated with rhythmic masticatory muscle activity.
- Sleep bruxism has a strong coexistence with sleep arousal, obstructive sleep apnea, gastroesophageal reflux, and the use or abuse of substances such as alcohol, coffee, tobacco, and some drugs.
- Currently, central pathophysiological factors are considered the most important in the development of sleep bruxism, displacing peripheral factors.

BACKGROUND

Sleep bruxism (SB) is a masticatory muscle activity during sleep, characterized as rhythmic (phasic) or nonrhythmic (tonic) muscle contraction.[1] In adults there is an estimated 8% SB prevalence,[2,3] whereas in the pediatric population it is 3.4% to 40.6%.[4] As reported by the International Classification of Sleep Disorders, 3rd edition (ICSD-3) of the American Academy of Sleep Medicine (AASM), SB is classified as a movement disorder during sleep.[5] However, in the latest international consensus it is proposed that SB occurs in healthy subjects, without a central movement disorder, or with any other sleep disorder.[1] Furthermore, it has been proposed to consider SB as a condition or activity, rather than a disease or risk factor for orofacial structures.[1,6] Accordingly, and depending on its pathophysiology, SB could be classified as a risk factor, a protective factor, or an innocuous factor.[1]

When considering a polysomnographic view point, a rhythmic masticatory muscle activity (RMMA) is seen as a motor manifestation of SB. Such RMMAs are also reported in 59.8% of subjects without SB.[7] Nevertheless, 90% of subjects with SB present RMMA,[8–10] and these events are characterized by greater amplitude and frequency,

and may be a severe manifestation of this action.[11] A cascade of physiologic events that make up the SB episode itself is described and includes (1) autonomic-cardiac activation, 4 to 8 minutes before RMMA/SB; (2) increase in electroencephalographic (EEG) activity 4 seconds before RMMA/SB; (3) tachycardia 1 second before RMMA/SB; and (4) increase in muscle tone of the suprahyoid muscles 0.8 seconds before RMMA/SB.[3,12] From a clinical point of view, SB presents mainly as teeth grinding[11,13] rather than clenching, the latter being closely related to awake bruxism.[12]

Because there is no consensus regarding the etiologic factors of SB, it is currently defined as a multifactorial disease.[3,14] Two types of risk factors related to SB development have been described, the peripheral risk factors (dental occlusion and orofacial bone anatomy) and the central risk factors (pathophysiological and psychological). While ruling out occlusal components as part of the SB etiology, central factors are currently considered to play a significant role.[15,16] Likewise, primary psychological aspects and anxiety have for years been the subject of debate. This should, however, be considered carefully because an etiologic relationship has not yet been established.[2,17–21] The aim of this article was to review the main and clinically relevant pathophysiological risk factors,

Department of Integral Adult Care Dentistry, Temporomandibular Disorder and Orofacial Pain Program, Sleep & Pain Research Group, Faculty of Dentistry, Universidad de La Frontera, Avenida Francisco Salazar 01145, Temuco, Chile.
* Corresponding author.
E-mail address: thomas.bornhardt@ufrontera.cl

Sleep Med Clin 16 (2021) 373–380
https://doi.org/10.1016/j.jsmc.2021.02.010
1556-407X/21/© 2021 Elsevier Inc. All rights reserved.

related to SB in adults and their diagnostic process.

PATHOPHYSIOLOGICAL FACTORS

Among the central and clinically important pathophysiological risk factors for SB recently identified, are phenomena related to sleep, gastroesophageal pH/gastroesophageal reflux, and substance use or abuse among others.

Phenomena Linked to Sleep

The most significant sleep-related phenomena that impact SB are sleep arousal (SA) and obstructive sleep apnea (OSA). SAs are observed during polysomnography and are defined as an abrupt shift of EEG frequency, including alpha, theta, and/or frequencies greater than the 16 Herz (but not spindles) that lasts at least 3 seconds, with at least 10 seconds of stable sleep preceding the change. Rapid eye movement (REM) sleep requires a concurrent increase in submental electromyography (EMG) lasting at least 1 second.[22] The relationship between RMMA/SB events and SA was initially documented in the late 1960s,[23,24] the specific relationship, however, remains unclear.[25] It has been remarked that the RMMA/SB phenomenon may be secondary to SA in approximately 79% of events and concomitant in 100% of these events.[8,26] It has further been suggested that the episode of RMMA/SB could be part of a generalized arousal phenomenon.[12] Experimental induction of SA is able to generate an RMMA/SB event, resulting in a response associated with teeth grinding in 7.5% of cases[25] and is 7 times greater in subjects with SB in comparison with control subjects.[25] Moreover and pending evaluation, studies agree that SA distribution that results in an RMMA/SB event is associated with A3 phase in the cyclic alternating pattern.[12,24,27]

For its part, OSA is characterized by repetitive episodes of complete (apnea) or partial (hypopnea) upper airway obstruction occurring during sleep. These events often result in reduced blood oxygen saturation and are usually terminated by brief SAs.[5] Prevalence of SB in patients with OSA varies between 33.3% and 50.0%, where subjects with OSA have an odds ratio of 1.8 to present RMMA/SB.[28–31] It is proposed that the position of the jaw can influence the upper airway (UA) lumen, affecting its patency and the possibility of collapse during sleep. Position of the hyoid bone is advanced and raised during mandibular closure, causing an increase/maintenance of the UA patency.[32] When presented with hypercapnia and the respiratory inspiratory threshold load, a direct proportional activation of the genioglossus and masseter muscles is generated; this is proposed as a method to stabilize the mandibular position, prompting hyoid position, thus achieving better control of the UA lumen.[33] These phenomena would explain the increased UA lumen as a result of the RMMA/SB episode,[9] and the improvement of its permeability.

In reference to respiratory events (REs) and SB, it has been reported that approximately 80.5% of RMMA/SB episodes occur on average 5 minutes following REs, and analyzing the 30-seconds interval, 86.8% occur between 0 and 10 seconds after the RE.[31] Because most REs are associated with OSA and with an SA, a common relationship with SB is suspected.[29,34] In this manner, rhythmic-type SB has been associated with SA phenomena, particularly those generated after RE.[29,35] It has been noted that an increase in the SA index related to RE would increase the possibility of prompting an RMMA/SB event by 5%.[30] Similarly, there could be a relationship between oxygen desaturation index and the presence of RMMA/SB.[30] An increase of 1 point in the index of spontaneous SA per hour of sleep, would decrease the probability of RMMA/SB event by 11%.[30] This coincides with the fact that an RMMA/SB episode could be triggered, in contrast to mild and transient states of hypoxia,[9,28] and that oxygen saturation values return to physiologic levels, seconds after RMMA/SB.[36] Reportedly, 54.9% of RMMA/SB occurs after REs, whereas 25.5% precede them.[31] Furthermore, a supine position during sleep increases the probability of an RE, and that position can also increase SB events.[37]

Regarding the number of REs per hour of sleep, RMMA/SB episodes are mostly associated with mild and moderate OSA.[28,35] Fifty-four percent of patients with mild OSA present RMMA/SB, whereas it has only been reported in 40% of moderate OSA.[38] It is proposed that most RMMA/SB associated with OSA would be at the cutoff point of 5.3 REs per hour of sleep, with a sensitivity of 0.533 and specificity 0.907.[28] It was further observed that 4 seconds before the RMMA/SB episode, respiratory amplitude increased between 8% and 23%, which would then increase when the suprahyoid muscle group was activated, reaching 60% to 82% amplitude. This would end with a respiratory amplitude increase of 108% to 206%, whereas the episode of RMMA/SB itself is being carried out. There appears to be a clear need to improve UA patency.[39] Finally, in episodes of RMMA/SB associated with SA, the respiratory amplitude is 11 times greater than when an isolated SA occurs.[39] Although a direct cause has not yet been defined, the effect of some RMMA/SB seems to be related to respiratory requirements during sleep and SA distribution.

Gastroesophageal pH and Gastroesophageal Reflux Disease

The evidence suggests that gastroesophageal reflux disease (GERD) is related to development of SA, dry mouth/digestive tract, greater number of swallows, and a supine position.[40] An important association between GERD and OSA has also been reported.[41] SB prevalence is noted in 73.7% of the patients with GERD,[42] including rhythmic episodes noted in 70% of the subjects and nonrhythmic events in 10%.[43] An odds ratio of 6.58 is estimated for the presence of SB in subjects with GERD[42]; in long-term GERD cases, SB is associated with severe dental wear.[44,45]

From an experimental point of view, a reduction of gastroesophageal (GE) pH causes an increase in the frequency of EMG bursts, RMMA episodes, RMMA with tooth grinding, swallowing, and SA events.[46] Thus, the episode of RMMA/SB associated with swallowing could result in GE pH increase.[46] Swallowing activity is associated with the amount of saliva present in the mouth, providing bicarbonate and the epidermal growth factor.[40] However, the amount of saliva and swallowing episodes decreases to one-tenth during sleep versus wakefulness.[40] Most swallows take place in N1-N2 stages of No REM sleep and sometimes during REM sleep, the latter being related to SA.[10] In subjects with SB, these swallows increase up to 7 times, especially in the N2 No REM stage.[10] It has also been observed that the supine position during sleep, is associated with a 70% increase in RMMA/SB and swallowing. On the other hand, it has been reported that a rapid drop in GE pH to 4 to 5 can trigger an RMMA/SB episode in a statistically significant manner; a pH of 4 or less in the GE tract induces an RMMA/SB event in 100% of cases.[40] When proton pump inhibitors have been used, a 40% reduction in EMG, RMMA, and RMMA bursts associated with tooth grinding is observed.[40,46]

In light of the preceding, it is proposed that SB and GERD share a common pathophysiological/etiologic mechanism[42] in which buffering and lubrication capacity of saliva would play an important role.[46] In addition, salivary secretion would be enhanced, as a result of periodontal mechanoreceptor stimulation during the RMMA/SB.[40] It is possible that the acidification itself of the gastroesophageal pathway would activate visceral vagal inputs at the trigeminal mesencephalic nucleus level, thus activating the masticatory muscles.[45]

Substance Use or Abuse

The evidence suggests a pathophysiological relationship between SB and the consumption of some substances, namely alcohol, coffee, tobacco, and certain drugs. It has been reported that subjects with SB have a higher intake of alcohol before going to bed[47] and also more SB events.[48–51] Furthermore, coffee is one of the most commonly used stimulating substances worldwide, and it is frequently associated with SB.[48,50] Tobacco consumption is also strongly related to SB occurrence.[47–49,51,52] Tobacco smokers have 5 times more SB episodes than nonsmokers, considering that along with an increased use of tobacco, the probability of presenting SB also increases.[52] In contrast, the use of stimulants in patients with excessive daytime sleepiness associated with OSA, mainly caffeine and nicotine, has frequently been reported and may also increase SB association. In reference to the use of drugs, the information is complex, due to methodological difficulties of the studies.[53] The use of antidepressants, barbiturates, and psychostimulant drugs has been associated with a higher risk of developing SB.[53–55] The use of botulinum toxin appears to reduce SB events, although adverse reactions have been described at the mandibular bone level.[51] Drugs such as clonazepam and clonidine have also been associated with fewer SB events. Nevertheless, there are severe adverse effects such as morning hypotension in the case of clonidine, or a high addiction profile with clonazepam.[51] The relationship between these substances and SB is described in greater detail in **Table 1**. Finally, illegal drugs were not considered in this review, however, the association with BS is difficult to determine due to reporting bias.

Other Associated Factors

There is growing research that identifies certain genetic factors that would predispose the development of SB. These include single nucleotide polymorphism (SNP) of HTR2A associated with the serotonergic system and of DRD3 (SNP rs6280, C allele) in the dopaminergic system.[56–58] In addition, a recent study observed that the HTR2A polymorphism rs2770304 could affect the association between SB and OSA.[58] Favorable outcomes have also been reported as to the relation between SB and coactivations between the central nervous system and the autonomic nervous system.[21,31,59]

DIAGNOSIS

The gold standard for SB diagnosis is polysomnography with audio/video recording.[13,60,61] However, because it is not always easily accessible, a clinical diagnosis is extremely important. The use

Table 1
Relation between substance use or abuse and sleep bruxism

Substance	Relation with Sleep Bruxism (SB)	Odds Ratio
Alcohol	Binge drinking and heavy drinking are closely related with SB development.	1.9
Coffee	Drinking 8 cups of coffee per day is related to weekly SB events.	1.5–1.9
Tobacco	Tobacco use could double the likelihood of SB.	2.8
	Heavy smokers have a greater probability of SB.	2.5
	The use of smokeless tobacco is also associated with SB.	2.05
Drugs	There is a relation between SB and use of the following:	
	• Paroxetine	3.63
	• Venlafaxine	2.28
	• Duloxetine	2.16
	• Methylphenidate	1.67
	• Fluoxetine, sertraline, citalopram, escitalopram, and some barbiturates.	–
	• Dopaminergic drugs (agonist and antagonist) present mixed results.	–
	• The use of botulinum toxin A, buspirone, clonazepam, clonidine, and gabapentin could reduce SB events.	–

of clinical diagnostic criteria proposed by ICSD-3 is accepted and also recommended.[62] These criteria take into account as necessary and essential, the presence of regular or frequent tooth grinding, sounds occurring during sleep, associated with at least 1 or more of the following: (1) abnormal tooth wear; (2) transient morning jaw muscle pain or fatigue; (3) temporary headache; or (4) jaw locking on awakening; all being consistent with reports of tooth grinding during sleep.[5] It is important to consider that over time the perception of these criteria has varied. For instance, dental wear is currently considered a poor indicator of current SB, although it may be an indicator of SB in the past.[63] Given the high association rate between GERD and dental wear,[64] it is important to exercise caution in the specific diagnosis of tooth wear. It is also suggested that SB events would not necessarily be a direct cause of muscle pain.[65] With regard to headaches in the temporal region, a temporomandibular disorder should be considered first as a possible cause for the headaches.[65,66] Hence, the morning headache is not only related to SB, there is also a variety of headaches that could be related (**Box 1**). Currently, the agreement for SB clinical diagnostic criteria is being evaluated via polysomnography, where the report of teeth grinding at least once per week, associated with muscle pain or fatigue, has a likelihood ratio of 6, a diagnostic odds ratio of 13.5, and a specificity of 90%.[62] Likewise, the

report of teeth grinding of at least 4 times per week associated with tooth wear shows a likelihood ratio of 6 and a diagnostic odds ratio of 13.6.[62] In addition, the use of portable 4-channel diagnostic devices is an alternative to the gold standard with acceptable validity,[67] and is a promising area in the future.

Finally, progress of SB studies has led to new requirements and proposals that resulted in the

Box 1
Main sleep bruxism differential diagnosis for morning headaches

I. Primary headaches with circadian rhythm

II. Secondary headaches that occur on waking:

Headache attributed to temporomandibular disorders (11.7)[a]

Sleep apnea headache (10.1.4)[a]

Medication overuse headache (8.2)[a]

Headache attributed to substance withdrawal (8.3)[a]

Some headaches attributed to nonvascular intracranial disorder (7)[a]

[a] Headache Classification Committee of the International Headache Society (IHS) The International Classification of Headache Disorders, 3rd edition. Cephalalgia. 2018;38(1):1-211. doi:10.1177/0333102417738202.

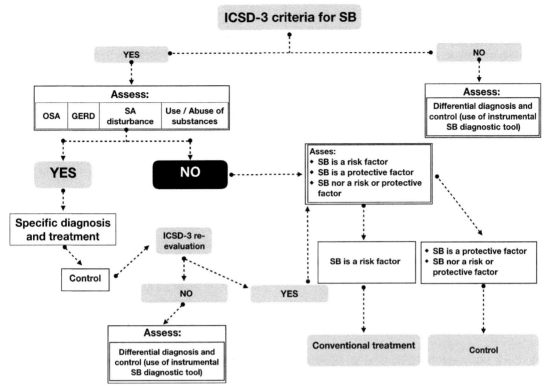

Fig. 1. Proposed algorithm for clinical approach of SB.

development of an SB classification system based on the diagnostic method applied. This classification includes possible SB (self-report of the subject), probable (clinical diagnosis with/without positive self-report), and definitive (instrumental diagnosis with or without self-report and/or positive clinical diagnosis).[1] It should be noted that as regards this classification, the vast majority of studies are based on probable SB. Definitive diagnosis of this disorder has improved in recent years with the aid of polysomnography.

SUMMARY

Evidently, SB is of great concern to clinicians, researchers, and patients. Therefore, in addition to a significant increase in related research, the concept of SB has also evolved.[21] SA, OSA, gastroesophageal pH/GERD and the use or abuse of certain substances have increasingly been cited as important pathophysiological or concomitant SB factors. It is worthwhile mentioning, that with adequate treatment of these disorders, a reduction and/or full recovery has also been reported.[46,68,69] Furthermore, clinical diagnosis is critical, given the difficulty of accessing a diagnostic gold standard. In this sense, the report of

tooth grinding during sleep remains the main clinical diagnostic criterion for SB.

In conclusion, **Fig. 1** proposes an algorithm to assist clinicians when SB is suspected, wherein the different central pathophysiological factors associated with SB are evaluated, allowing for an adequate diagnosis and individualized treatment program.

CLINICS CARE POINTS

- In adults the estimated prevalence of SB is 8% and RMMA is its motor manifestation.

- RMMA/SB phenomenon may be secondary to SA in approximately 79% of events and concomitant in 100% of these events.

- The RMMA/SB seems to be more related to mild OSA than moderate or severe OSA.

- A reduction of GE pH causes an increase in the frequency of EMG bursts, RMMA episodes, RMMA with tooth grinding, swallowing, and SA events.

- There is growing research identifying genetic factors related to SB.

- The most agreement for SB clinical diagnostic criteria were the report of tooth grinding at least once per week, associated with muscle pain or fatigue; and grinding of the teeth at least 4 times per week associated with tooth wear.

- Tooth wear alone is not a good predictor of current SB.

DISCLOSURE

The authors have nothing to disclose.

REFERENCES

1. Lobbezoo F, Ahlberg J, Raphael KG, et al. International consensus on the assessment of bruxism: report of a work in progress. J Oral Rehabil 2018; 45(11):837–44.
2. Maluly M, Andersen ML, Dal-Fabbro C, et al. Polysomnographic study of the prevalence of sleep bruxism in a population sample. J Dent Res 2013; 92(7 Suppl):97S–103S.
3. Carra MC, Huynh N, Fleury B, et al. Overview on sleep bruxism for sleep medicine clinicians. Sleep Med Clin 2015;10(3):375–xvi.
4. Manfredini D, Restrepo C, Diaz-Serrano K, et al. Prevalence of sleep bruxism in children: a systematic review of the literature. J Oral Rehabil 2013; 40(8):631–42.
5. American Academy of Sleep Medicine. International classification of sleep disorders. 3rd edition. Darien (IL): American Academy of Sleep Medicine; 2014.
6. Raphael KG, Santiago V, Lobbezoo F. Is bruxism a disorder or a behaviour? Rethinking the international consensus on defining and grading of bruxism. J Oral Rehabil 2016;43(10):791–8.
7. Lavigne GJ, Rompré PH, Poirier G, et al. Rhythmic masticatory muscle activity during sleep in humans. J Dent Res 2001;80(2):443–8.
8. Miki H, Minakuchi H, Miyagi M, et al. Association of masticatory muscle activity with sleep arousal and other concomitant movements during sleep. J Oral Rehabil 2020;47(3):281–8.
9. Dumais IE, Lavigne GJ, Carra MC, et al. Could transient hypoxia be associated with rhythmic masticatory muscle activity in sleep bruxism in the absence of sleep-disordered breathing? A preliminary report. J Oral Rehabil 2015;42(11):810–8.
10. Miyawaki S, Lavigne GJ, Pierre M, et al. Association between sleep bruxism, swallowing-related laryngeal movement, and sleep positions. Sleep 2003; 26(4):461–5.
11. Lavigne GJ, Kato T, Kolta A, et al. Neurobiological mechanisms involved in sleep bruxism. Crit Rev Oral Biol Med 2003;14(1):30–46.
12. Lavigne GJ, Huynh N, Kato T, et al. Genesis of sleep bruxism: motor and autonomic-cardiac interactions. Arch Oral Biol 2007;52(4):381–4.
13. Lavigne GJ, Rompré PH, Montplaisir JY. Sleep bruxism: validity of clinical research diagnostic criteria in a controlled polysomnographic study. J Dent Res 1996;75(1):546–52.
14. Castroflorio T, Bargellini A, Rossini G, et al. Sleep bruxism and related risk factors in adults: a systematic literature review. Arch Oral Biol 2017;83:25–32.
15. Lobbezoo F, Naeije M. Bruxism is mainly regulated centrally, not peripherally. J Oral Rehabil 2001; 28(12):1085–91.
16. Lobbezoo F, Ahlberg J, Manfredini D, et al. Are bruxism and the bite causally related? J Oral Rehabil 2012;39(7):489–501.
17. Manfredini D, Lobbezoo F. Role of psychosocial factors in the etiology of bruxism. J Orofac Pain 2009; 23(2):153–66.
18. Haraki S, Tsujisaka A, Nonoue S, et al. Sleep quality, psychologic profiles, cardiac activity, and salivary biomarkers in young subjects with different degrees of rhythmic masticatory muscle activity: a polysomnography study. J Oral Facial Pain Headache 2019;33(1):105–13.
19. Ohlmann B, Bömicke W, Habibi Y, et al. Are there associations between sleep bruxism, chronic stress, and sleep quality? J Dent 2018;74:101–6.
20. Polmann H, Domingos FL, Melo G, et al. Association between sleep bruxism and anxiety symptoms in adults: a systematic review. J Oral Rehabil 2019; 46(5):482–91.
21. Klasser GD, Rei N, Lavigne GJ. Sleep bruxism etiology: the evolution of a changing paradigm. J Can Dent Assoc 2015;81:f2.
22. Berry RB, Quan SF, Abreu AR, et al, for the American Academy of Sleep Medicine. The AASM manual for the scoring of sleep and associated events: rules, terminology and technical specifications. Version 2.6. Darien (IL): American Academy of Sleep Medicine; 2020.
23. Reding GR, Zepelin H, Robinson JE Jr, et al. Nocturnal teeth-grinding: all-night psychophysiologic studies. J Dent Res 1968;47(5):786–97.
24. Huynh N, Kato T, Rompré PH, et al. Sleep bruxism is associated to micro-arousals and an increase in cardiac sympathetic activity. J Sleep Res 2006;15(3): 339–46.
25. Kato T, Montplaisir JY, Guitard F, et al. Evidence that experimentally induced sleep bruxism is a consequence of transient arousal. J Dent Res 2003; 82(4):284–8.
26. Kato T, Rompré P, Montplaisir JY, et al. Sleep bruxism: an oromotor activity secondary to micro-arousal. J Dent Res 2001;80(10):1940–4.
27. Macaluso GM, Guerra P, Di Giovanni G, et al. Sleep bruxism is a disorder related to periodic arousals during sleep. J Dent Res 1998;77(4):565–73.

28. Martynowicz H, Gac P, Brzecka A, et al. The relationship between sleep bruxism and obstructive sleep apnea based on polysomnographic findings. J Clin Med 2019;8(10):1653.

29. Hosoya H, Kitaura H, Hashimoto T, et al. Relationship between sleep bruxism and sleep respiratory events in patients with obstructive sleep apnea syndrome. Sleep Breath 2014;18(4):837–44.

30. Tan MWY, Yap AU, Chua AP, et al. Prevalence of sleep bruxism and its association with obstructive sleep apnea in adult patients: a retrospective polysomnographic investigation. J Oral Facial Pain Headache 2019;33(3):269–77.

31. Saito M, Yamaguchi T, Mikami S, et al. Temporal association between sleep apnea-hypopnea and sleep bruxism events. J Sleep Res 2013. https://doi.org/10.1111/jsr.12099.

32. Pancherz H, Winnberg A, Westesson PL. Masticatory muscle activity and hyoid bone behavior during cyclic jaw movements in man. A synchronized electromyographic and videofluorographic study. Am J Orthod 1986;89(2):122–31.

33. Hollowell DE, Bhandary PR, Funsten AW, et al. Respiratory-related recruitment of the masseter: response to hypercapnia and loading. J Appl Physiol (1985) 1991;70(6):2508–13.

34. Kostrzewa-Janicka J, Jurkowski P, Zycinska K, et al. Sleep-related breathing disorders and bruxism. Adv Exp Med Biol 2015;873:9–14.

35. Tsujisaka A, Haraki S, Nonoue S, et al. The occurrence of respiratory events in young subjects with a frequent rhythmic masticatory muscle activity: a pilot study. J Prosthodont Res 2018;62(3):317–23.

36. Manfredini D, Guarda-Nardini L, Marchese-Ragona R, et al. Theories on possible temporal relationships between sleep bruxism and obstructive sleep apnea events. An expert opinion. Sleep Breath 2015;19(4):1459–65.

37. Phillips BA, Okeson J, Paesani D, et al. Effect of sleep position on sleep apnea and parafunctional activity. Chest 1986;90(3):424–9.

38. Sjöholm T, Lehtinen II, Helenius H. Masseter muscle activity in diagnosed sleep bruxists compared with non-symptomatic controls. J Sleep Res 1995;4(1):48–55.

39. Khoury S, Rouleau GA, Rompré PH, et al. A significant increase in breathing amplitude precedes sleep bruxism. Chest 2008;134(2):332–7.

40. Miyawaki S, Tanimoto Y, Araki Y, et al. Association between nocturnal bruxism and gastroesophageal reflux. Sleep 2003;26(7):888–92.

41. Wetselaar P, Manfredini D, Ahlberg J, et al. Associations between tooth wear and dental sleep disorders: a narrative overview. J Oral Rehabil 2019; 46(8):765–75.

42. Mengatto CM, Dalberto Cda S, Scheeren B, et al. Association between sleep bruxism and gastroesophageal reflux disease. J Prosthet Dent 2013;110(5):349–55.

43. Miyawaki S, Tanimoto Y, Araki Y, et al. Relationships among nocturnal jaw muscle activities, decreased esophageal pH, and sleep positions. Am J Orthod Dentofacial Orthop 2004;126(5):615–9.

44. Li Y, Yu F, Niu L, et al. Associations among bruxism, gastroesophageal reflux disease, and tooth wear. J Clin Med 2018;7(11):417.

45. Li Y, Yu F, Niu L, et al. Association between bruxism and symptomatic gastroesophageal reflux disease: a case-control study. J Dent 2018;77:51–8.

46. Ohmure H, Kanematsu-Hashimoto K, Nagayama K, et al. Evaluation of a proton pump inhibitor for sleep bruxism: a randomized clinical trial. J Dent Res 2016;95(13):1479–86.

47. Ohayon MM, Li KK, Guilleminault C. Risk factors for sleep bruxism in the general population. Chest 2001;119(1):53–61.

48. Bertazz-Silveira E, Kruger CM, Porto De Toledo I, et al. Association between sleep bruxism and alcohol, caffeine, tobacco, and drug abuse: a systematic review. J Am Dent Assoc 2016;147(11): 859–66.e4.

49. Itani O, Kaneita Y, Ikeda M, et al. Disorders of arousal and sleep-related bruxism among Japanese adolescents: a nationwide representative survey. Sleep Med 2013;14(6):532–41.

50. Rintakoski K, Kaprio J. Legal psychoactive substances as risk factors for sleep-related bruxism: a nationwide Finnish Twin Cohort study. Alcohol Alcohol 2013;48(4):487–94.

51. de Baat C, Verhoeff M, Ahlberg J, et al. Medications and addictive substances potentially inducing or attenuating sleep bruxism and/or awake bruxism [published online ahead of print, 2020 Jul 27]. J Oral Rehabil 2020. https://doi.org/10.1111/joor.13061.

52. Rintakoski K, Ahlberg J, Hublin C, et al. Tobacco use and reported bruxism in young adults: a nationwide Finnish Twin Cohort Study. Nicotine Tob Res 2010; 12(6):679–83.

53. Winocur E, Gavish A, Voikovitch M, et al. Drugs and bruxism: a critical review. J Orofac Pain 2003;17(2): 99–111.

54. Melo G, Dutra KL, Rodrigues Filho R, et al. Association between psychotropic medications and presence of sleep bruxism: a systematic review. J Oral Rehabil 2018;45(7):545–54.

55. Singh H, Kaur S, Shah A. Antidepressant induced bruxism: a literature review. J Psychiatr Intensive Care 2019;15(1):37–44.

56. Oporto GH 5th, Bornhardt T, Iturriaga V, et al. Single nucleotide polymorphisms in genes of dopaminergic pathways are associated with bruxism. Clin Oral Investig 2018;22(1):331–7.

57. Oporto GH 5th, Bornhardt T, Iturriaga V, et al. Genetic polymorphisms in the serotonergic system

are associated with circadian manifestations of bruxism. J Oral Rehabil 2016;43(11):805–12.

58. Wieckiewicz M, Bogunia-Kubik K, Mazur G, et al. Genetic basis of sleep bruxism and sleep apnea-response to a medical puzzle. Sci Rep 2020;10(1): 7497.

59. Nukazawa S, Yoshimi H, Sato S. Autonomic nervous activities associated with bruxism events during sleep. Cranio 2018;36(2):106–12.

60. Palinkas M, De Luca Canto G, Rodrigues LA, et al. Comparative capabilities of clinical assessment, diagnostic criteria, and polysomnography in detecting sleep bruxism. J Clin Sleep Med 2015;11(11): 1319–25.

61. de Holanda TA, Castagno CD, Barbon FJ, et al. Sleep architecture and factors associated with sleep bruxism diagnosis scored by polysomnography recordings: a case-control study. Arch Oral Biol 2020;112:104685.

62. Stuginski-Barbosa J, Porporatti AL, Costa YM, et al. Agreement of the International Classification of Sleep Disorders Criteria with polysomnography for sleep bruxism diagnosis: a preliminary study. J Prosthet Dent 2017;117(1):61–6.

63. Manfredini D, Lombardo L, Visentin A, et al. Correlation between sleep-time masseter muscle activity and tooth wear: an electromyographic study. J Oral Facial Pain Headache 2019;33(2):199–204.

64. Watanabe M, Nakatani E, Yoshikawa H, et al. Oral soft tissue disorders are associated with gastroesophageal reflux disease: retrospective study. BMC Gastroenterol 2017;17(1):92.

65. Castrillon EE, Exposto FG. Sleep bruxism and pain. Dent Clin North Am 2018;62(4):657–63.

66. Headache Classification Committee of the International Headache Society (IHS). The International Classification of Headache Disorders, 3rd edition. Cephalalgia 2018;38(1):1–211.

67. Casett E, Réus JC, Stuginski-Barbosa J, et al. Validity of different tools to assess sleep bruxism: a meta-analysis. J Oral Rehabil 2017;44(9):722–34.

68. Martinot JB, Borel JC, Le-Dong NN, et al. Bruxism relieved under CPAP treatment in a patient with OSA syndrome. Chest 2020;157(3):e59–62.

69. Oksenberg A, Arons E. Sleep bruxism related to obstructive sleep apnea: the effect of continuous positive airway pressure. Sleep Med 2002;3(6): 513–5.

Restless Sleep Disorder

Lourdes M. DelRosso, MD[a],*, Rosalia Silvestri, MD[b], Raffaele Ferri, MD[c]

KEYWORDS

- Restless sleep • Restless sleep disorder • Children

KEY POINTS

- Restless sleep disorder (RSD0 involves large movements during sleep and daytime function impairment.
- Video-PSG is necessary for the diagnosis of RSD.
- Secondary causes of restless sleep need to be ruled out prior to the diagnosis of RSD.
- Iron supplementation is the only treatment option so far.

INTRODUCTION

Decades of research have proven the importance of a good night's sleep. Sleep has restorative functions that are key for overall health and wellbeing. These functions include memory consolidation, hormone regulation, growth, and sympathetic/parasympathetic balance. A good night's sleep can be assessed quantitatively and qualitatively. The American Academy of Sleep Medicine (AASM) states that in order to promote optimal health, adults and children must sleep an adequate amount of time and has published guidelines for daily sleep duration.[1] National and international organizations for sleep have increased their efforts to bring awareness to the adverse impact of lack of sleep.[2] The quality of sleep has also been studied over the years; inadequate sleep has been associated with a feeling that sleep was restless or of poor quality.[3] Nonrestorative sleep and restless sleep are terms that have been used to identify the opposite to a good night of sleep. It is well known that nonrestorative sleep results in daytime impairment, fatigue, excessive sleepiness, return to napping, and daytime microsleeps.[4] In children, a poor night of sleep has also been associated with behavioral problems, mood changes, inattention, impulsivity, and poor academic performance.[5]

The first international classification of sleep disorders defined restlessness during sleep as "persistent or recurrent body movements, arousals, and brief awakenings that occur in the course of sleep."[6] The current version, the International Classification of Sleep Disorders, 3rd edition,[7] does not include this definition anymore; however, restless sleep continues to be a common sleep complaint, particularly in pediatric sleep medicine.[8] In fact, the concern about movements during sleep in children is not new to the sleep medicine literature; early studies identified a group of children aged 8 to 12 years with increased number of movements at night who were called hyperkinetic children. At the time, the authors proposed that increased restlessness during sleep was associated with overactivity during wakefulness.[9]

More recently, research on children with restless sleep has identified that restlessness can be secondary to other conditions but also can be a primary sleep disorder.[8,10,11] Expert consensus has identified the diagnostic criteria of restless sleep disorder (RSD). This article discusses the clinical characteristics of children with RSD, the current

The authors do not have any commercial or financial conflict of interest to declare.
[a] University of Washington, Seattle Washington, Seattle Children's Hospital, 4800 Sand Point Way NE, Seattle, WA 98105, USA; [b] Sleep Medicine Center, Department of Clinical and Experimental Medicine, University of A. O.U.G. Martino - Pad. H, 1o piano, Via Consolare Valeria, 1, 98125 Messina (ME), Italy; [c] Oasi Research Institute – IRCCS, Via C Ruggero 73, 94018 Troina, Italy
* Corresponding author.
E-mail address: Lourdesdelrosso@me.com

diagnostic criteria, recommended evaluation, and treatment options.

CLINICAL CHARACTERISTICS

RSD has been identified in children and adolescents presenting with a chief complaint of restless sleep. When asked to describe what restless sleep meant, the parents used terms as "moving all night", "trashing the bed", or "moving like a fish." In some instances the child had fallen out of bed or the bedroom arrangement was changed for the child's safety (sleeping on a mattress on the floor). The parents identified the restless sleep as the cause of daytime fatigue, sleepiness, or behavioral problems. The authors' first publication describing RSD clinically and polysomnographically evaluated children aged 6 to 18 years and compared them with children with restless legs syndrome (RLS) and controls. In this publication, the authors further characterized the clinical parental complaints that included frequent nocturnal body movements such as repositioning, moving large muscle groups during sleep, no difficulty falling asleep, no symptoms of RLS, or nocturnal awakenings associated with daytime impairment such as excessive sleepiness, decreased school performance, or some hyperactivity. Parents also stated that the movements occurred almost every night and at any hour of the night.[10] The parents identified the pattern of sleep in their children with RSD to be different from sleep in their siblings in that children with RSD were "restless" all night.[10] Full clinical and polysomnographic evaluation did not reveal a known sleep disorder or other medical condition. In this initial report, the authors showed objective PSG findings demonstrating that children with RSD had decreased total sleep time and increased awakenings compared with controls. The sleep disruption was comparable to children with RLS but without the increased leg movements. Because parents complained that movements occurred all night, regardless of the time of the night, the authors designed a second study to identify the movements and assess the movement index across the night. **Box 1** summarizes the clinical findings in children with RSD. Laboratory evaluation showed that children with RSD had low ferritin levels (average 20).

In their second publication, the authors used synchronized video-polysomnography (vPSG) to describe and count the nocturnal movements in children with RSD. The authors demonstrated that RSD children, compared to children with RLS and controls, showed increased total body movement, arm movements, and leg movements (not qualifying for PLMS). The total movement index, obtained by summing together all types of movements in each subject and dividing it by the total sleep time, was higher in children with RSD and statistically significantly different than the total movement index in children with RLS and controls. The movement index was different in all sleep stages. Movement duration was similar in all groups, with an approximate mean movement duration of 8 seconds. The authors also analyzed the sleep disruption caused by the movements and found that children with RSD had a higher number of movements ending in wakefulness than controls. They also demonstrated that the parental concern of "moving all night long" was indeed true. The authors showed that the movements of children with RSD occurred after sleep onset and persisted through the night.

These 2 initial studies identified the clinical and polysomnographic presentation of children with RSD. The authors found out that RSD is a condition characterized by frequent recurrent motor movements during sleep involving large muscle groups often described by parents as frequent repositioning or disruption of the bed sheets.[10,11] The movements, occurring throughout the night, are sleep related and cause significant daytime impairment.[10] Polysomnographically, children had decreased sleep efficiency, increased awakenings, and no evidence of increased leg movement activity. Children with RSD also demonstrated a movement index of at least 5 per hour in vPSG.[8,11] RSD was found to have a prevalence of 7.7% in a population referred to a sleep center.[8]

PATHOPHYSIOLOGY

The pathophysiology of RSD is still unknown, although the authors have postulated the following mechanisms that may act simultaneously and in synergy: iron deficiency, sleep instability, and increased sympathetic activation.

Research on iron deficiency has shown that it alters patterns of neurotransmission impacting motor activity both during the day and at night.[12] The low ferritin levels identified in children with RSD seem to support this evidence. Furthermore, iron supplementation in children with RSD has shown to improve symptoms of both sleep and daytime impairment (discussed in the treatment section).

Sleep instability is an attractive potential pathophysiologic mechanism based on the polysomnographic evidence of sleep disruption (reduced total sleep time and increased number of awakenings)

Box 1
Summary of clinical and polysomnographic characteristics of restless sleep disorder

Clinical symptoms	Frequent large body movement during sleep Daytime symptoms of excessive sleepiness, mood changes, and hyperactivity
Ferritin levels	Decreased
Polysomnography	Decreased total sleep time Increased awakenings Movements > 5/h

but also on the daytime consequences of sleepiness, fatigue, or inattention.[11]

Cyclic alternating pattern (CAP) is a physiologic rhythm detected in polysomnography during non-rapid eye movement (NREM) sleep and is recognized to be a physiologic marker of NREM sleep instability. CAP is formed by the recurrent occurrence of transient events with specific characteristics and formed by cycles with 2 phases. Phase A is comprised of transient electrocortical activations, while phase B is comprised of the background electroencephalogram (EEG) activity (interrupted by Phase A).[13] Phases A and B repeat cyclically during the night in a recurrent pattern and are interrupted by the presence of stable sleep periods without oscillations, called non-CAP (NCAP).[14] CAP rate refers to the percentage of CAP time to NREM sleep time.[15] CAP A phases are further subdivided into: A1, A2 and A3, based on their EEG frequency content,[16,17] with A1 containing a preponderance of slow waves and A3 a preponderance of fast arousal-related EEG activities (A2 is an admixture of slow and fast EEG activities). A recent study showed that children with RSD demonstrate a lower percentage of A3 subtypes than controls, accompanied by shorter duration of the B phase of the CAP cycle and shorter CAP cycle. In the same study, the authors also assessed the correlation between the total number of movements per hour in children with RSD and some CAP variables and were unable to find any significant correlation showing that CAP is not specifically associated with the movements in RSD. This finding is particularly interesting, as the authors found that movements tended to occur during NCAP periods, but when occurring within CAP sequences, they were most often associated with the CAP A2 and A3 subtypes. These CAP events largely overlap with arousals.[17] In that sense, the authors' study corroborated that movements in children with RSD can and are in some instances followed by arousals and awakenings, and, therefore,

contributing to sleep disruption.[11] These findings confirm that frequent movements in RSD are associated with sleep disruption and are likely involved in nonrestorative sleep and daytime symptoms.

To test their third hypothesis about sympathetic activation in children with RSD, the authors analyzed hear rate variability (HRV) from the electrocardiogram obtained during polysomnography. HRV provides information about the balance in autonomic nervous system. The interaction between the sympathetic and parasympathetic systems orchestrates each heart beat and heart rate. HRV has been studied in association with sympathetic/parasympathetic predominance in various sleep disorders. The analysis of HRV includes 2 domains: the time domain and the frequency domain, which is further subdivided into high-frequency band (HF) and low-frequency band (LF). The HF band represents mainly parasympathetic activity, while the low frequency (LF) band is a marker of sympathetic and vagal modulation.[18]

When transitioning from wakefulness to sleep, there is a shift from sympathetic to parasympathetic predominance, with a subsequent slowing in heart rate mainly secondary to parasympathetic predominance with sleep onset.[19] Healthy NREM sleep is therefore characterized by a slower stable heart rate[20] and REM shifts to a sympathetic predominance.[21] Other sleep disorders such as obstructive sleep apnea,[22,23] periodic limb movements sleep disorder,[24] and other conditions associated with increased sleep fragmentation[25] have shown changes in HRV.[26]

HRV in children with RSD showed a longer RR interval during stage N3 than in children with RLS. Frequency domains showed more changes. The very low frequency band during N3 was higher in children with RSD than controls or children with RLS; the LF band was higher in RSD compared with controls. During REM sleep, the LF/HF ratio was higher in RSD and RLS. The conclusion of this study was that children with RSD have increased sympathetic activation during sleep, particularly N3 and REM, compared with controls. Children with RSD did not show abnormalities in HRV during relaxed wakefulness preceding sleep.

In conclusion current research in children with RSD is demonstrating that iron deficiency can play a role as well as sleep instability and increased sympathetic predominance during sleep.

DIAGNOSIS

The International RLS Study Group formed a taskforce composed of 10 sleep experts to evaluate the evidence for RSD. Based on the medical literature and expert clinical experience, the task force found sufficient evidence for RSD and established 8 essential criteria for diagnosis of RSD (**Box 2**).[27] The diagnosis of RSD includes clinical symptoms of restless sleep consisting of large movements during sleep, a duration of symptoms for more than 3 months and more than 3 nights a week, and, importantly, video-polysomnographic evidence of 5 or more large body movements per hour. Children with RSD must have daytime impairment: either sleepiness, behavioral concerns or cognitive deficits.[27] Because all the research has been done in children aged 6 to 18 years, the taskforce established the criteria for children in this age range. Exclusion of mimics and other medical conditions needs to be part of the initial evaluation and will be discussed in the next session.

EVALUATION

The evaluation of a child with suspected RSD must include exclusion of mimics. Restless sleep is seen in 80% of children with RLS and 89% of children with periodic leg movements of sleep (PLMS).[28] A review of the literature on restless sleep has identified a list of medical or sleep disorders that can present with restless sleep. **Box 3** lists some of these disorders that need to be excluded (eg, acute otitis media, asthma, pain, and bruxism). Because restless sleep in children is commonly seen in association with other medical or sleep disorders, it is recommended to initiate the

evaluation with a complete medical history and physical examination.

Synchronized video-polysomnography is required for the diagnosis of RSD. Its utility is twofold: it can identify another sleep disorder such as obstructive sleep apnea or periodic limb movements disorder,[29,30] nocturnal seizures,[31] and eczema,[32] among other disorders that can be associated with restless sleep. The AASM Scoring Manual[33] recommends an accuracy of at least 1 video frame per second when recording video PSG and recommends the use for video for the identification of sleep-associated movements such as those seen in REM sleep behavior disorder (RBD) and rhythmic movement disorders (RMDs). The diagnosis of RSD requires the demonstration of at least 5 movements per hour during vPSG.[10] **Fig. 1** summarizes our proposed algorithm to evaluate a child with restless sleep. **Fig. 2** shows typical movement artifacts during PSG.

THERAPEUTIC OPTIONS

There are currently no recommendations for the treatment of RSD in children. Although the mechanism of the frequent movements during sleep is not fully elucidated, an association with iron deficiency has been identified. Iron is important in the synthesis of dopamine, a neurotransmitter that impacts motor activity.[12] RLS is the most studied sleep disorder in association with iron deficiency.[34] The International RLS Study Group has published guidelines recommending iron supplementation as first-line treatment for adults with RLS and supports the use of intravenous iron infusion for RLS.[34] Cho and colleagues suggested a dose-dependent improvement in symptoms after intravenous ferric carboxymaltose,[35] with symptoms of RLS improving for up to 24 weeks after the infusion.[36]

Expert consensus recommends iron supplementation in children when serum ferritin is less than 50 μg/L.[34] Iron supplementation in children with RLS and PLMD is usually the first line

---

Box 2
Consensus diagnostic criteria for restless sleep disorder

Criteria A-H must be met

A. "Restless sleep" reported by the patient's parent or caregiver

B. Restless sleep defined by large movements

C. The movements occur during sleep

D. 5 or more movements per hour of sleep identified in video PSG

E. Restless sleep at least 3 times per week

F. Restless sleep for at least 3 months

G. Restless sleep causes clinically significant daytime impairment

H. Restless sleep is not better explained by another disorder or substance

Adapted from DelRosso LM, Ferri R, Allen RP, et al. Consensus diagnostic criteria for a newly defined pediatric sleep disorder: restless sleep disorder (RSD). Sleep Med 2020;75:335-40.

Box 3
Secondary causes of restless sleep

Medical	Asthma
	Otitis media
	Pain
Neurologic	Migraine
	Seizure
Psychiatric	Anxiety
	Depression
Sleep	Obstructive sleep apnea
	Restless legs syndrome
	Periodic leg movement disorder

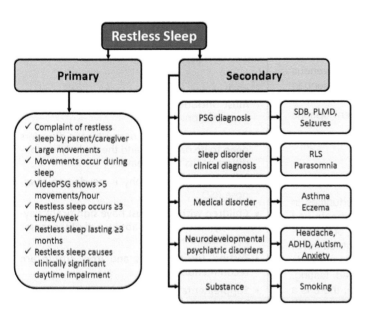

Fig. 1. Proposed algorithm to evaluate a child with restless sleep.

treatment as well, accepted by most pediatric sleep physician.[37]

The authors have treated children with RSD with iron supplementation, both oral and intravenous.[38] Oral iron supplementation for 3 months involved ferrous sulfate 325 mg tablet daily or liquid 3 mg/kg/d if children could not swallow a tablet.

Children given intravenous ferric carboxymaltose received 15 mg/kg f they weighted less than 50 kg and a 750 mg single dose if they weighted over 50 kg. The authors found out that serum ferritin increased significantly from baseline with both oral and intravenous iron, and clinical symptoms improved in both groups, including fewer

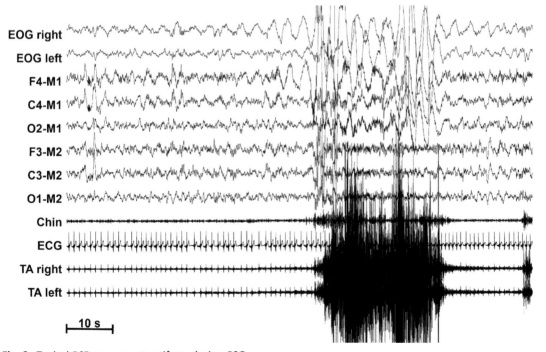

Fig. 2. Typical RSD movement artifacts during PSG.

movements during sleep, fewer awakenings, and less sleepiness during the day. Generally, oral iron had as side effects constipation and poor compliance. Children who underwent intravenous infusion with ferric carboxymaltose experienced no significant side effects.

More research is needed on treatment options for children with RSD.

FUTURE DIRECTIONS

There are still a lot of research opportunities in RSD. There is a need to assess movements and symptoms in children with RSD outside of the current age group of 6 to 18 years. The contribution of restless sleep to daytime symptomatology needs to be assessed formally with validated testing. The natural history of RSD is unknown; there is a need to identify what happens to children with RSD when they become adults, and there is a need to study if RSD is also present in adults and how does it manifest including the presence of RSD in the elderly. Other methods to identify RSD beyond PSG also can be studied, including actigraphy, home video monitoring, and smart device technology.

SUMMARY

RSD is a pediatric sleep disorder characterized by parental complaint of frequent large movements, repositioning, and sleep disruption that cause significant daytime impairment. Consensus diagnostic criteria have been published and include symptoms persisting for more than 3 months and occurring more than 3 nights per week, and at least 5 movements per hour occurring during polysomnography. Nocturnal movements must result in impairment in daytime function (sleepiness, school performance, irritability or hyperactivity), and the condition is not better explained by behavioral or medical disorders or medication effect. The prevalence of RSD has been estimated to be 7.7% of children referred to a sleep center.[8] Children with RSD usually have ferritin levels below 50 μg/L (mean 20.8),[10] which may point toward a common underlying pathway similar to RLS.[39] Although there are currently no US Food and Drug Administration approved medications for the management of restless sleep in children, iron supplementation has shown to be beneficial in children with RSD. The diagnosis of RSD involves exclusion of mimics, because restless sleep can be secondary to a medical or sleep comorbidity such as RLS and PLMS.[28]

CLINICS CARE POINTS

- Evaluation of children with restless sleep must include a full history and physical examination.
- Other medical, sleep, or psychiatric disorders need to be ruled out, and the underlying condition needs to be treated.
- Video-polysomnography is needed to diagnose RSD.
- Children with RSD must have significant daytime symptoms in the absence of other causes of restless sleep.
- Testing ferritin levels and iron profile are recommended.
- Supplementation with oral or intravenous iron should occur if ferritin is less than 50 ng/mL.

REFERENCES

1. Paruthi S, Brooks LJ, D'Ambrosio C, et al. Pediatric sleep duration consensus statement: a step forward. J Clin Sleep Med 2016;12(12):1705–6.
2. Watson NF, Badr MS, Belenky G, et al. Recommended amount of sleep for a healthy adult: a joint consensus statement of the American Academy of sleep medicine and sleep research society. Sleep 2015;38(6):843–4.
3. Ohayon MM. Prevalence and correlates of nonrestorative sleep complaints. Arch Intern Med 2005; 165(1):35–41.
4. Kothare SV, Kaleyias J. The clinical and laboratory assessment of the sleepy child. Semin Pediatr Neurol 2008;15(2):61–9.
5. Kotagal S. Hypersomnia in children: interface with psychiatric disorders. Child Adolesc Psychiatr Clin N Am 2009;18(4):967–77.
6. Medicine AAoS. Diagnostic classification of sleep and arousal disorders first edition. Sleep 1979;2: 1–154. Association of Sleep Disorders Centers and the Association for the Psychophysiological Study of Sleep; 1979.
7. American Academy of Sleep M. In: Sateia M, editor. International classification of sleep disorders. 3rd edition. Darien, IL: American Academy of Sleep Medicine; 2014.
8. DelRosso LM, Ferri R. The prevalence of restless sleep disorder among a clinical sample of children and adolescents referred to a sleep centre. J Sleep Res 2019;e12870.

9. Busby K, Firestone P, Pivik RT. Sleep patterns in hyperkinetic and normal children. Sleep 1981;4(4):366–83.

10. DelRosso LM, Bruni O, Ferri R. Restless sleep disorder in children: a pilot study on a tentative new diagnostic category. Sleep 2018;41(8).

11. DelRosso LM, Jackson CV, Trotter K, et al. Videopolysomnographic characterization of sleep movements in children with restless sleep disorder. Sleep 2019;42(4): zsy269.

12. Angulo-Barroso RM, Peirano P, Algarin C, et al. Motor activity and intra-individual variability according to sleep-wake states in preschool-aged children with iron-deficiency anemia in infancy. Early Hum Dev 2013;89(12):1025–31.

13. Terzano MG, Mancia D, Salati MR, et al. The cyclic alternating pattern as a physiologic component of normal NREM sleep. Sleep 1985;8(2):137–45.

14. Terzano MG, Parrino L, Spaggiari MC. The cyclic alternating pattern sequences in the dynamic organization of sleep. Electroencephalogr Clin Neurophysiol 1988;69(5):437–47.

15. Parrino L, Ferri R, Bruni O, et al. Cyclic alternating pattern (CAP): the marker of sleep instability. Sleep Med Rev 2012;16(1):27–45.

16. Terzano MG, Parrino L, Smerieri A, et al. Atlas, rules, and recording techniques for the scoring of cyclic alternating pattern (CAP) in human sleep. Sleep Med 2001;2:537–53.

17. Parrino L, Smerieri A, Rossi M, et al. Relationship of slow and rapid EEG components of CAP to ASDA arousals in normal sleep. Sleep 2001;24(8):881–5.

18. Ferri R, Parrino L, Smerieri A, et al. Cyclic alternating pattern and spectral analysis of heart rate variability during normal sleep. J Sleep Res 2000;9(1):13–8.

19. Snyder F, Hobson JA, Morrison DF, et al. Changes in respiration, heart rate, and systolic blood pressure in human sleep. J Appl Physiol 1964;19:417–22.

20. Boudreau P, Yeh WH, Dumont GA, et al. Circadian variation of heart rate variability across sleep stages. Sleep 2013;36(12):1919–28.

21. Glos M, Fietze I, Blau A, et al. Cardiac autonomic modulation and sleepiness: physiological consequences of sleep deprivation due to 40 h of prolonged wakefulness. Physiol Behav 2014;125:45–53.

22. Kwok KL, Yung TC, Ng DK, et al. Heart rate variability in childhood obstructive sleep apnea. Pediatr Pulmonol 2011;46(3):205–10.

23. Nisbet LC, Yiallourou SR, Nixon GM, et al. Nocturnal autonomic function in preschool children with sleep-disordered breathing. Sleep Med 2013;14(12):1310–6.

24. Manconi M, Ferri R, Zucconi M, et al. Effects of acute dopamine-agonist treatment in restless legs syndrome on heart rate variability during sleep. Sleep Med 2011;12(1):47–55.

25. Antelmi E, Plazzi G, Pizza F, et al. Impact of acute administration of sodium oxybate on heart rate variability in children with type 1 narcolepsy. Sleep Med 2018;47:1–6.

26. Sforza E, Pichot V, Cervena K, et al. Cardiac variability and heart-rate increment as a marker of sleep fragmentation in patients with a sleep disorder: a preliminary study. Sleep 2007;30(1):43–51.

27. DelRosso LM, Ferri R, Allen RP, et al. Consensus diagnostic criteria for a newly defined pediatric sleep disorder: restless sleep disorder (RSD). Sleep Med 2020;75:335–40.

28. Picchietti DL, Rajendran RR, Wilson MP, et al. Pediatric restless legs syndrome and periodic limb movement disorder: parent-child pairs. Sleep Med 2009;10(8):925–31.

29. Medicine AAoS. International classification of sleep disorders. 3rd edition. Darien, IL: American Academy of Sleep Medicine; 2014.

30. Walter LM, Nixon GM, Davey MJ, et al. Differential effects of sleep disordered breathing on polysomnographic characteristics in preschool and school aged children. Sleep Med 2012;13(7):810–5.

31. Wang X, Marcuse LV, Jin L, et al. Sleep-related hypermotor epilepsy activated by rapid eye movement sleep. Epileptic Disord 2018;20(1):65–9.

32. Camfferman D, Kennedy JD, Gold M, et al. Sleep and neurocognitive functioning in children with eczema. Int J Psychophysiol 2013;89(2):265–72.

33. Berry RB, Gramaldo CE, et al. For the American Academy of sleep medicine, . The AASM Manual for the Scoring of sleep and associated events. Darien (IL): AASM; 2017.

34. Allen RP, Picchietti DL, Auerbach M, et al. Evidence-based and consensus clinical practice guidelines for the iron treatment of restless legs syndrome/Willis-Ekbom disease in adults and children: an IRLSSG task force report. Sleep Med 2018;41:27–44.

35. Cho YW, Allen RP, Earley CJ. Efficacy of ferric carboxymaltose (FCM) 500 mg dose for the treatment of restless legs syndrome. Sleep Med 2018;42:7–12.

36. Allen RP, Adler CH, Du W, et al. Clinical efficacy and safety of IV ferric carboxymaltose (FCM) treatment of RLS: a multi-centred, placebo-controlled preliminary clinical trial. Sleep Med 2011;12(9):906–13.

37. Picchietti DL. Restless legs syndrome/Willis-Ekbom disease and periodic limb movement disorder in children. In: Basow DS, editor. UpToDate. Waltham (MA): UpToDate; 2020.

38. DelRosso LM, Picchietti DL, Ferri R. Comparison between oral ferrous sulfate and intravenous ferric carboxymaltose in children with restless sleep disorder. Sleep 2021;44(2): zsaa155.

39. Connor JR, Patton SM, Oexle K, et al. Iron and restless legs syndrome: treatment, genetics and pathophysiology. Sleep Med 2017;31:61–70.

Sleep and Epilepsy, Clinical Spectrum and Updated Review

Ting Wu, MD[a], Alon Y. Avidan, MD, MPH[b],*, Jerome Engel Jr, MD, PhD[c]

KEYWORDS

- Epilepsy • Interictal discharges • Sleep-related hypermotor epilepsy • Parasomnias
- Sleep-related movement disorder

KEY POINTS

- Among the epilepsy syndromes, self-limited epilepsy with centrotemporal spikes and Panayiotopoulos syndrome have seizures that occur more often during sleep whereas seizures associated with juvenile myoclonic epilepsy (JME) occur in general within 2 hours of awakening.
- Disturbed sleep as manifested by reduced sleep efficiency and decreased percentage of slow wave sleep commonly is found in patients with Lennox-Gastaut syndrome as well as focal epilepsy.
- Non–rapid eye movement parasomnia preferentially arise out of stage N3, do not manifest with hyperkinetic automatism, are not stereotyped, and are much less frequent compared with seizures associated with sleep-related hypermotor epilepsy.
- Blowing, deep inspiration, sniffling, coughing, and changes in respiratory rate and volume were seen more often with seizures than with rapid eye movement sleep behavior disorder (RBD), whereas dream recollection is more suggestive of RBD.

INTRODUCTION

Recording of brain wave patterns during sleep often is essential in the evaluation of patients presenting for complex nocturnal behaviors. It is helpful particularly when sleep-related epilepsy is on the differential diagnosis. This is because for certain epilepsy syndromes, the awake electroencephalogram (EEG) may be entirely normal during the day, with epileptiform discharges and/or seizures manifesting only during sleep. In this review, the role of sleep in facilitating the activation of epileptiform discharges is discussed briefly. This is followed by examining, in more detail, those epilepsy types and syndromes whose presentation are strongly influenced by the sleep-wake cycle. Finally, in the last part, clinical manifestations of parasomnias and sleep-related movement disorders are contrasted with typical semiology of sleep-related hypermotor seizures.

SLEEP AND INTERICTAL DISCHARGES

In general, epileptiform discharges are more common and facilitated during non–rapid eye movement (NREM) sleep compared with rapid eye movement (REM) sleep. Spikes have been shown to exhibit homeostatic pattern similar to that of slow waves of sleep, occurring with greater density in the first few cycles of sleep and decreasing in frequency and abundance as sleep continues.[1,2] Although coupling with slow wave is noted in most epilepsies, coupling of interictal discharges with spindles also has been reported, for example, in self-limited epilepsy with centrotemporal spikes.[3] The preponderance of epileptiform discharges

a Ronald Reagan Medical Center, David Geffen School of Medicine at UCLA, 710 Westwood Plaza, Room 1-240, Los Angeles, CA 90095, USA; b UCLA Sleep Disorders Center, UCLA Department of Neurology, David Geffen School of Medicine at UCLA, 710 Westwood Boulevard, RNRC, C153, Mail Code 176919, Los Angeles, CA, USA; c UCLA Seizure Disorder Center, Brain Research Institute, David Geffen School of Medicine at UCLA, 10833 Le Conte Avenue, Los Angeles, CA 90095, USA
* Correspnding author.
E-mail address: avidan@mednet.ucla.edu

Sleep Med Clin 16 (2021) 389–408
https://doi.org/10.1016/j.jsmc.2021.02.011

during NREM sleep has been attributed to hypersynchrony. In particular, during NREM sleep, there is reduced input from the brainstem reticular activating system, which results in progressive hyperpolarization and synchronization of the thalamocortical circuits.[4] This state of synchronization facilitates the occurrence of epileptiform discharges. On the other hand, although seen much more rarely, epileptiform discharges also may occur during REM sleep, where the EEG is desynchronized, and muscle tone is attenuated. Studies have found that ictal discharges persisting during REM sleep more diagnostic valuable for seizure localization.[5,6]

SLEEP AND SELECT EPILEPSY SYNDROMES

Approximately 12% to 20% of seizures occur exclusively at night.[1,7,8] This section reviews in brief the epilepsy syndromes whose seizures have a strong correlation with sleep, focusing mostly on the role sleep plays in the clinical or EEG manifestations of these seizures.

Self-limited Epilepsy with Centrotemporal Spikes

Self-limited epilepsy with centrotemporal spikes, previously known as benign rolandic epilepsy or benign epilepsy with centrotemporal spikes, is one of the most common childhood epilepsy syndromes (**Fig. 1**). Onset usually is between ages 3 years and 13 years, with remission before the age of 16.[9–12] Paresthesia involving cheeks, tongue, and lips may precede the seizure. Three types of semiology have been described[13]: (1) hemifacial seizures with speech arrest and

drooling with preserved awareness; (2) hemifacial seizures with loss of awareness, gurgling-grunting, and postictal emesis; and (3) hemibody tonic-clonic seizures. On EEG, high-amplitude spike or spike-and-wave discharges with a transverse dipole in the centrotemporal region, which may shift or spread from side to side, are activated by drowsiness and NREM sleep.[7–9] Work by Varotto and colleagues[9] was suggestive that a state of reduced local connectivity and diffuse disconnection during light sleep may be responsible for epileptogenesis. Although remission rate is high, behavioral and neuropsychological problems are reported and may be correlated with intermittent slow waves noted during wakefulness and high number of spikes in the first hour of sleep as well as high index of multiple asynchronous bilateral spike waves in the first hours of sleep.[14]

Panayiotopoulos Syndrome

Panayiotopoulos syndrome primarily affects children between 1 year and 14 years of age, with 76% of the cases between ages 3 years and 6 years[15]; 70% of the seizures occur during sleep, with another 13% upon awakening.[16] More than 80% have nausea, retching, and emesis with preserved consciousness at the beginning of a seizure. Autonomic symptoms, such as pallor, flushing, cyanosis, incontinence, hypersalivation, mydriasis or miosis, temperature dysregulation, and cardiorespiratory irregularities, also are common. These may be followed by loss of consciousness, eye and head deviation, speech arrest, hemifacial convulsions, or visual hallucinations, which may proceed into hemibody or generalized convulsions. Prolonged seizures, some lasting for

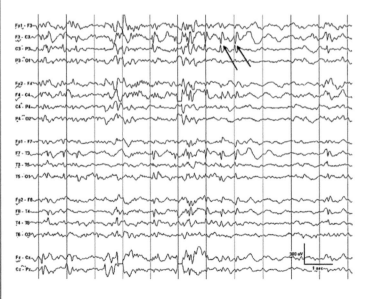

Fig. 1. Repetitive centrotemporal spikes (*arrows*) in an 8-year-old boy with benign rolandic epilepsy. (From Bazil, Carl W. "Effects of Sleep on the Postictal State." Epilepsy & Behavior 19, no. 2 (2010): 146 to 50. https://doi.org/10.1016/j.yebeh.2010.06.022. http://www.sciencedirect.com/science/article/pii/S1525505010004439" (requires permission).)

more than 30 minutes and even hours, may be common.[15] Interictal EEG may demonstrate multi-focal spike with a shifting focus, with occipital spikes the most commonly encountered (76%), followed by discharges in temporal (24%), parietal (16%), central (14%), and frontal (10%) regions, either alone or in combination.[16] Occasionally, no interictal discharges are present. A majority of patients have fewer than 5 seizures prior to remission, which usually is within 1 year to 2 years of onset.[15] **Fig. 2** illustrates an EEG notable for occipital spikes from a patient who presented with the typical autonomic symptoms.

West Syndrome

West syndrome is characterized by triad of infantile spasm, intellectual disability and a specific EEG pattern, termed *hypsarrhythmia* (**Fig. 3**). An electrodecremental response characterized by relative diffuse attenuation may be noted with spasms. Onset usually is between 3 months to 12 months of age and presents clinically with brief postarousal, synchronous spasms of head, trunk, and limbs,

which often occur in clusters and may be associated with a stereotypical cry.[7,8] Studies have shown that hypsarrhythmia interferes with the physiologic decrease in slow waves in NREM sleep throughout the night and consequently disrupts memory consolidation that normally takes place during sleep.[17]

Lennox-Gastaut Syndrome

With Lennox-Gastaut syndrome, the typical onset is between 3 years and 5 years of age. Characteristically, multiple seizure types may be present, including tonic, tonic-clonic, myoclonic, atonic, and atypical absences.[18,19] On EEG, slow spikes and sharp waves (**Fig. 4**) as well as polyspikes are common. Disruptions in sleep include reduced sleep efficiency and increased number of awakenings as well as increased NREM stages N1 and N2 and decreased slow wave sleep. Studies have found that the number of interictal discharges peak during the first 3 hours and decrease throughout the night, possibly related to the natural homeostatic process of sleep.[20] Lifelong intellectual disability is common.

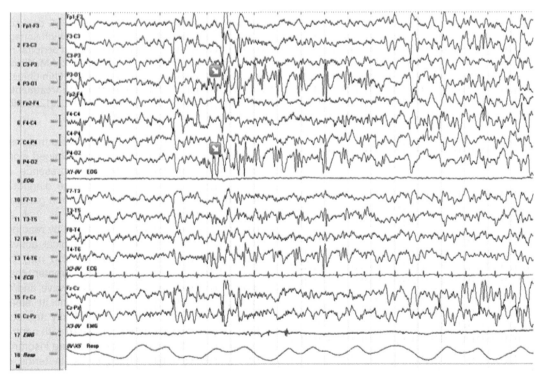

Fig. 2. Panayiotopoulos syndrome: this is an EEG from a toddler who presented with episodes before going to bed, of nausea and vomiting followed by loss of consciousness, clonic movements of lower extremities, tonic deviation of gaze, and fecal incontinence. The sleep EEG is noted for numerous spike-and-wave paroxysms in that predominate in occipital regions (*arrows*) with spread to anterior region (time constant: 0.3 s; high-frequency filter: 35 Hz). (From Martín del Valle, F., A. Díaz Negrillo, G. Ares Mateos, F. J. Sanz Santaeufemia, T. Del Rosal Rabes, and F. J. González-Valcárcel Sánchez-Puelles. "Panayiotopoulos Syndrome: Probable Genetic Origin, but Not in Scn1a." European Journal of Pediatric Neurology 15, no. 2 (2011): 155-57. https://doi.org/10.1016/j.ejpn.2010.08.002 http://www.sciencedirect.com/science/article/pii/S1090379810001510" (requires permission).)

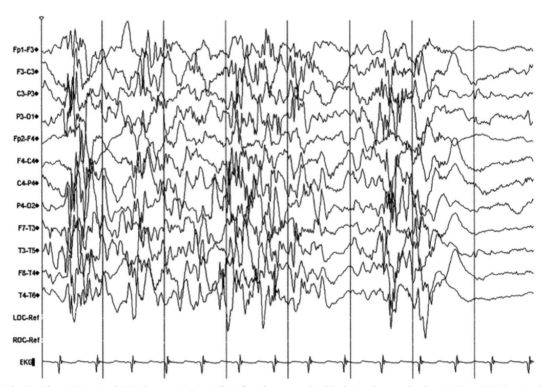

Fig. 3. Classic interictal EEG in a patient with infantile spasm highlighting hypsarrhythmia. The EEG depicted multifocal or generalized spikes, intermixed with a rather chaotic and asynchronous mixture of high-voltage slow wave activity and sharp waves. Focal slow activity is apparent on the right centrotemporal and occipital regions. Attenuated slow waves may be noted intermittently. (From: Journal of Experimental & Clinical Medicine. Kuo, Yung-Ting, Ying-Tzu Chen, Geng-Chang Yeh, Hsiao-Feng Chou, Chuan-Yu Wang, and Chuang Chin Chiueh. "Theta Power Spectral Analysis of Electroencephalography in Infantile Spasms: Before and after Acth Treatment." Journal of Experimental & Clinical Medicine 4, no. 6 (2012): 330-33. https://doi.org/10.1016/j.jecm.2012.10.009. http://www.sciencedirect.com/science/article/pii/S1878331712001325. (requires permission).)

Childhood Absence Epilepsy

Most common between the ages of 4 years and 14 years, absence epilepsy is characterized by brief (usually <10 seconds) pauses in activity, sometimes with associated eyelid fluttering. The EEG demonstrates characteristic "typical 3 Hz Spike-and-wave complexes (SWC)" discharges are pathognomonic (**Fig. 5**). Particularly during the first cycle of sleep, generalized spike waves are common, and polyspikes as well as focal spike waves with frontal predominance also may be seen.[7,8] Studies have suggested these interictal discharges may have preference for the transition periods between wakefulness to sleep as well as between stages of NREM sleep.[21,22]

Juvenile Myoclonic Epilepsy

Juvenile myoclonic epilepsy (JME) has onset between 8 years and 26 years of age and is characterized by seizures generally within 2 hours of awakening.[7,8] Common triggers include sleep deprivation and sudden arousals.[18,19] Prior to a first-time seizure, brief myoclonic jerks, especially affecting the upper extremities, but also that may affect the lower extremities, with retained consciousness may be reported; the presence of myoclonus is essential to making the diagnosis (**Fig. 6**).[23] Other than the most common generalized tonic-clonic seizures, absence as well as perioral reflex myoclonia (precipitated by reading, speaking, and other neuropsychological activation) and praxis-induced seizures also may be seen. EEG is characterized by greater than 3.5 Hz (on average) spike and slow wave and/or polyspike discharges, more frequent at sleep onset or on arousal (**Fig. 7**).[18,19] Mekky and colleagues[24] have shown that compared with control population, JME patients reported more insomnia and excessive daytime sleepiness. In terms of sleep parameters, reduced sleep efficiency, increased wake after sleep onset, prolonged REM latency, and, interestingly, prolonged REM duration were reported. The arousal index during both NREM and REM sleep also was significantly higher compared with control, in line with significantly disrupted sleep.[24] Other studies have confirmed these findings except that REM

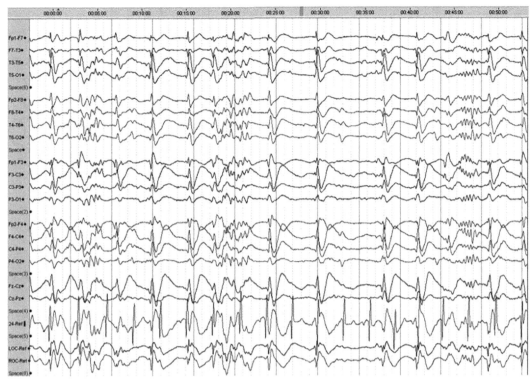

Fig. 4. Representative electroencephalogram of Lennox-Gastaut syndrome, demonstrating the characteristic slow spike-and-wave complexes. (From: VanStraten, Amanda F., and Yu-Tze Ng. "Update on the Management of Lennox-Gastaut Syndrome." *Pediatric Neurology* 47, no. 3 (2012): 153-61. https://doi.org/10.1016/j.pediatrneurol.2012.05. 001. http://www.sciencedirect.com/science/article/pii/S0887899412002147. (Requires permission).)

percentage generally was decreased compared with control.[24,25] A majority of patients have no reported neuropsychiatric deficits.

Electrical Status Epilepticus During Slow Wave Sleep

Electrical status epilepticus during slow wave sleep (ESES) and continuous spike-and-wave discharges during sleep (CSWS) are used interchangeably and described by the International League Against Epilepsy as follows: "Epilepsy with continuous spike-and-waves during slow sleep results from the association of various seizure types, partial or generalized, occurring during sleep, and atypical absences when awake. Tonic seizures do not occur, differentiating this from Lennox-Gastaut syndrome. The characteristic EEG pattern consists of continuous diffuse spike-and-waves during slow wave sleep. Duration varies from months to years. Despite the usually benign evolution of seizures, prognosis is guarded because of the appearance of neuropsychologic disorders."[26] Onset usually is between 2 months to 2 years of age with peak between 2 years to 4 years of age.[27] The absence of tonic seizures differentiates this from Lennox-

Gastaut syndrome. On EEG, there is a characteristic increase with sleep onset of bilateral high amplitude 1.5-Hz to 2.5-Hz slow spike-and-wave discharges, at times with anterior predominance (**Fig. 8**). Classically, a spike-and-wave index (SWI) of greater than 85% during NREM sleep has been used.[27] Gencpinar and colleagues[28,29] have demonstrated that the physiologic decrease in slow waves throughout the night is disturbed in patients with ESES/CSWS with a higher SWI, resulting in a greater degree of sleep disruption. Malformations or cortical lesions may be found in approximately half of the patients with ESES/CSWS.[30] Mutations in GR1N2A, which encodes for the GLuN2A subunit of the *N*-methyl D-aspartate receptor, have been found in patients with ESES/CSWS, self-limited epilepsies with centrotemporal spikes, and Landau-Kleffner syndrome, suggesting the 3 entities may be related as continuation on a spectrum.[31,32] Attention deficits and hyperactivity are common, although the overall prognosis depends on the etiology, duration of ESES, and treatment response. Behavioral deficits can recover soon after normalization of EEG, although long-term cognitive deficits may remain.[33]

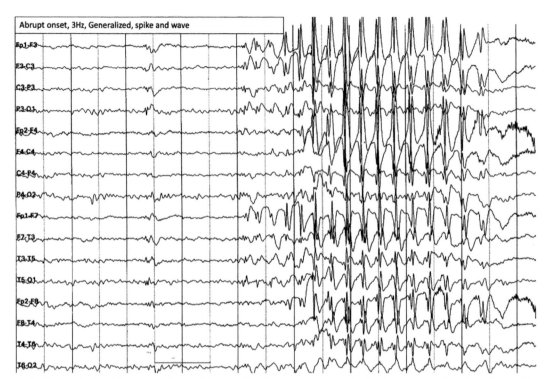

Fig. 5. Illustrative EEG from a patient with juvenile absence epilepsy; the ictal recording showing abrupt 3-Hz spike and slow wave discharges. (From: Zeliha Matur, Betül Baykan, Nerses Bebek, Candan Gürses, Ebru Altındağ, Ayşen Gökyiğit, The evaluation of interictal focal EEG findings in adult patients with absence seizures, Seizure, Volume 18, Issue 5, 2009, Pages 352-358, ISSN 1059-1311, https://doi.org/10.1016/j.seizure.2009.01.007. http://www.sciencedirect.com/science/article/pii/S1059131109000041 (Requires permission).)

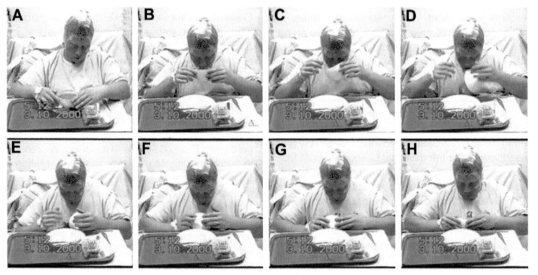

Fig. 6. The figure depict nocturnal polygraphic recording lasting 2 seconds of an 18-year-old man with juvenile myoclonic epilepsy (JME). The panel illustrates the patient following and early morning provoked awakening during breakfast. The patient is seen lifting a cup of beverage (*A,B*), a myoclonic jerk event (*C*) makes him drop his cup of coffee (*D-H*). The patient also experiences mild extension and elevation of his hands (*D-F*). He quickly picks it up again (*F-H*). The whole sequence lasts 2 seconds. (From Pierre Genton, Pierre Thomas, Dorothee G.A. Kasteleijn-Nolst Trenité, Marco Tulio Medina, Javier Salas-Puig, Clinical aspects of juvenile myoclonic epilepsy, Epilepsy & Behavior, Volume 28, Supplement 1, 2013, Pages S8-S14, ISSN 1525-5050, https://doi.org/10.1016/j.yebeh.2012.10.034. (http://www.sciencedirect.com/science/article/pii/S152550501300005X) (Requires permission).)

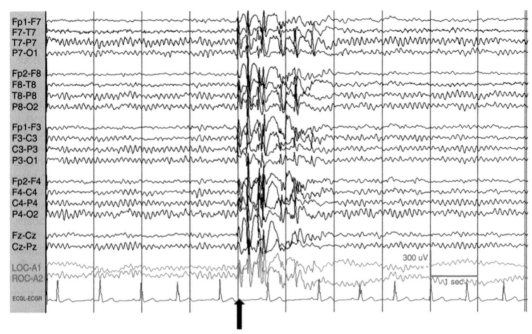

Fig. 7. Representative EEG in a 17-year-old girl with JME, highlighting the generalized irregular 4-Hz spike and polyspike and wave (*arrow*) in the setting of a normal background. The arrow highlights an episode of a jerk document by the technician during this discharge. (From: Marcuse, Lara V, MD; Fields, Madeline C, The EEG and epilepsy, Pages 121-155. In Rowan's Primer of EEG Second Edition © 2016, Elsevier. (Requires permission).)

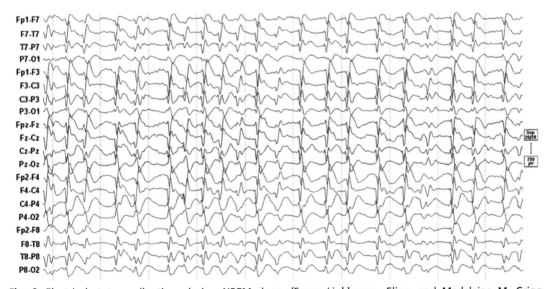

Fig. 8. Electrical status epilepticus during NREM sleep. (From: Liukkonen, Elina, and Madeleine M. Grigg-Damberger. "Electrical Status Epilepticus in Sleep." Sleep Medicine Clinics 7, no. 1 (2012): 147-56. https://doi.org/10.1016/j.jsmc.2011.12.003. http://www.sciencedirect.com/science/article/pii/S1556407X11001159 (Requires permission).)

Landau-Kleffner Syndrome

Landau-Kleffner syndrome, or acquired epileptic aphasia, has onset generally between 3 years and 9 years of age.[18,19] EEG is characterized by continuous spike-and-waves during NREM sleep, often with SWI of less than 85% (**Fig. 9**).[7,8] Brain imaging is normal.[34] Prior to onset, patients were developing normally and reaching language milestones appropriately. With onset, acute or gradual language regression is essential to diagnosis. Seizures often are focal onset with or without secondary generalization or atypical absence; approximately 20% to 30% of the patients may not have any seizures. Aphasia was thought to be related to hearing agnosia and may improve with normalization of EEG although there may be residual language and cognitive deficits.

Focal Epilepsies

In general, seizures arising out of the temporal lobes occur more frequently during wakefulness whereas those with onset in the frontal and to a lesser extend parietal lobes occur more often during early NREM sleep.[35] Miller and colleagues[36] found that compared with healthy controls, patients with focal epilepsy averaged less slow wave sleep, especially in the first hour of sleep, and the presence (not the number of) nocturnal discharges was associated with a longer REM latency. In their work studying ripples (80–150 Hz) occurring during sleep, Song and colleagues[37] found that there was a preferred phase angle of coupling between ripples and slow waves between areas of seizure onset in the frontal and parietal lobes versus areas not involved in seizure onset. Their work is based on the theory that trough to peak transition is mediated by synchronous summation of miniature excitatory postsynaptic potentials whereas peak to trough transitions are mediated by hyperpolarization of large neuronal networks.[38] Rates of trough to peak transitions were increased in the seizure-onset zone whereas rates of peak to trough transitions were not increased in the same area.

Among the frontal lobe seizures, those arising from the supplementary motor area may occur in both sleep and wakefulness whereas those arising

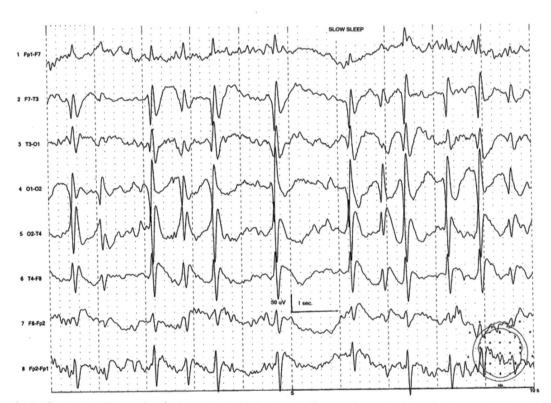

Fig. 9. Illustrative EEG recording from a patient with Landau-Kleffner syndrome depicting the characteristic continuous spike-and-wave activity in more than 85% of slow sleep. (From: Roberto Horacio Caraballo, Natalia Cejas, Noelia Chamorro, María C. Kaltenmeier, Sebastian Fortini, Ana María Soprano, Landau–Kleffner syndrome: A study of 29 patients, Seizure, Volume 23, Issue 2, 2014 Pages 98-104, ISSN 1059-1311, https://doi.org/10.1016/j.seizure.2013.09.016 .(http://www.sciencedirect.com/science/article/pii/S105913111300277X) (Requires permission).

from the prefrontal region, including anterior frontomesial, anterior frontolateral, and orbitofrontal cortices occur more often during NREM sleep.[21] In their review of orbitofrontal epilepsies, Chibane and colleagues[39] found that approximately 50% of the patients had sleep-related seizures, 56% either did not have an aura or reported nonspecific auras, and 62.5% had hypermotor manifestations, mostly of the hyperkinetic type. Semiology also may include autonomic disturbance, fear/anxiety, oroalimentary automatism, vocalization, and so forth, depending on propagation pathway. Epileptiform discharges in frontal and temporal leads can be seen on EEG.[39]

Nocturnal frontal lobe epilepsy (NFLE), renamed sleep-related hypermotor epilepsy (SRHE),[40] usually has onset in the second decade of life, although adult onset also has been reported.[41]

The change in name was an effort to bring to attention the key features of this clinical entity, namely the association of the seizures with sleep (rather than circadian rhythm of the day), the possibility of having onset external to the frontal lobes, and its distinct hypermotor semiology.[40] Temporal and insular-opercular are the most common regions of seizure onset after the frontal lobes, although onset from parietal, posterior cingulate, and occipital regions also has been reported.[42–44] Initially, seizure frequency may be high, with mean 3 ±3 seizures per night and 20 ±11 seizures per month.[45] Nearly all seizures occur during NREM sleep, particularly during stage 2 sleep.[45] Interictal EEG may be normal, and at times surface EEG may fail to capture any abnormality during an ictal event, which contributes to the difficulty in differentiating these from sleep disorders. Several

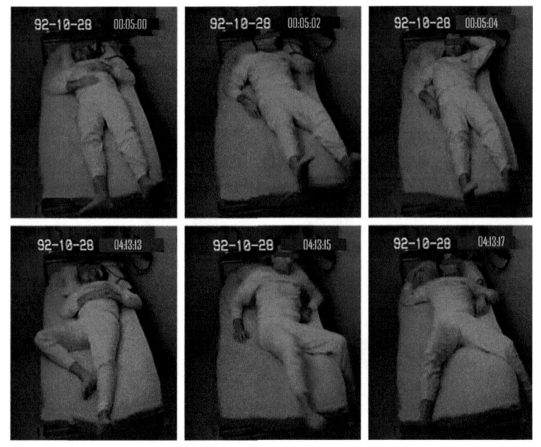

Fig. 10. Paroxysmal arousals in SRHE. The photographic sequences list still images taken at regular intervals during the video sequence), highlighting the semiology of the episode: simple paroxysmal arousals consisting of abrupt/sudden awakening, followed with sitting up on the bed and extending the head and trunk with the arms raised forward, facial grimacing demonstrating frightened expression, proceeding to ballistic and choreoathetotic movements. (From: Provini, Federica, Francesca Bisulli, and Paolo Tinuper. "Nocturnal Frontal Epilepsies: Diagnostic and Therapeutic Challenges for Sleep Specialists." *Sleep Medicine Clinics* 7, no. 1 (2012): 105-12. https://doi.org/10.1016/j.jsmc.2011.12.007. http://www.sciencedirect.com/scicence/article/pii/S1556407X11001196. (Requires permission).)

genetic mutations have been found to be associated, including mutations involving genes (CHRNA4 and CHRNB2) that encode for the subunits of the heteromeric neuronal nicotinic acetylcholine receptors, in which the autosomal dominant form is the most well-known (ADNFLE), although a recessive form due to mutation in PRIMA1 gene also has been described.[41,46,47] PRIMA1 is a transmembrane protein anchoring acetylcholinesterase to neuron membranes; the mutation results in an increase in cholinergic response.[47] Mutations in other genes (KCNT1 and DEPDC5) also have been reported.[48,49] Based on the known mutations involving the acetylcholine system in ADNFLE, Halász and colleagues[21] examined the role of arousal and sleep in the activation of seizures of absence epilepsy and NFLE. Acetylcholine activating the frontal cortex is essential to arousal and with SRHE, an overactive cholinergic system results in abnormal arousals, which often are noted on EEG prior to an attack.

Therefore, this raises the possibility that SRHE may be an epilepsy related to pathology of the ascending reticular activating system.[21]

SEMIOLOGY OF SLEEP-RELATED HYPERMOTOR EPILEPSY AND PARASOMNIAS

The semiology of SRHE is grouped into 3 categories, with increasing levels of complexity.[21,45] Paroxysmal arousals are frequent, abrupt, and brief (ranging 2–20 seconds), during which patients suddenly open their eyes, raise their heads or sit up in bed, often with dystonic posture of limbs; have a frightened or surprised expression; and scream (**Fig. 10**). Following the event, patients may return to sleep quickly. Minimal motor events with stereotyped movements of the limbs, axial muscles, and/or the head lasting 2 seconds to 4 seconds is another variant. The second type is paroxysmal dystonia, which usually begins with paroxysmal arousal, followed by hypermotor

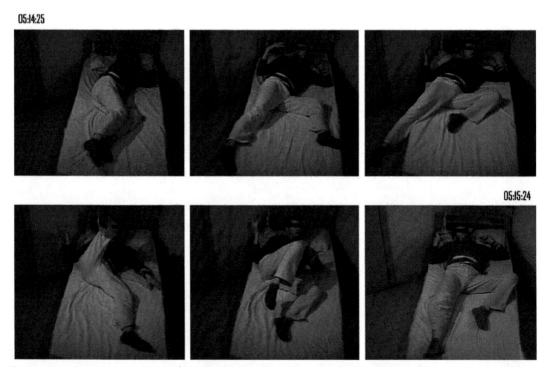

Fig. 11. Complex paroxysmal arousals in the setting of SRHE (previously classified as nocturnal paroxysmal dystonia because the episodes were thought to represent a movement disorder). Episodes are characterized by more rapid, vigorous, bordering on appearing combative involving the extremities (legs > arms) and along with dystonic asymmetric posturing, unintelligible vocalizations, cursing, whistling, or spitting. Epileptic nocturnal wandering is the most complex type of seizure and consists of abrupt dystonic posturing, dyskinetic gesticulation, displacement from bed, ambulation, dystonic postures jumping, yelling, and assuming an expression of dread. The episodes are on the differential diagnosis of somnambulism. (From: Provini, Federica, Francesca Bisulli, and Paolo Tinuper. "Nocturnal Frontal Epilepsies: Diagnostic and Therapeutic Challenges for Sleep Specialists." *Sleep Medicine Clinics* 7, no. 1 (2012): 105-12. https://doi.org/10.1016/j.jsmc.2011.12.007. http://www.sciencedirect.com/science/article/pii/S1556407X11001196. (Requires permission).)

behavior, which may include dystonic posturing, ballistic movement, body rocking, kicking, cycling, automatism, and head or eye deviation (**Fig. 11**). The episodes usually last between 20 seconds and 2 minutes. Awareness may be retained. The third type is episodic nocturnal wandering, in which the patients may exhibit various combination of stereotyped, agitated ambulation with sudden changes in direction, jumping and screaming, or other unintelligible vocalization, lasting 1 minute to 3 minutes in duration. Autonomic fluctuations in heart rate and respiratory rate also may be present. The events are highly stereotypical in the same patient, although all 3 types may manifest during different times. The variability in semiology may be due to the duration and length of the propagation pathway from the seizure-onset zone.[40]

EPILEPSY VERSUS NON–RAPID EYE MOVEMENT PARASOMNIAS

Clinical manifestation of SRHE may overlap with parasomnias, in particular confusional arousal (CA), sleep terror, and sleepwalking (somnambulism). Common features shared by the 3 most common NREM parasomnias include initiation from stage N3 sleep, relatively brief duration (although may be as long as 15–20 minutes in children), and absence of higher cognitive functions, such as attention, intent, social interactions, and so forth. Patients often are difficult to arouse during the event and likely to be confused or aggressive when awakened; amnesia of the event is a universal feature.[50] According to the *International Classification of Sleep Disorders – Third Edition*

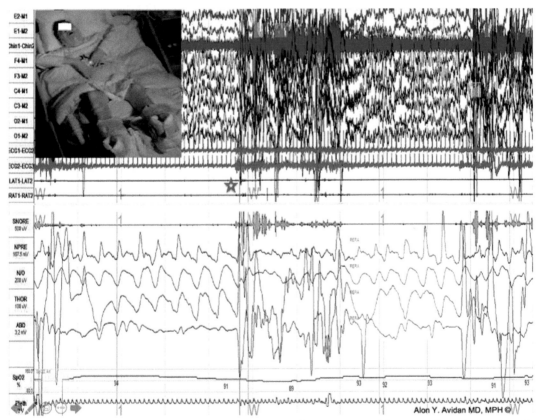

Fig. 12. A 120-second epoch of a diagnostic polysomnogram from a 54-year-old man conducted to evaluate for arousals with confusion and singing behavior. The figure highlights one of the patient's representative events depicted in an embedded video during his event illustrating an arousal from stage N3 sleep, as demarcated by the star, with the patient's arms abducted (flapping his arms and described by the technicians to be "quacking like a duck"). Channels are as follows: electro-oculogram (left: E1-M2; right: E2-M1), chin electromyogram (chin1-chin2), EEG (left: frontal-F3, central-C3, occipital-O1, left mastoid-M1; right: frontal-F4, central-C4, occipital-O2, right mastoid-M2), 2 ECG channels, 2 limb electromygram (LAT and RAT), snore channel, nasal-oral airflow (N/O), nasal pressure signal (NPRE), respiratory effort (thoracic, abdominal), and oxygen saturation (Sao2). LAT, left anterior tibialis electromyogram; RAT, right anterior tibialis electromyogram. (Previously published in: Avidan, A.Y. and N. Kaplish, The parasomnias: epidemiology, clinical features, and diagnostic approach. Clin Chest Med, 2010. 31(2): p. 353-70. Source: Alon Y. Avidan, MD, MPH © Copyright to remain with author.)

(*ICSD-3*), CA (as illustrated in **Fig. 12**) is characterized by "mental confusion or confused behavior that occurs while the patient is in bed. There is an absence of terror or ambulation outside of the bed. There is typically a lack of autonomic arousal such as mydriasis, tachycardia, tachypnea, and diaphoresis during an episode."[50] Patients with sleep terror present with an abrupt scream, autonomic activation, confusion, and inconsolability, and attempts at consolation may prolong the episode and may result in injury because the patient may become more aggresive.[51] The diagnostic criteria for sleep terror are as follows: "the arousals are characterized by episodes of abrupt terror, typically beginning with an alarming vocalization such as a frightening scream. There is intense fear and signs of autonomic arousal, including mydriasis, tachycardia, tachypnea, and diaphoresis during an episode."[50] In adults, bolting out of bed and violent behaviors may be observed. With sleepwalking, complex and amnestic ambulation may occur along with highly inappropriate behaviors, such as urinating into a waste basket. A subtype of sleep walking is sleep-related eating disorder, which includes somnambulism along with amnestic sleep eating, often of inappropriate food items, such as a cat food/dish soap sandwich.

There are a few key features used to differentiate parasomnias from epilepsy. Parasomnias usually occur less frequently, averaging a few times per week, rarely more than once per night, and generally less than 4 times a month. This is in contrast with nocturnal seizures, which may occur multiple times per night. Although both conditions have onset in childhood, NREM parasomnias usually manifest at a younger age and are seen much less commonly among the adult patient population (where they are likely facilitated through sleep deprivation, sleep apnea, and central nervous system active medications, in particular hypnotics and antidepressants).[50] Finally, compared with the epileptic episodes, NREM parasomnias preferentially arise out of stage N3 (in particular the first few hours), do not manifest with hyperkinetic automatism (such as kicking, rocking, or cycling movements), and are not stereotyped.[51–53] Dystonic posturing can occur in both epilepsy and NREM parasomnias. REM parasomnias, occurring during the second half of the night, are likely to manifest with abnormalities in dream content and muscle tone (augmentation in the setting of REM sleep behavior disorder [RBD] and persistent atonia/paralysis in isolated sleep paralysis).

Peter-Derex and colleagues[54] retrospectively analyzed the nocturnal recordings of 50 patients, 10 each among temporal lobe epilepsy (TLE), frontal lobe epilepsy (FLE), nocturnal terrors (NTs), CA, and normal arousal (NA). Their primary objective

A

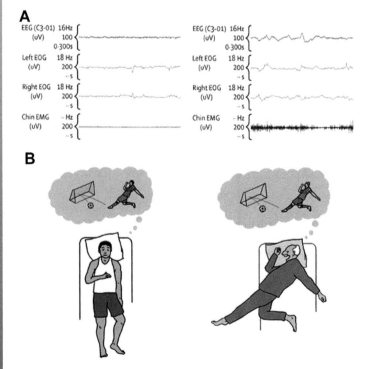

B

Fig. 13. (*A*) REM RSWA is depicted by a tonic and phasic muscle tone augmentation on the EMG signals of the polysomnography; normal REM sleep (*left*) depicts normal muscle atonia (paralysis) the chin in contrast to the abnormal muscle tone in the setting of RBD. (*B*) The corresponding dream enactment of hitting a soccer ball (*right*) in contrast to the normal sleeper who essentially is paralyzed and remains quiet and relaxed while dreaming of scoring a goal (*left*). Too often, patients with RBD have more aggressive dreaming (such as defending themselves against intruders, leading to injury). EMG, electromyography; EOG, electrooculography. (Francesca Siclari, Katja Valli, Isabelle Arnulf, Dreams and nightmares in healthy adults and in patients with sleep and neurological disorders, The Lancet Neurology, Volume 19, Issue 10, 2020, Pages 849-859, ISSN 1474-4422; with permission.)

was to study the beat-to-beat RR interval (RRI) as well as heart rate variability over a period of 60 heart beats before and after the first motor manifestation. Although the RRI was significantly lower for TLE compared with the other conditions, analysis of the slope demonstrated faster cardiac change in NTs and FLE compared with TLE and NA. There was no significant difference between NTs and FLE.

The relationship between parasomnias and epilepsy has been examined in a few studies. Provini and colleagues,[45] in their review of 100 cases of NFLE, found that approximately 40% of the patients had at least 1 first-degree relative with probable parasomnia. In a prospective familial aggregation study, the lifetime prevalence of sleep-walking, sleep terror, or CA was significantly higher among NFLE probands as well as their healthy relatives compared with control

population.[55] Cornejo-Sanchez and colleagues[56] studied the prevalence of sleep walking and sleep paralysis among Colombian patients with genetic epilepsy (including, JME, juvenile absence epilepsy, childhood absence epilepsy, and genetic epilepsy with febrile seizures plus). The prevalence of sleep walking was 11.6% in patients with epilepsy; this compared with a prevalence in the general Colombian population of 12.3% and 9% in 2004 and 2008, respectively. In addition, 46.3% of the patients with genetic generalized epilepsy reported having at least 1 relative with sleepwalking. Examining the microstructure of sleep have provided a potential explanation for the higher prevalence of parasomnias among epilepsy patients and their families. Two commonly used parameters used to characterize sleep microstructure are the arousal index and cyclic alternating pattern (CAP). The arousal index is

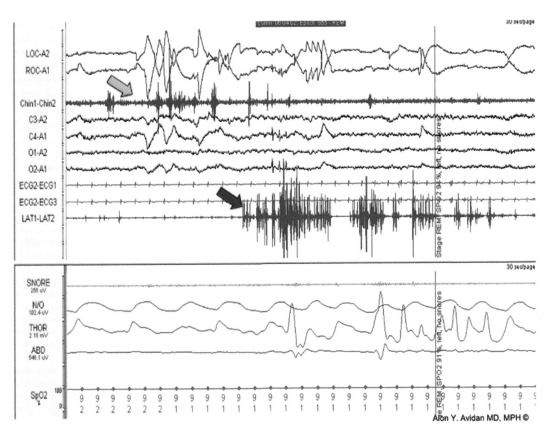

Fig. 14. A 30-second epoch from the diagnostic polysomnogram of an 80-year-old man who was referred to the sleep disorders clinic for evaluation of recurrent violent nighttime awakenings. Illustrated in this figure is a typical spell that this patient was experiencing. He was noted to yell, jump from bed, and have complex body movements. RSWA was noted in both the chin (*green arrow*) as well as the anterior tibialis electromyography (EMG) (*blue arrow*). Channels are as follows: electrooculogram (left: LOC-A2; right: ROC-A1), chin EMG, EEG (left central, right central, left occipital, and right occipital), 2 ECG channels, limb EMG (LAT), snore channel, nasal-oral airflow, respiratory effort (thoracic, abdominal), and oxygen saturation (Sao2). (*Source:* Alon Y. Avidan, MD, MPH © Copyright to remain with author.)

defined as the number of arousal per hour of sleep whereas CAP is periodic EEG activity during NREM, where the CAP rate is the percentage ratio of CAP time to total NREM sleep time.[57] Patients with SRHE have a high CAP rate, which translates into more microarousal and disturbed sleep.[58] NREM parasomnias also have been found to be associated with significant NREM fragmentation and instability.[59] Therefore, a dysfunction in the mechanism that normally balances arousal and sleep maintenance is likely to be present in both disorders.

Electrodes implanted intracranially for the evaluation of medically refractory epilepsy have offered insight into NREM parasomnias when both happen to be present in the same patient. This was reviewed in detail by Gibbs and colleagues.[60] The key finding is the presence of electrophysiologically diverse local states occurring simultaneously during sleep. Specifically, fast wake–like activity is recorded in certain regions, for example, motor and cingulate cortices, whereas delta sleep–like activity continues in other regions for example, frontal cortex. This discrepancy may be missed on surface EEG, where traditionally, only generalized slow wave and/or muscle and movement artifacts are captured during NREM parasomnias.[61] This differential activation of select brain regions may help explain certain features of

NREM parasomnias, for example, activation of amygdala results in emotional response whereas deactivation of hippocampus results in amnesia of the event afterward.[62]

EPILEPSY VERSUS RAPID EYE MOVEMENT SLEEP BEHAVIOR DISORDER

Although much less common, seizures also may occur during REM sleep. Nguyen-Michel and colleagues[63] compared dream-enactment motor events in the setting of REM sleep behavior disorders (RBDs) with those of sleep-related seizures (arising out of either REM or NREM). They found that during epileptic events, patients more often woke up abruptly, opened their eyes, raised head/trunk, had whole-body movements or dystonic posturing, and interacted with objects in the environment, whereas patients with RBD were more likely to have their eyes closed and exhibited more jerky, nonstereotypical movements. Blowing, deep inspiration, sniffling, coughing, and changes in respiratory rate and volume were seen more often with seizures than with RBD. Semiology was similar between seizures arising out of NREM and REM, although the latter occurred more often during the second half of the night, similar to RBDs. Among the seizures associated with REM sleep, 88% occurred during

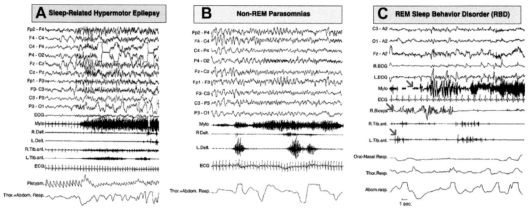

Fig. 15. Polysomnographic epochs highlighting (A) the unique features of SRHE; (B) an NREM parasomnia, sleep terror type; and (C) an episode of DEB and REM RSWA in the setting of RBD. (A) The EEG channels depict an ictal paroxysmal EEG discharge, mainly over the frontal regions during the seizure. (B) The abrupt arousal during the NREM parasomnia event of sleep terror highlights a nonepileptiform diffuse hypersynchronous activity that defines the underlying sleep-state instability, a hallmark of NREM parasomnias. (C) RBD is demarcated by the mixed frequency EEG pattern of REM stage. Instead of the expected EEG atonia, however, the patient's polysomnogram illustrates RSWA (*arrows*) during the DEB episode. From the polysomnographic perspective, the epileptic seizure manifests as stereotyped motor activation. The SRHE as well as NREM parasomnia, sleep terror type, will present with autonomic activation. (From: Nocturnal frontal lobe epilepsy to Sleep-Related Hypermotor Epilepsy: A 35-year diagnostic challenge Seizure: Paolo Tinuper, Francesca Bisulli, From nocturnal frontal lobe epilepsy to Sleep-Related Hypermotor Epilepsy: A 35-year diagnostic challenge, Seizure, Volume 44, 2017, Pages 87-92, ISSN 1059-1311, https://doi.org/10.1016/j.seizure.2016.11.023. (http://www.sciencedirect.com/science/article/pii/S1059131116302916). © 2016. Requires Permissions)

or near bursts of REMs noted in the anterior frontal leads. Another key feature for distinguishing RBD from seizures is dream recollection associated with the former. Specifically, when awakened during an episode of RBD, patients often are able to recount the dream immediately prior to arousal. The dreams are related to the patients' need to protect themselves against intruders or animals. In the process of defending themselves, patients may demonstrate behaviors, such as punching and kicking, that may result in injury to the patient or bed partner. Although such dreams are the majority, a minority of patients with RBD experience spots dreams or more adventurous dreaming.

On polysomnography, substantially augmented phasic or tonic muscle activity can be seen on electromyography channels during polysomnography (**Figs. 13** and **14**). REM sleep without atonia

(RSWA) corresponding to the dream enactment behavior (DEB) is required to make the diagnosis of RBD, although DEB may be diagnoses based solely on observation during the polysomnogram or on clinical history by a bed partner.

Autonomic activation usually is only mild or entirely absent.[53] Upon awakening, alertness usually is immediate, which may help differentiate from seizures, where often a postictal state may be present. Unlike NREM parasomnias and sleep-related epilepsy, RBD usually affects patients older than 50 years of age, where there is strong association with neurodegenerative conditions, such as parkinsonism.

Fig. 15 summarizes the polysomnographic signature markers of sleep-related epilepsy, NREM parasomnias (disorders of arousal), and REM parasomnias (such as RBD).

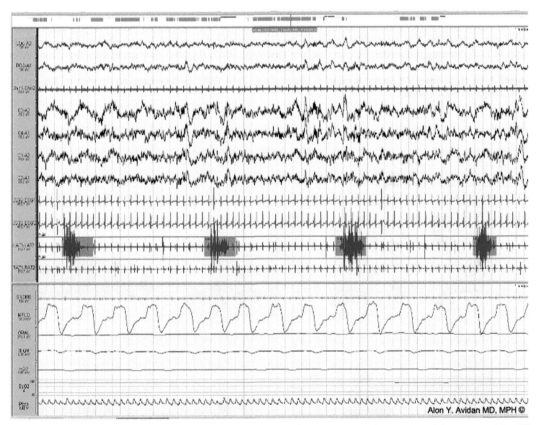

Alon Y. Avidan MD, MPH ©

Fig. 16. This is a 60-second sleep epoch from a diagnostic polysomnogram of a 66-year-old woman with difficulties falling asleep, excessive daytime sleepiness, and uncomfortable sensation in her legs associated with an irresistible urge to move her legs. Her husband reports that she has frequent night-time kicking and jerking movements, which disrupt his sleep. Illustrated in this figure is a succession of 5 periodic limb movements occurring in the right and left anterior tibialis muscles. Channels are as follows: electrooculogram (left: LOC-A2; right: ROC-A1), chin electromyography (EMG) (chin-chin), EEG (left central [C3-A2], right central [C4-A1], left occipital [O1-A2], right occipital [O2-A1]), electrocardiogram (ECG), limb EMG (left leg [LAT], right leg [RAT]), patient position, snoring (SNORE), nasal-oral airflow (N/O), respiratory effort (thoracic [THOR], abdominal [ABD]), nasal pressure (NPRE), and oxygen saturation (Spo_2) and plethysmography channel. (Source: Alon Y. Avidan, MD, MPH © Copyright to remain with author.)

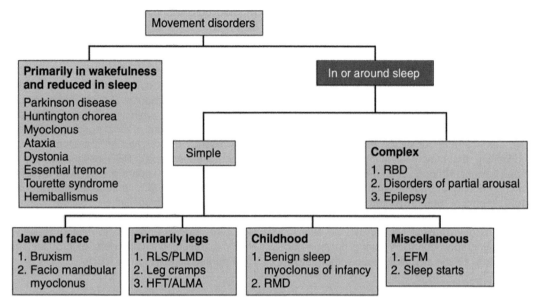

Fig. 17. Flowchart for the approach to the differential diagnosis of sleep-related movement disorders. ALMA, alternating leg muscle activation; EFM, excessive fragmentary myoclonus; HFT, hypnagogic foot tremor; PLMD, periodic limb movement disorder; RLS, restless legs syndrome; RMD, rhythmic movement disorder. (From: Allen, R, Salas, R and Gamaldo, C Movement Disorders in Sleep, in Atlas of Clinical Sleep Medicine, Second Edition Kryger, Meir H., Avidan, AY, Berry, R editors, Copyright © 2014, 2010 by Saunders, an imprint of Elsevier Inc. p.162 Requires Permissions.)

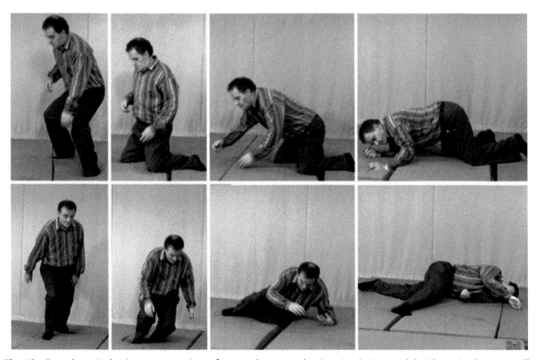

Fig. 18. Cataplexy. A classic representation of a complete cataplectic episode in an adult. The episodes generally follow a strong emotional stimulus, such as laughter. The example demonstrates the gradual onset of buckling of the knees and falling to the floor. (From: Ruoff C, Mignot, E. Central Nervouss System Hypersomnias, in Atlas of Clinical Sleep Medicine, Second Edition Kryger, Meir H., Avidan, AY, Berry, R editors, Copyright © 2014, 2010 by Saunders, an imprint of Elsevier Inc. p.16 Requires Permissions.)

Epilepsy versus Select Sleep-related Movement Disorders

Sleep starts or hypnic jerks are described by *ICSD-3* as "sudden, brief, simultaneous contractions of the body or one or more body segments occurring at sleep onset."[50] Compared with epileptic myoclonus, sleep starts often are associated with perception of falling or less frequently, pain, or tingling. Other sensory features, including banging, snapping noises, flashing lights, or hypnagogic dreams, also have been reported.[50] Intense jerks may be followed by brief autonomic activation. On EEG, sleep starts usually are associated with characteristic features of drowsiness or stage N1 sleep; this is in contrast to the typical spike-and-wave discharges associated with epileptic myoclonus.

Periodic limb movements of sleep (PLMSs) are depicted in **Fig. 16** and are characterized as abrupt, stereotyped, and repetitive, occurring in a sequence of 2 movements in series with amplitude greater than or equal to 8 microvolts, lasting 0.5 seconds to 10 seconds in duration, and recurring every 5 seconds to 90 seconds.[50] The Periodic Limb Movement Index, which assesses the frequency of PLMSs, is the number of PLMSs per hour of total sleep time. Because these limb movements can occur during wakefulness or sleep, they are referred to as PLMSs when they occur during sleep and periodic limb movements

of wakefulness when they occur during wakefulness. Movements also may occur in the arms but generally are limited to the legs. Periodic limb movement disorder of sleep requires polysomnographic conformation of PLM index greater than 15/h in adults and greater than 5/h in children with clinical sleep disturbance, such as insomnia/hypersomnia, and exclusion of other sleep disorder.

Propriospinal myoclonus is characterized by jerks beginning in spinal innervated axial muscles of neck, check, or abdomen propagating rostrally and caudally to more peripheral areas. There is a strong correlation with sleep onset. Unlike an epileptic event, these may be suppressed with sleep onset (appearance of spindles on EEG) or mental stimulation.[50,53]

Sleep-related rhythmic movements are defined by *ICSD-3* as "repetitive, stereotyped and rhythmic motor behaviors involving large muscle groups."[50] Example movements include head banging, head rolling, body rocking, body rolling, and leg banging.[64] The movements usually have frequency of 0.5 Hz to 2 Hz and can be associated with humming or other inarticulate sounds. Compared with epileptic events, environmental disturbance, including being spoken to, may result in cessation of the movements. These typically are not considered pathologic unless there are associated clinical consequences, which may include disturbance to normal sleep, impairment in

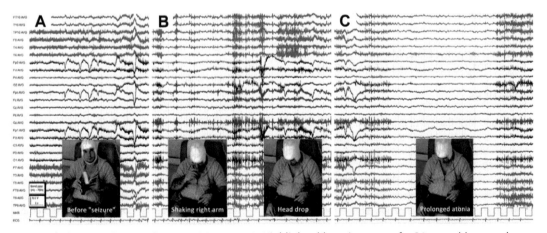

Fig. 19. "Shaking" without epileptic activity on EEG. Highlighted here is a case of a 24-year-old man, who presented with recurrent episodes of "shaking" of his right upper extremity. The patient was treated incorrectly for epilepsy for a few years. Additional work-up, with video-EEG monitoring during his spell, revealed cataplectic attacks. (*A*) Demonstrate muscles artifacts before the "seizure" subsequently followed by onset of cataplexy. (*B*) "Shaking" of the right upper extremely corresponds to the negative myoclonus of upper limbs and head during partial cataplexy, with intermittently attenuation of muscle activity. (*C*) Prolonged muscle atonia with abolished muscle artifacts without epileptic activity. (FROM: V. Dinkelacker and colleagues / Sleep Medicine 36 (2017) 119e121Vera Dinkelacker, Vi-Huong Nguyen-Michel, Lionel Thivard, Vincent Navarro, Claude Adam, Olivier Pallanca, Isabelle Arnulf, "I feel my arm shaking": partial cataplexy mistaken for drug-resistant focal epilepsy, Sleep Medicine, Volume 36, 2017, Pages 119-121, ISSN 1389-9457, https://doi.org/10.1016/j.sleep.2017.05.003.(http://www.sciencedirect.com/science/article/pii/S138994571730206X) Requires Permissions.)

daytime function, or injury.[50] The movements also may be observed during quiet wakefulness.

Fig. 17 highlights a conceptualized flowchart in the approach to the differential diagnosis of sleep-related movement disorders.

Cataplexy refers to an abrupt but brief (<2 minutes) loss or decrease of voluntary skeletal muscle tone with retained consciousness precipitated by strong emotions, such as anger, laughter, joy, elation, or surprise[65–67] (**Figs. 17–19**). It is estimated to be present in 65% to 75% of patients with narcolepsy[68,69] and is the most specific symptom of narcolepsy type I.

SUMMARY

Much progress has been made in elucidating the relationship between epilepsy and sleep. This review seeks to summarize the current state of understanding of the interplay between the 2, from the preponderance of epileptiform discharges during NREM sleep to the sleep-related electrophysiologic manifestations of multiple epilepsy types and syndromes. In addition, certain key features for differentiating parasomnias from SRHE also are discussed. Because sleep disorders and epilepsy are not exclusive of each other, familiarity with these conditions is essential to both sleep specialist and neurologist for the appropriate diagnosis and management of the affected patient population.

DISCLOSURE

Wu: None.
   Avidan: Harmony, Eisai, Merck.
   Engel: R01 NS033310 and U54 NS100064.

REFERENCES

1. Terzano MG, Parrino L, Smerieri A, et al. CAP and arousals are involved in the homeostatic and ultradian sleep processes. J Sleep Res 2005;14:359–68.
2. Halász P, Bódizs R, Ujma PP, et al. Strong relationship between NREM sleep, epilepsy and plastic functions - a conceptual review on the neurophysiology background. Epilepsy Res 2019;150:95–105.
3. Nobili L, Ferrillo F, Baglietto MG, et al. Relationship of sleep interictal epileptiform discharges to sigma activity (12-16 Hz) in benign epilepsy of childhood with Rolandic spikes. Clin Neurophysiol 1999;110:39–46.
4. Steriade M, Contreras D, Amzica F. Synchronized sleep oscillation and paroxysm development. Trend Neurosci 1994;17:199–208.
5. Malow BA, Aldrich MS. Localizing value of rapid eye movement sleep in temporal lobe epilepsy. Sleep Med 2000;1:57–60.
6. Okanari K, Baba S, Otsubo H, et al. Rapid eye movement sleep reveals epileptogenic spikes for resective surgery in children with generalized interictal discharges. Epilepsia 2015;56:1445–53.
7. Schmitt B. Sleep and epilepsy syndromes. Neuropediatrics 2015;46(3):171–80.
8. Xu L, Guo D, Liu YY, et al. Juvenile myoclonic epilepsy and sleep. Epilepsy Behav 2018;80:326–30.
9. Varotto G, Franceschetti S, Caputo D, et al. Network characteristics in benign epilepsy with centrotemporal spikes patients indicating defective connectivity during spindle sleep: a partial directed coherence study of EEG signals. Clin Neurophysiol 2018;129(11):2372–9.
10. Bouma PA, Bovenkerk AC, Westendorp RG, et al. The course of benign partial epilepsy of childhood with centrotemporal spikes: a meta-analysis. Neurology 1997;48:430–7.
11. Callenbach PM, Bouma PA, Geerts AT, et al. Long-term outcome of benign childhood epilepsy with centrotemporal spikes: Dutch Study of Epilepsy in Childhood. Seizure 2010;19:501–6.
12. Kellaway P. The electroencephalographic features of benign centrotemporal (rolandic) epilepsy of childhood. Epilepsia 2000;41:1053–6.
13. Lerman P. Benign partial epilepsy with centrotemporal spikes. In: Roger J, Dravet C, Bureau M, et al, editors. Epileptic syndromes in infancy, childhood and adolescence. London and Paris: John Libbey Eurotext Ltd; 1985. p. 150–8.
14. Nicolai J, van der Linden I, Arends JB, et al. EEG characteristics related to educational impairments in children with benign childhood epilepsy with centrotemporal spikes. Epilepsia 2007;48(11):2093–100.
15. Panayiotopoulos CP, Michael M, Sanders S, et al. Benign childhood focal epilepsies: assessment of established and newly recognized syndromes. Brain 2008;131(Pt 9):2264–86.
16. Specchio N, Trivisano M, Di Ciommo V, et al. Panayiotopoulos syndrome: a clinical, EEG, and neuropsychological study of 93 consecutive patients. Epilepsia 2010;51(10):2098–107.
17. Fattinger S, Schmitt B, Bölsterli Heinzle BK, et al. Impaired slow wave sleep downscaling in patients with infantile spasms. Eur J Paediatr Neurol 2015;19(2):134–42.
18. Carreño M, Fernández S. Sleep-related epilepsy. Curr Treat Options Neurol 2016;18(5):23.
19. Tinuper P, Bisulli F. From nocturnal frontal lobe epilepsy to Sleep-Related Hypermotor Epilepsy: a 35-year diagnostic challenge. Seizure 2017;44:87–92.
20. Sforza E, Mahdi R, Roche F, et al. Nocturnal interictal epileptic discharges in adult Lennox-Gastaut syndrome: the effect of sleep stage and time of night. Epileptic Disord 2016;18(1):44–50.

21. Halász P, Kelemen A, Szűcs A. The role of NREM sleep micro-arousals in absence epilepsy and in nocturnal frontal lobe epilepsy. Epilepsy Res 2013; 107(1–2):9–19.

22. Halász P, Dévényi É. Petit mal absence in night-sleep withspecial reference to transitional sleep and REM periods. Actamed Acad Sci Hung 1974;31:31–45.

23. Kasteleijn-Nolst Trenite DG, Schmitz B, Janz D, et al. Consensus on diagnosis and management of JME: from founder's observations to current trends. Epilepsy Behav 2013;28(Suppl 1):S87–90.

24. Mekky JF, Elbhrawy SM, Boraey MF, et al. Sleep architecture in patients with juvenile myoclonic epilepsy. Sleep Med 2017;38:116–21.

25. Roshan S, Puri V, Chaudhry N, et al. Sleep abnormalities in juvenile myoclonic epilepsy–a sleep questionnaire and polysomnography based study. Seizure 2017;50:194–201.

26. Commission on Classification and Terminology of the International League Against Epilepsy. Proposal for revised classification of epilepsies and epileptic syndromes. Epilepsia 1989;30(4):389–99.

27. Tassinari CA, Rubboli G, Volpi L, et al. Electrical status epilepticus during slow sleep (ESES or CSWS) including acquired epileptic aphasia (Landau-Kleffner syndrome). In: Roger J, Bureau M, Dravet C, et al, editors. Epileptic syndromes in infancy, childhood and adolescence. London and Paris: John Libbey Eurotext Ltd; 2005. p. 295–314.

28. Bölsterli BK, Schmitt B, Bast T, et al. Impaired slow wave sleep downscaling in encephalopathy with status epilepticus during sleep (ESES). Clin Neurophysiol 2011;122(9):1779–87.

29. Gencpinar P, Dundar NO, Tekgul H. Electrical status epilepticus in sleep (ESES)/continuous spikes and waves during slow sleep (CSWS) syndrome in children: an electroclinical evaluation according to the EEG patterns. Epilepsy Behav 2016;61:107–11.

30. Galanopoulou AS, Bojko A, Lado F, et al. The spectrum of neuropsychiatric abnormalities associated with electrical status epilepticus in sleep. Brain Dev 2000;22(5):279–95.

31. Carvill GL, Regan BM, Yendle SC, et al. GRIN2A mutations cause epilepsy-aphasia spectrum disorders. Nat Genet 2013;45(9):1073–6.

32. Lemke JR, Lal D, Reinthaler EM, et al. Mutations in GRIN2A cause idiopathic focal epilepsy with rolandic spikes. Nat Genet 2013;45(9):1067–72.

33. Pera MC, Brazzo D, Altieri N, et al. Long-term evolution of neuropsychological competences in encephalopathy with status epilepticus during sleep: a variable prognosis. Epilepsia 2013;54(Suppl 7):77–85.

34. Caraballo RH, Cejas N, Chamorro N, et al. Landau-Kleffner syndrome: a study of 29 patients. Seizure 2014;23(2):98–104.

35. Herman ST, Walczak TS, Bazil CW. Distribution of partial seizures during the sleep–wake cycle: differences by seizure onset site. Neurology 2001; 56:1453–9.

36. Miller LA, Ricci M, van Schalkwijk FJ, et al. Determining the relationship between sleep architecture, seizure variables and memory in patients with focal epilepsy. Behav Neurosci 2016;130(3):316–24.

37. Song I, Orosz I, Chervoneva I, et al. Bimodal coupling of ripples and slower oscillations during sleep in patients with focal epilepsy. Epilepsia 2017;58(11):1972–84.

38. Timofeev IV, Grenier F, Steriade M. Disfacilitation and active inhibition in the neocortex during the natural sleep-wake cycle: an intracellular study. Proc Natl Acad Sci USA 2001;98:1924–9.

39. Chibane IS, Boucher O, Dubeau F, et al. Orbitofrontal epilepsy: case series and review of literature. Epilepsy Behav 2017;76:32–8.

40. Tinuper P, Bisulli F, Cross JH, et al. Definition and diagnostic criteria of sleep-related hypermotor epilepsy. Neurology 2016;86(19):1834–42.

41. Scheffer IE, Bhatia KP, Lopes-Cendes I, et al. Autosomal dominant nocturnal frontal lobe epilepsy. A distinctive clinical disorder. Brain 1995;118(Pt 1): 61–73.

42. Mai R, Sartori I, Francione S, et al. Sleep related hyperkinetic seizures: always a frontal onset? Neurol Sci 2005;26(Suppl 3):s220–4.

43. Enatsu R, Bulacio J, Nair DR, et al. Posterior cingulate epilepsy: clinical and neurophysiological analysis. J Neurol Neurosurg Psychiatry 2014;85:44–50.

44. Montavont A, Kahane P, Catenoix H, et al. Hypermotor seizures in lateral and mesial parietal epilepsy. Epilepsy Behav 2013;28:408–12.

45. Provini F, Plazzi G, Tinuper P, et al. Nocturnal frontal lobe epilepsy. A clinical and polygraphic overview of 100 consecutive cases. Brain 1999;122(Pt 6): 1017–31.

46. Berkovic SF, Scheffer IE. Genetics of the epilepsies. Epilepsia 2001;42:16–23.

47. Hildebrand MS, Tankard R, Gazina EV, et al. PRIMA1 mutation: a new cause of nocturnal frontal lobe epilepsy. Ann Clin Transl Neurol 2015;2:821–30.

48. Heron SE, Smith KR, Bahlo M, et al. Missense mutations in the sodium-gated potassium channel gene KCNT1 cause severe autosomal dominant nocturnal frontal lobe epilepsy. Nat Genet 2012;44(11):1188–90.

49. Picard F, Makrythanasis P, Navarro V, et al. DEPDC5 mutations in families presenting as autosomal dominant nocturnal frontal lobe epilepsy. Neurology 2014;82(23):2101–6.

50. American Academy of Sleep Medicine. International Classification of sleep disorders. 3rd edition. Darien, IL: American Academy of Sleep Medicine; 2014.

51. Tinuper P, Provini F, Bisulli F, et al. Movement disorders in sleep: guidelines for differentiating epileptic from non-epileptic motor phenomena arising from sleep. Sleep Med Rev 2007;11(4):255–67.

52. Ekambaram V, Maski K. Non-rapid eye movement arousal parasomnias in children. Pediatr Ann 2017; 46(9):e327–31.

53. Bisulli F, Vignatelli L, Provini F, et al. Parasomnias and nocturnal frontal lobe epilepsy (NFLE): lights and shadows–controversial points in the differential diagnosis. Sleep Med 2011;12(Suppl 2):S27–32.

54. Peter-Derex L, Catenoix H, Bastuji H, et al. Parasomnia versus epilepsy: an affair of the heart? Neurophysiol Clin 2018;48(5):277–86.

55. Bisulli F, Vignatelli L, Naldi I, et al. Increased frequency of arousal parasomnias in families with nocturnal frontal lobe epilepsy: a common mechanism. Epilepsia 2010;51:1852–60.

56. Cornejo-Sanchez DM, Carrizosa-Moog J, Cabrera-Hemer D, et al. Sleepwalking and sleep paralysis: prevalence in Colombian families with genetic generalized epilepsy. J Child Neurol 2019;34(9): 491–8.

57. Parrino L, Grassi A, Milioli G. Cyclic alternating pattern in polysomnography: what is it and what does it mean? Curr Opin Pulm Med 2014;20:533–41.

58. Parrino L, Halasz P, Tassinari CA, et al. CAP, epilepsy and motor events during sleep: the unifying role of arousal. Sleep Med Rev 2006;10:267–85.

59. Espa F, Ondze B, Deglise P, et al. Sleep architecture, slow wave activity, and sleep spindles in adult patients with sleepwalking and sleep terrors. Clin Neurophysiol 2000;111:929–39.

60. Gibbs SA, Proserpio P, Terzaghi M, et al. Sleep-related epileptic behaviors and non-REM-related parasomnias: insights from stereo-EEG. Sleep Med Rev 2016;25:4–20.

61. Schenck CH, Pareja JA, Patterson AL, et al. Analysis of polysomnographic events surrounding 252 slow-wave sleep arousals in thirty eight adults with injurious sleepwalking and sleep terrors. J Clin Neurophysiol 1998;15: 159–66.

62. Nobili L, De Gennaro L, Proserpio P, et al. Local aspects of sleep: observations from intracerebral recordings in humans. Prog Brain Res 2012;199: 219–32.

63. Nguyen-Michel VH, Solano O, Leu-Semenescu S, et al. Rapid eye movement sleep behavior disorder or epileptic seizure during sleep? A video analysis of motor events. Seizure 2018;58:1–5.

64. Woolfe M, Prime D, Tjoa L, et al. Nocturnal motor events in epilepsy: is there a defined physiological network? Clin Neurophysiol 2019;130(9):1531–8.

65. Slowik JM, Collen JF, Yow AG. Narcolepsy. Treasure Island, FL: StatPearls; 2020.

66. Reading PJ. Update on narcolepsy. J Neurol 2019; 266(7):1809–15.

67. Nallu S, Guerrero GY, Lewis-Croswell J, et al. Review of narcolepsy and other common sleep disorders in children. Adv Pediatr 2019;66:147–59.

68. Leschziner G. Narcolepsy: a clinical review. Pract Neurol 2014;14(5):323–31.

69. Akintomide GS, Rickards H. Narcolepsy: a review. Neuropsychiatr Dis Treat 2011;7:507–18.

Moving?

Make sure your subscription moves with you!

To notify us of your new address, find your **Clinics Account Number** (located on your mailing label above your name), and contact customer service at:

Email: journalscustomerservice-usa@elsevier.com

800-654-2452 (subscribers in the U.S. & Canada)
314-447-8871 (subscribers outside of the U.S. & Canada)

Fax number: 314-447-8029

Elsevier Health Sciences Division
Subscription Customer Service
3251 Riverport Lane
Maryland Heights, MO 63043

*To ensure uninterrupted delivery of your subscription, please notify us at least 4 weeks in advance of move.

9780323813679